AF515169

Psychological, Emotional, Social and Cognitive Aspects of Implantable Cardiac Devices

Riccardo Proietti • Gian Mauro Manzoni
Giada Pietrabissa • Gianluca Castelnuovo
Editors

Psychological, Emotional, Social and Cognitive Aspects of Implantable Cardiac Devices

Springer

Editors
Riccardo Proietti
Cardiac Center, Morriston Hospital
University of Swansea
Swansea
UK

Giada Pietrabissa
Department of Psychology
Università Cattolica del Sacro Cuore
Milano
Italy

Gian Mauro Manzoni
eCampus University Faculty of Psychology
Novedrate (Como)
Italy

Gianluca Castelnuovo
Department of Psychology
Università Cattolica del Sacro Cuore
Milano
Italy

ISBN 978-3-319-55719-9   ISBN 978-3-319-55721-2 (eBook)
DOI 10.1007/978-3-319-55721-2

Library of Congress Control Number: 2017945678

© Springer International Publishing AG 2017
This work is subject to copyright. All rights are reserved by the Publisher, whether the whole or part of the material is concerned, specifically the rights of translation, reprinting, reuse of illustrations, recitation, broadcasting, reproduction on microfilms or in any other physical way, and transmission or information storage and retrieval, electronic adaptation, computer software, or by similar or dissimilar methodology now known or hereafter developed.
The use of general descriptive names, registered names, trademarks, service marks, etc. in this publication does not imply, even in the absence of a specific statement, that such names are exempt from the relevant protective laws and regulations and therefore free for general use.
The publisher, the authors and the editors are safe to assume that the advice and information in this book are believed to be true and accurate at the date of publication. Neither the publisher nor the authors or the editors give a warranty, express or implied, with respect to the material contained herein or for any errors or omissions that may have been made. The publisher remains neutral with regard to jurisdictional claims in published maps and institutional affiliations.

Printed on acid-free paper

This Springer imprint is published by Springer Nature
The registered company is Springer International Publishing AG
The registered company address is: Gewerbestrasse 11, 6330 Cham, Switzerland

Preface

In 1989 I was a young research registrar at St George's Hospital London. These were exciting times as within a few months of my arrival we started implanting the first generation of transvenous implantable defibrillator (ICD), which no longer required a thoracotomy. This change had the potential to make ICD therapy available to a much wider group of patients. Psychological and emotional issues were not uppermost in our minds as we grappled with the technical challenges of these new devices with their limited shock outputs and sometimes marginal defibrillation thresholds. However, within two years I had lost two patients, one teenager to a gruesome suicide following an appropriate shock therapy, and another older patient to severe depression following over 40 inappropriate shocks for atrial fibrillation. Following these events the importance of psychological and emotional factors in ICD patients was very clear to me and my practice since then has always included pre-implant counselling and access to post-implant support.

Since the 1990s there have been many technical developments in ICD therapy including biphasic shocks, improved detection algorithms, vastly increased arrhythmia event storage capability, and remote monitoring. However the risk of inappropriate therapies, whilst reduced, remains and appropriate shock therapy is still the main means of sudden death prevention by the device. In addition the occurrence of a number of high profile manufacturer's advisories, relating to leads and devices, has highlighted concerns about reliability. That the ICD remains an imperfect therapy, preventing sudden death only by waiting for it to be imminent and then striking with shock therapy, is not in question.

Meanwhile the indications for device therapy have broadened with more than a million people worldwide living with an ICD. Many of these new ICD recipients are receiving the devices for primary prevention of sudden death having never suffered an arrhythmia, their potential mortality drawn starkly to their attention. Many of these patients will survive for decades as their risk of sudden death is low. To allow them to continue to lead active working, social and sexual lives requires careful consideration of and preparation for the impact of ICD therapy. The impact of device therapy spreads far beyond the patient, affecting partners and families too.

In this book Proietti and colleagues have brought together a wide range of expertise in Psychological, Emotional, Social and Cognitive Aspects of Implantable Cardiac Device therapy to create a standard reference on this important topic. We owe it to all of our implantable device patients to consider this vital aspect of their care.

Morriston, Swansea, UK Mark Anderson

Contents

Contributors

Abdullah Alabdulgader, MD, DCH (I), DCH (Edin.). Prince Sultan Cardiac Center, Al Hassa, Saudi Arabia

Ahmed AlTurki, M.D. McGill University Health Center, Montreal, QC, Canada

Gian Andrea Bertone Division of Cardiological Rehabilitation, Ospedale San Giuseppe, IRCCS Istituto Auxologico Italiano, Oggebbio (VCO), Italy

Francesco Borgia Department of Psychology, Università Cattolica del Sacro Cuore, Milan, Italy

Gianluca Castelnuovo Psychology Research Laboratory, Ospedale San Giuseppe, IRCCS Istituto Auxologico Italiano, Oggebbio (VCO), Italy

Department of Psychology, Università Cattolica del Sacro Cuore, Milan, Italy

Audrey Charneux, M.A. Research Center, Montreal Heart Institute, Montréal, QC, Canada

Wendy Churchouse, BEM, MSc, RGN, Dip N, En(G). Cardiac Centre, Morriston Hospital, Swansea, UK

Bianca D'Antono, Ph.D. Research Center, Montreal Heart Institute, Montréal, QC, Canada

Department of Psychology, Université de Montréal, Montréal, QC, Canada

Martin Eisenberger, M.D., Ph.D. Faculty of Health and Social Studies, University of South Bohemia in České Budějovice, České Budějovice, Czech Republic

Mauro Feola, M.D., F.E.S.C. Cardiovascular Rehabilitation-Heart Failure Unit, Ospedale SS Trinità, Fossano, CN, Italy

Luca Alessandro Gondoni Division of Cardiological Rehabilitation, Ospedale San Giuseppe, IRCCS Istituto Auxologico Italiano, Oggebbio (VCO), Italy

Tal Hasin, M.D. Department of Cardiology, Shaare Zedek Medical Center, Jerusalem, Israel

Jochen Jordan Department of Psychocardiology, Kerckhoff Clinic, Bad Nauheim, Germany

Alena Kajanová, Ph.D. Faculty of Health and Social Studies, University of South Bohemia in České Budějovice, České Budějovice, Czech Republic

Teresa Kus, M.D., Ph.D. Cardiology Department, Hôpital du Sacré-Cœur de Montréal, Montréal, QC, Canada

Pharmacology Department, Université de Montréal, Montréal, QC, Canada

William R. Lewis, M.D. Department of Medicine, MetroHealth Campus of Case Western Reserve University, Cleveland, OH, USA

Gian Mauro Manzoni Psychology Research Laboratory, Ospedale San Giuseppe, IRCCS Istituto Auxologico Italiano, Oggebbio (VCO), Italy

Faculty of Psychology, eCampus University, Novedrate, Como, Italy

Mariella Montano Department of Cardiology, Ospedale Castelli, Verbania, Italy

Ferruccio Nibbio Division of Cardiological Rehabilitation, Ospedale San Giuseppe, IRCCS Istituto Auxologico Italiano, Oggebbio (VCO), Italy

Ludmila Peregrinova Department of Psychocardiology, Kerckhoff Clinic, Bad Nauheim, Germany

Giada Pietrabissa Psychology Research Laboratory, Ospedale San Giuseppe, IRCCS Istituto Auxologico Italiano, Oggebbio (VCO), Italy

Department of Psychology, Università Cattolica del Sacro Cuore, Milan, Italy

Riccardo Proietti Department of Cardiology, Ospedale Luigi Sacco, Milan, Italy

McGill University Health Center, Montreal, QC, Canada

Cardiac Center, Morriston Hospital, University of Swansea, Swansea, UK

Moshe Rav Acha, M.D., Ph.D. Department of Cardiology, Shaare Zedek Medical Center, Jerusalem, Israel

Zuzana Řimnáčová Faculty of Health and Social Studies, University of South Bohemia in České Budějovice, České Budějovice, Czech Republic

Serena Santagostino Department of Psychology, Università Cattolica del Sacro Cuore, Milan, Italy

Mitzi M. Saunders, R.N., Ph.D., A.C.N.S-.B.C. University of Detroit Mercy, Detroit, MI, USA

Arjun D. Sharma, M.D., F.A.C.C. , St Paul, MN, USA

Marzia Testa, M.D. School of Geriatry, Università degli Studi di Torino, Torino, Italy

Ingela Thylén, R.N., Ph.D. Department of Cardiology and Department of Medical and Health Sciences, Linköping University, Linköping, Sweden

Anna Maria Titon Division of Cardiological Rehabilitation, Ospedale San Giuseppe, IRCCS Istituto Auxologico Italiano, Oggebbio (VCO), Italy

Vilma Torres, M.D. Department of Medicine, MetroHealth Campus of Case Western Reserve University, Cleveland, OH, USA

Paolo Valore, Ph.D. Department of Philosophy, University of Milan, Milan, Italy

Chapter 1
Cognitive Functioning in Implantable Cardioverter Defibrillator/Pacemaker Recipients

Mauro Feola and Marzia Testa

Abstract Cognitive impairment (CI) is one of the most common recurring chronic conditions among elderly people. Congestive heart failure (CHF) is recognised as an important cause of CI, not only in the elderly but also in younger people. Cardiac devices such as cardiac resynchronization therapy (CRT), implantable cardioverter defibrillator (ICD) and pacemaker (PM) are frequently used in HF patients and might modify cognitive functioning in different ways.

This chapter describes how cardiac devices could influence cognitive functioning in HF patients and how CI could impact the management of heart failure.

Keywords Cognitive impairment • Heart failure • Cardiac devices

Heart Failure and Cognitive Impairment (CI)

Cognition is a superior cortical function that involves multiple brain processes it allows individuals to perceive information, learn and acquire specific knowledge and subsequently use it for problem solving and daily life action planning. Brain functioning covers different specific cognitive domains such as brief and long-term memory, attention/working memory, executive functioning, psychomotor speed, language/speech and visuo-spatial ability, all of which can be measured by several neuropsychological tests.

A significant decline in one or more cognitive functions determines a cognitive impairment (CI), which is one of the most common recurring chronic conditions among elderly people, such as diabetes, hypertension, chronic kidney disease, congestive heart

---

M. Feola, M.D., F.E.S.C. (✉)
Cardiovascular Rehabilitation-Heart Failure Unit, Ospedale SS Trinità, Via Ospedale 4, 12045 Fossano (CN), Italy
e-mail: m_feola@virgilio.it

M. Testa, M.D.
School of Geriatry, Università degli Studi di Torino, Torino, Italy

© Springer International Publishing AG 2017
R. Proietti et al. (eds.), *Psychological, Emotional, Social and Cognitive Aspects of Implantable Cardiac Devices*, DOI 10.1007/978-3-319-55721-2_1

failure. The most common causes of CI are Alzheimer's, fronto-temporal, Lewy body and cerebrovascular diseases. Moreover, there are a number of reversible causes of CI such as hypothyroidism, vitamin B12 deficiency, sleep apnea, anticholinergic drugs, depression, infections, hearing and visual disturbances and space occupying lesions [1].

Congestive heart failure (CHF) is an ulterior condition that could lead to CI not only in the elderly but also in younger people [2–4].

Impairments of memory, attention, executive functioning and psychomotor speed can affect the ability of CHF patients to manage their disease, to recognize if symptoms are worsening, to make appropriate choices about their health and to adhere to specific, often complex therapeutic regimens [5]. CI may also increase mortality and be related to higher rates of hospital admission and functional impairment [6–8].

Prevalence of CI in CHF

The prevalence rate of CI in CHF patients varies from study to study, ranging from 25 to 70–80%. This heterogeneity depends largely on differences in the sampling methods of these studies. In the study by Harkness et al., a CI, defined as a Montreal Cognitive Assessment (MOCA) score <26, was detected in >70% of CHF patients with NYHA class III or IV [9]. Similar results were obtained in a randomized controlled trial by Davis et al. [10]. In a study on 515 hospitalized elderly patients, a CI was seen in 57.9% of patients with NYHA class III-IV and 43% of NYHA class II [11]. In 2012 Gure et al. [12] studied 6189 CHF patients and found prevalence rates of mild cognitive impairment and dementia in 24% and 15% of patients respectively. Finally, the systematic review of Vogels et al. [2] compared a pooled sample of 2937 CHF patients to 14,848 controls and found that the risk of CI was 1.62 times greater in the CHF group.

Pathophysiology

Cerebral blood flow (CBF) reduction can determine brain changes which affect people with HF. CBF depends on several variables such as cerebrovascular reactivity, cardiac output (CO) and blood pressure. Low cardiac output, low systolic blood pressure and impaired auto regulatory mechanisms might impair CBF and determine neuroanatomic and neuropsychological changes [13].

A significant reduction of blood flow velocity at middle cerebral arteries, subsequent to carbon dioxide, was demonstrated to be correlated with NYHA class severity and left ventricular ejection fraction (LVEF) [14] in CHF patients. In a group of elderly patients with stable cardiovascular disease, patients with lower CO (<4.0 L/min) performed worse than normal CO subjects (≥4.0 L/min) in tests of executive functioning including sequencing and planning. Moreover, arterial hypotension was found to be associated with CI in older CHF patients [15]. In a large Italian study involving 13,635 patients (1583 of whom affected by CHF), systolic blood pressure below 130 mmHg predicted CI only in patients with CHF and any increase of 10 mmHg had a protective effect against CI with an OR = 0.78 (95% CI: 0.71–0.86) [16]. According to available data, lower systolic blood pressure resulted to be related not only to CI because of cerebral hypoperfusion, chronic hypotension and antihypertensive drugs, but also with increased mortality [17–19]. Moreover, a diastolic blood pressure <70 mmHg was shown to play an additive role in predicting the development of dementia in CHF patients [20].

Poor cerebral autoregulation in older patients is further worsened by heart failure through hypoperfusion, which in turn leads to the occurrence of local ischemia and the release of vasodilators and cytokines [21]. Considered together these mediators contribute to the development of CI far beyond the increase of the amyloid precursor protein (APP) and the deposition of the amyloid-beta protein.

Left ventricular ejection fraction was demonstrated to be correlated with the Mini Mental State Examination (MMSE) in a small sample of older CHF patients [17]. A significant relationship between neuropsychological test scores (the MMSE or the Repeatable Battery for the Assessment of Neuropsychological Status or the Cambridge Cognition Test) and LVEF in CHF patients was also observed in other clinical experiences [22–24]. However, there are studies in which, after adjusting for different variables, the correlation between low ejection fraction and CI did not result to be statistically significant [25, 26].

Among laboratory tests, B-type natriuretic peptide has been demonstrated to be predictive of cognitive impairment in a general elderly population [27, 28], in individuals with cardiovascular disease [29] and in patients with CHF [30].

Other data linked cognition and functional status as assessed by NYHA class or the 6-min walking test (6MWT). In two studies [27, 31], CHF patients with a NYHA class III-IV showed impaired cognition. In a group of stable CHF out-patients, their results at the 6MWT resulted to be positively related to their MMSE scores even after adjusting for different variables (e.g. demographic features, indexes of disease severity, comorbidities, level of disability and quality of life) [32].

Atrial fibrillation, including paroxysmal atrial fibrillation, was shown to be strongly related to cognitive and functional declines independently of the presence of a clinical stroke in the patient's history [33–35].CI due to atrial fibrillation is not only determined by micro-emboli, but also by a reduction in the ventricular rate response and a decline in cerebral perfusion [36].

Recently, obesity and depression have been added as additional risk factors for poor cognitive performance in older adults with CHF. An interaction between hypoperfusion and obesity has a particularly adverse effect on attention and executive functions [37, 38], whereas depression has been shown to be a determining factor in producing memory impairment in CHF patients [39].

Furthermore, a number of reversible causes of CI such as hypothyroidism, vitamin B12 deficiency, anemia, undernutrition, sleep apnea, anticholinergic drugs, infections, hearing and vision disturbances, seem to be frequently associated with heart failure.

Consequences of Cognitive Impairment in CHF Patients

Adherence to specific and often complex therapeutic regimens, recognizing symptoms of exacerbation, respecting scheduled appointments and making appropriate decisions about health can be affected by the impairment of memory, attention and executive functioning in CHF patients [5].

In a study on 251 CHF patients, a CI was found in 58% of subjects and the greatest cognitive deficits were found in verbal learning, immediate memory and delayed verbal memory. These deficits were significantly associated with poorer medication adherence [40]. Moreover, CHF patients who showed a CI by scoring <26 at the Montreal Cognitive Assessment (MOCA) were found to have a lower self-management ability in comparison to patients with a normal MOCA score (>26) [41]. This relationship was shown to be consistent because it was confirmed by other studies that used different neuropsychological tests [42–44].

CI is also a strong predictor of mortality, hospital admission and functional decline. In 1113 elderly patients admitted for heart failure, the in-hospital mortality rate was higher in the group of impaired patients (18%) than in the group of patients without CI (3%); also the 1-year mortality rate was higher among cognitive impaired patients (27% versus 15%, $p < 0.0001$). In a multivariate model, having a cognitive impairment was associated with an almost fivefold increase of mortality in CHF patients [6]. Also McLennan et al. [3] found that cognitively impaired CHF patients were more likely to experience an unplanned hospitalization and/or death within 5 years.

In another study enrolling 166 stable CHF patients, poorer scores in general cognition (MMSE), working memory, psychomotor speed and executive functioning were shown to be significant predictors of mortality [7].

However, as shown in a study by Dodson et al. [8], the assessment and documentation of CI in CHF patients is likely to have an almost paradoxical effect. Indeed, Dodson et al. found that cognitively impaired patients with a documented CI did not have a significantly higher 6-month mortality or hospital readmission risk in comparison with patients without CI, while the risk was significantly higher in impaired patients whose CI was not reported.

Cognitive Impairment and Cardiac Devices

CRT (Cardiac Resynchronization Therapy)

In recent decades, new therapeutic strategies for CHF have been developed, cardiac resynchronization therapy (CRT) is presently the most innovative therapy for CHF. Approximately 30% of patients with CHF present significant ventricular dyssynchrony and conduction disturbances [45] (e.g. left bundle branch block—LBBB); CRT is a cardiac device that improves the mechanical efficiency of the heart by “resynchronizing” ventricular contraction. CRT uses a biventricular pacemaker with two wires located in the lower chambers of the heart that deliver simultaneous or near simultaneous electrical impulses to both lower heart chambers (the right and left ventricles), causing the heart to beat in a more synchronized, efficient manner. According to the current guidelines [46], CRT is recommended in patients in sinus rhythm with a QRS duration of ≥120 ms, LBBB QRS morphology and an EF ≤35%. Patients receiving CRT are expected to survive with good functional status for >1 year, reducing the risk of CHF hospitalization and of premature death.

In multiple clinical trials, CRT was shown to improve 6-min walking distance, NYHA functional class, quality of life (QoL), left ventricle ejection fraction (LVEF), mortality and time to first hospitalization [47, 48]. The few studies that evaluated the effect of CRT on cognitive functioning gave contrasting results [49–51]. Dixit et al. [50] demonstrated that cognitive functioning had significantly improved in patients responding to CRT, specifically in the domains of attention, working memory and speed of processing. On the contrary, Hoth et al. [51] did not find any significant improvement in the cognitive measures, except when patients were divided into two groups according to the improvement in LVEF. Patients who manifested a LVEF improvement (≥15%) had a significant amelioration in executive functions and visuospatial skills. However, in a recent systematic review by Proietti et al. [52], which includes the two studies mentioned above, CRT demonstrated a non significant overall effect on cognition. It should be noted that these studies used different methods to define cognitive impairment and the majority of participants did not have CI before CRT implantation. Therefore, it might be concluded that CRT is not likely to improve cognitive function but it could be effective in maintaining normal cognitive performance in implanted CHF recipients.

ICD (Implantable Cardioverter Defibrillator)

Approximately half of the deaths in patients with HF, especially in those with milder symptoms, occurs suddenly and unexpectedly, and many, if not most, of these are related to ventricular arrhythmias. Prevention of sudden death is therefore an important goal in CHF. ICDs play an important role in reducing the risk of death from ventricular arrhythmias in primary prevention. ICD implantation is recommended in primary prevention for patients with symptomatic CHF (NYHA class II–III) and EF ≤35%, despite ≥3 months of treatment with optimal pharmacological therapy. Implanted patients are expected to survive for >1 year with good functional status [53].

A significant correlation between ICD implantation and depression or anxiety has been demonstrated in many studies [54], whereas cognitive performance has been examined just in a pair of them.

In our single-centre observational study which included 318 CHF patients implanted with an ICD for primary prevention, we observed similar anxiety and depression levels as well as similar cognitive performance (measured with MMSE) in comparison to non-ICD implanted subjects [55]. These surprising results might be due to the low rate of electrical intervention of the devices (appropriate or non-appropriate). In another prospective study on 77 ICD-patients, no significant changes in psychomotor speed and executive functioning were observed over a 12 month period, whereas over time significant declines were found in total memory and in delayed memory recall [56].

PM (Pacemaker)

Cardiac pacemaker (PM) is a frequently implanted device in CHF patients for the treatment of bradyarrhythmias. It is normally implanted in patients with conduction disturbances such as sinus node dysfunction and/or complete atrioventricular block. These disturbances frequently occur in older people and also in patients with CHF, the main clinical symptoms are syncopes, presyncopes and dizziness (Fig. 1.1 compares a PM with an ICD).

It has been suggested that patients suffering from bradyarrhythmias may show intellectual decline and that treatment with an artificial pacemaker may improve their cognitive functioning [57–60]. However, the studies do not present conclusive

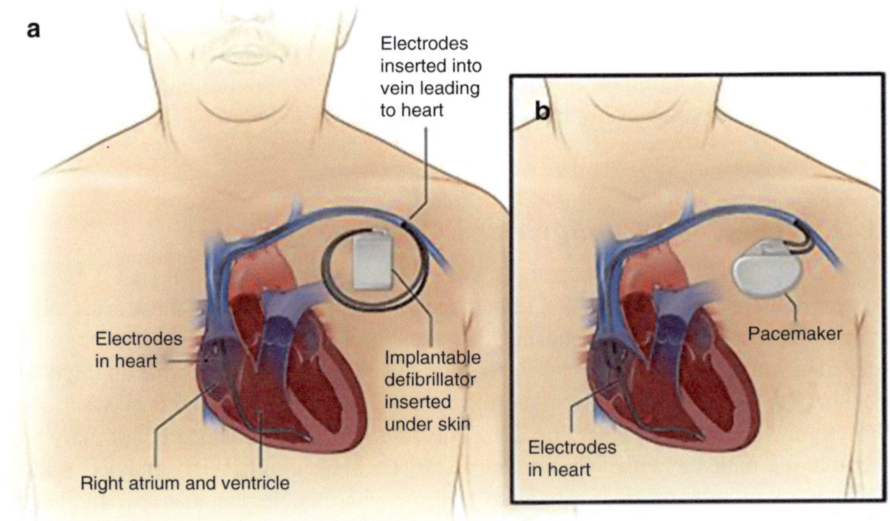

Fig. 1.1 The image compares an ICD with a pacemaker. (**a**) Shows the location and general size of an ICD in the upper chest. The wires with electrodes on the ends are inserted into the heart through a vein in the upper chest. (**b**) Shows the location and general size of a pacemaker in the upper chest. The wires with electrodes on the ends are inserted into the heart through a vein in the upper chest

results because most of them are based on small samples or very short follow-ups or are not controlled studies. Koide et al. [57] found an improvement in cerebral blood flow and verbal cognitive functions after PM implantation in 14 severe bradycardic patients, whereas in a similar study by Rockwood et al. [58] on 19 elderly patients, this correlation was not demonstrated even 6 and 12 months after implantation.

In a recent case-control study by Barbe et al. [60] based on 26 patients, cognitive assessment was made before PM implantation and compared with a 5 day and 6 month follow-up. On average, initial cognitive performances were no different between the two groups, whereas a slight improvement in cognitive performance was observed at the 6-month follow-up.

In conclusion, even if studies were limited by small sample size, there is consistent evidence that cognitive functioning in bradycardic older patients may improve after PM implantation.

The main characteristics of the studies that were examined are summarized in Table 1.1.

Table 1.1 Major characteristics of the studies examined

	No. patients	Age	Cognitive measures
CRT			
Conti et al. (2007)	10	52 ± 11	Hopkins verbal learning test, digit span and symbol digit subtest of the WAIS-III
Dixit et al. (2010)	20	54.8 ± 11.9	Digit span and symbol digit subtest of the WAIS-III, controlled oral word association test, TMT part A and B
Hoth et al. (2010)	27	68.4 ± 9.0	RBANS (delayed and immediate memory, language, global cognition, visuospatial skills, executive functioning)
ICD			
Kim et al. (2013)	77	64.8 ± 9.1	Memory (total and delayed recall), psychomotor speed, executive function
Feola et al. (2013)	318	71.6 ± 9.9	MMSE, 6MWT
PM			
Koide et al. (1994)	14	75.2	Verbal cognitive function
Rockwood et al. (1992)	19	65+	Immediate memory, language learning of abstract materials
Jabourian et al. (1995)	450	77.8 ± 10.2	MMSE, Benton, Rey copy and memory
Barbe et al. (2002)	26	75.0 ± 6.1	MMSE, Wechsler memory scale, word fluency, cube drawing

RBANS repeatable battery for the assessment of neuropsychological status, *MMSE* mini mental state examination, *6MWT* 6-min walking test

Conclusion

CI is a clinical condition frequently associated with CHF. It has shown to be a significant predictor of mortality, hospital admission and functional decline, and could affect the ability of CHF patients to manage their disease. The challenge for clinicians is not only the effective treatment of CHF but also the identification and management of CI in order to prevent further complications. Unfortunately, there is no definitive consensus on what could be the best comprehensive and standardized tool to identify cognitive changes in CHF patients.

As far as the use of cardiac devices in HF patients and their influence on CI, there are even more doubts due to: (a) a low number of studies on this matter; (b) the different methods used to define CI in these studies.

According to the literature it seems that bradycardic older patients implanted with a PM device showed a slight improvement in cognitive functioning. In CHF patients who received CRT, significant improvements in visuospatial skills and executive functions were found only in subjects whose LVEF improved. Finally, evidence on the effect of ICD devices on cognitive performances is still inconclusive, which indicates that more randomized controlled studies are needed in order to explore and study the impact of cardiac devices on cognitive functioning in CHF patients.

References

1. Morley JE. Mild cognitive impairment: a treatable condition. J Am Med Dir Assoc. 2014;15:1–5.
2. Vogels RLC, Scheltens P, et al. Cognitive impairment in heart failure: a systematic review of the literature. Eur J Heart Fail. 2007;9:440–9.
3. McLennan SN, Pearson SA, Cameron J, Stewart S. Prognostic importance of cognitive impairment in chronic heart failure patients: does specialist management make a difference? Eur J Heart Fail. 2006;8:494–501.
4. Leto L, Feola M. Cognitive impairment in heart failure patients. J Geriatr Cardiol. 2014;11(4):316–28.
5. Gaviria M, Pliskin N, Kney A. Cognitive impairment in patients with advanced heart failure and its implication on decision-making capacity. Congest Heart Fail. 2011;17:175–9.
6. Zuccalà G, Pedone C, Cesari M, et al. The effects of cognitive impairment on mortality among hospitalized patients with heart failure. Am J Med. 2003;115:97–103.
7. Pressler SJ, Kim JS, Riley P, et al. Memory dysfunction, psychomotor slowing and decreased executive function predict mortality in patients with heart failure and low ejection fraction. J Card Fail. 2010;16:750–60.
8. Dodson JA, Tuyet-Trinh NT, Towle VR, et al. Cognitive impairment in older adults with heart failure: prevalence, documentation and impact on outcomes. Am J Med. 2013;126:120–6.
9. Harkness K, Demers C, et al. Screening for cognitive deficits using the Montreal cognitive assessment tool in outpatients ≥ 65 years of age with heart failure. Am J Cardiol 2011;107:1203–1207.
10. Davis K, Mintzer M, Himmelfarb CRD, et al. Targeted intervention improves knowledge but not self-care or readmissions in heart failure patients with mild cognitive impairment. Eur J Heart Fail 2012;14:1041–104.

11. Trojano L, Antonelli Incalzi R, Acanfora D, Picone C, Mecocci P, Rengo F. Cognitive impairment: a key feature of congestive heart failure in the elderly. J Neurol. 2003;250:1456–63.
12. Gure TR, Blaum CS, The LKM. Prevalence of cognitive impairment in older adults with heart failure. J Am Geriatr Soc. 2012;60:1724–9.
13. Bauer LC, Johnson JK, Pozehl BJ. Cognition in heart failure: an overview of the concepts and their measures. J Am Acad Nurse Pract. 2011;23:577–85.
14. Georgiadis D, Sievert M, Cencetti S, et al. Cerebrovascular reactivity is impaired in patients with cardiac failure. Eur Heart J. 2000;21:407–13.
15. Jefferson AL, Poppas A, Paul RH, et al. Systemic hypoperfusion is associated with executive dysfunction in geriatric cardiac patients. Neurobiol Aging. 2007;28:477–83.
16. Zuccalà G, Onder G, Pedone C, et al. Hypotension and cognitive impairment: selective association in patients with heart failure. Neurology. 2001;57:1986–92.
17. Zuccalà G, Cattel C, Manes-Gravina E, et al. Left ventricular dysfunction: a clue to cognitive impairment in older patients with heart failure. J Neurol Neurosurg Psychiatry. 1997;63:509–12.
18. Cacciatore F, Abete P, Ferrara N, et al. Congestive heart failure and cognitive impairment in an older population. J Am Geriatr Soc. 1998;46:1343–8.
19. Zuccalà G, Marzetti E, Cesari M, et al. Correlates of cognitive impairment among patients with heart failure: results of a multicenter survey. Am J Med. 2005;118:496–502.
20. Qiu C, Winblad B, Marengoni A, et al. Heart failure and risk of dementia and Alzheimer disease. Arch Intern Med. 2006;166:1003–8.
21. De la Torre JC. Cardiovascular risk factors promote brain hypoperfusion leading to cognitive decline and dementia. Cardiovasc Psychiatry Neurol. 2012;2012:367516.
22. Moser DJ, Cohen RA, Clark MM, et al. Neuropsychological functioning among cardiac rehabilitation patients. J Cardpulm Rehabil. 1999;19:91–7.
23. Steinberg G, Lossnitzer N, Schellberg D, et al. Peak oxygen uptake and left ventricular ejection fraction, but not depressive symptoms, are associated with cognitive impairment in patients with chronic heart failure. Int J Gen Med. 2011;4:879–87.
24. Festa JR, Jia X, Cheung K, et al. Association of low ejection fraction with impaired verbal memory in older patients with heart failure. Arch Neurol. 2011;68:1021–6.
25. Vogels RLC, Oosterman JM, van Harten B, et al. Profile of cognitive impairment in chronic heart failure. J Am Geriatr Soc. 2007;55:1764–70.
26. Van den Hurk K, Reijmer YD, ven den Berg E, et al. Heart failure and cognitive function in the general population: the Hoorn Study. Eur J Heart Fail. 2011;13:1362–9.
27. Kerola T, Nieminen T, Hartikainen S, et al. B-type natriuretic peptide as a predictor of declining cognitive function and dementia – a cohort study of an elderly general population with a 5-year follow-up. Ann Med. 2010;42:207–15.
28. Daniels LB, Laughlin GA, Kritz-Silverstein D, et al. Elevated natriuretic peptide levels and cognitive function in community-dwelling older adults. Am J Med. 2011;124:670e1–8.
29. Gunstad J, Poppas A, Smeal S, et al. Relation of brain natriuretic peptide levels to cognitive dysfunction in adults >55 years of age with cardiovascular disease. Am J Cardiol. 2006;98:538–40.
30. Feola M, Garnero S, Vallauri P, et al. Relationship between cognitive function, depression/ anxiety and functional parameters in patients admitted for congestive heart failure. Open Cardiovasc Med J. 2013;7:54–60.
31. Debette S, Bauters C, Leys D, et al. Prevalence and determinants of cognitive impairment in chronic heart failure patients. Congest Heart Fail. 2007;13:205–8.
32. Baldasseroni S, Mossello E, Romboli B, et al. Relationship between cognitive function and 6-minute walking test in older outpatients with chronic heart failure. Aging Clin Exp Res. 2010;22:308–13.
33. Ball J, Carrington MJ, Stewart S, Safety investigators. Mild cognitive impairment in high-risk patients with chronic atrial fibrillation: a forgotten component of clinical management? Heart. 2013;99:542–7.
34. Peters R, Beckett N. Atrial fibrillation is associated with an increased risk of cognitive and functional decline. Evid Based Med. 2013;18:e16.

35. Marzona I, O'Donnell M, Teo K, Gao P, Anderson C, Bosch J, Yusuf S. Increased risk of cognitive and functional decline in patients with atrial fibrillation: results of the ONTARGET and TRANSCEND studies. CMAJ. 2012;184:E329–36.
36. Cacciatore F, Testa G, Langellotto A, Galizia G, Della-Morte D, Gargiulo G, Vevilacqua A, Del Genio MT, Canonico V, Rengo F, Abete P. Role of ventricular rate response on dementia in cognitively impaired elderly subjects with atrial fibrillation: a 10-year study. Dement Geriatr Cogn Disord. 2012;34:143–8.
37. Alosco ML, Spitznagel MB, Gunstad J. Obesity as a risk factor for poor neurocognitive outcomes in older adults with heart failure. Heart Fail Rev. 2014;19:403–11.
38. Alosco ML, Spitznagel MB, Raz N, et al. Obesity interacts with cerebral hypoperfusion to exacerbate cognitive impairment in older adults with heart failure. Cerebrovasc Dis Extra. 2012;2:88–98.
39. Hanon O, Vidal JS, de Groote P, Galinier M, Isnard R, Logeart D, Komajda M. Prevalence of memory disorders in ambulatory patients aged ≥70 years with chronic heart failure (from the EFICARE study). Am J Cardiol. 2014;113:1205–10.
40. Hawkins LA, Kilian S, Firek A, et al. Cognitive impairment and medication adherence in outpatients with heart failure. Heart Lung. 2012;41:572–82.
41. Harkness K, Heckman GA, Akhtar-Danesh N, Demers C, Gunn E, McKelvie RS. Cognitive function and self-care management in older patients with heart failure. Eur J Cardiovasc Nurs. 2014;13:277–84.
42. Cameron J, Worrall-Carter L, Page K, et al. Does cognitive impairment predict poor self-care in patients with heart failure? Eur J Heart Fail. 2010;12:508–12.
43. Cameron J, Ski CF, McLennan SN, et al. Development of the heart failure screening tool (Heart-FAST) to measure barriers that impede engagement in self-care. Eur J Cardiovasc Nurs. 2014;13:408–17.
44. Davis KK, Dennison Himmelfarb CR, Szanton SL, et al. Predictors of heart failure self-care in patients who screened positive for mild cognitive impairment. J Cardiovasc Nurs. 2015;30(2):152–60.
45. Bradley DJ, Bradley EA, Baughman KL, et al. Cardiac resynchronization and death from progressive heart failure: a meta-analysis of randomized controlled trials. JAMA. 2003;289:730–40.
46. Priori SG, Blomström-Lundqvist C, Mazzanti A, et al. 2015 ESC guidelines for the management of patients with ventricular arrhythmias and the prevention of sudden cardiac death: the task force for the management of patients with ventricular arrhythmias and the prevention of sudden cardiac death of the European Society of Cardiology (ESC). Endorsed by: Association for European Paediatric and Congenital Cardiology (AEPC). Eur Heart J. 2015;36(41):2793–867.
47. Abraham WT, Fisher WG, Smith AL, Delurgio DB, Leon AR, Loh E, Kocovic DZ, et al. Cardiac resynchronization in chronic heart failure. N Engl J Med. 2002;346:1845–53.
48. Cleland JG, Daubert JC, Erdmann E, Freemantle N, Gras D, Kappenberger L, Tavazzi L. The effect of cardiac resynchronization on morbidity and mortality in heart failure. N Engl J Med. 2005;352:1539–49.
49. Conti JB, Sears SF. Cardiac resynchronization therapy: can we make our heart failure patients smarter? Trans Am Clin Climatol Assoc. 2007;118:153–64.
50. Dixit NK, Vazquez LD, Cross NJ, Kuhl EA, Serber ER, Kovacs A, Dede DE, et al. Cardiac resynchronization therapy: a pilot study examining cognitive change in patients before and after treatment. Clin Cardiol. 2010;33:84–8.
51. Hoth KF, Poppas A, Ellison KE, Paul RH, Sokobin A, Cho Y, Cohen RA. Link between change in cognition and left ventricular function following cardiac resynchronization therapy. J Cardiopulm Rehabil Prev. 2010;30:401–8.
52. Proietti R, Manzoni GM, Cravello L, Castelnuovo G, Bernier ML, Essebag V. Can cardiac resynchronization therapy improve cognitive function? A systematic review. Pacing Clin Electrophysiol. 2014;37(4):520–30.

53. McMurray JJ, Adamopoulos S, Anker SD, et al. ESC guidelines for the diagnosis and treatment of acute and chronic heart failure 2012: the task force for the diagnosis and treatment of acute and chronic heart failure 2012 of the European Society of Cardiology. Developed in collaboration with the Heart Failure Association (HFA) of the ESC. Eur Heart J. 2012;33(14):1787–847.
54. Freedenberg V, Thomas SA, Friedmann E. Anxiety and depression in implanted cardioverter-defibrillator recipients and heart failure: a review. Heart Fail Clin. 2011;7(1):59–68.
55. Feola M, Vallauri P, Salvatico L, et al. Neuropsychological impact of implantable cardioverter defibrillator in congestive heart failure patients. Int J Cardiol. 2013;166:275–6.
56. Kim J, Pressler SJ, Groh WJ. Change in cognitive function over 12 months among patients with an implantable cardioverter-defibrillator. J Cardiovasc Nurs. 2013;28(6):E28–36.
57. Koide H, Kobayashi S, Kitani M, Tsunematsu T, Nakazawa Y. Improvement of cerebral blood flow and cognitive function following pacemaker implantation in patients with bradycardia. Gerontology. 1994;40(5):279–85.
58. Rockwood K, Dobbs AR, Rule BG, Howlett SE, Black WR. The impact of pacemaker implantation on cognitive functioning in elderly patients. J Am Geriatr Soc. 1992;40(2):142–6.
59. Jabourian AP. Cognitive functions, EEG and gait disorders in cardiac arrhythmias, one day before and eight days after pacemaker implantation. Ann Med Psychol (Paris). 1995;153(2):89–105.
60. Barbe C, Puisieux F, Jansen I, Dewailly P, Klug D, Kacet S, DiPompeo C. Improvement of cognitive function after pacemaker implantation in very old persons with bradycardia. J Am Geriatr Soc. 2002;50(4):778–80.

Chapter 2
Neuropsychological Functioning After Implantable Cardioverter-Defibrillator Surgery

Abdullah Alabdulgader

Abstract Basic philosophy of medical practice is to preserve life around the globe irrespective of culture and civilization. But the perception and preference of life varies from person to person with respect to quality and span of life. This historical perspective to human life is in concordance to implantable cardiovertor-defibrillators (ICDs) i.e. an invention which has revolutionized the care of patients at risk of life threatening arrhythmias. Although, the evidence of the superiority of after implantable cardioverter-defibrillators (AICDs) over medications in overcoming the ventricular arrhythmias is beyond the scope of this chapter, yet the studies carried over the last decade strongly supports this choice. This chapter establishes new visionary approach for the new era demands. It consolidate new and Intelligent conceptualization for proper perspective and management options for the newly emerging ICD subjects problems and complaints. Smart anticipation of ICD subjects psychosocial and cognitive difficulties based in previous experience, as adjunct to optimizing their rhythm control will be discussed with global perspective aiming toward treating rhythm disorder in the human beings within the physical and biological diversities and cosmos around them. This chapter is a concise scientific back up for all those working in rhythm management and ICD to support them making critical decisions in the case of emergency situation, looks into the cerebral injury in ICD patients, providing knowledge in prevalence and impact of psychological distress in (ICD) patients, with special focus in PTSD in ICD. Quality of Life (QOL) in ICD patients has been given special attention. The new perspective correlating anxiety, depression and autonomic dysfunction and the viscous cycle for shock continuum as well as the benefits of spiritual well being has been discussed. The newly documented relation of solar and geomagnetic activity (SGA) to human heart rhythm and the sensitivity of the autonomic nervous system to SGA is also discussed. Novel preventive and therapeutic approaches has been discussed. Awareness of the magnitude of psychophysiological distress in ICD patients as a very

The original version of this chapter was revised. An erratum to this chapter can be found at DOI 10.1007/978-3-319-55721-2_19

A. Alabdulgader, M.D, MRCP (UK), FRCP (Edin)
Prince Sultan Cardiac Centre, Hofuf, Alhasa 31982, Saudi Arabia
e-mail: kidsecho@yahoo.com

© Springer International Publishing AG 2017
R. Proietti et al. (eds.), *Psychological, Emotional, Social and Cognitive Aspects of Implantable Cardiac Devices*, DOI 10.1007/978-3-319-55721-2_2

important step in patients overall management was given concern. The intelligent life style using non pharmacological modalities to prevent ventricular arrhythmias including device programming, cardiac rehabilitation and the intelligent idea of sparing shock with positive emotion illustrating the beneficial outcome of cardiac coherence are discussed. Special emphasis has been given to Cognitive behavioral therapy (CBT) and the increasing weight of evidence of its favorable psychophysiological out come in ICD patients. Acute and long term pharmacological treatment has been mentioned. Finally future directions for the new era related to Technical aspects of the device and System NeuroPsychoBiological approach and The new NeuroPsychoBiological Perspective: from Genes to Galaxies and Neurobiology of PTSD as well as special statement in Transcranial Magnetic Stimulation in Post-Traumatic Stress Disorder has been discussed.

Keywords Implantable cardioverter-defibrillator (ICD) • Neuropsychological functioning • Psychosocial distress • Post traumatic stress disorder (PTSD) • Cerebral electrical injury • Quality of life (QOL) • Anxiety • Depression • Autonomic dysfunction • Electrical shock • Heart rate variability • Emotion • Cardiac coherence • Psychotherapy • Cognitive behavioral therapy (CBT) • Neurobiology • Transcranial magnetic stimulation (TMS)

Introduction

Preservation of life is the core and top priority of medical practice in all human civilizations and cultures. Nevertheless, there are different perceptions and preferences between people as far as length and quality of life are concerned. This historical perspective to human life is in concordance to defibrillators (ICDs): an invention which has revolutionized the care of patients at risk of life threatening arrhythmias. The evidence of the superiority of AICDs over medications in aborting ventricular arrhythmias is beyond the scope of this chapter, but the voluminous literature of the last decade strongly supports this choice [1, 2]. This historic success in defeating sudden death, has allowed research and clinical care to focus more on patients centered outcomes, such as quality of life, device acceptance, psychological wellbeing and trauma reactions [3]. AICDs patients are typically seen by the electrophysiologist during a time in which they are accumulating increasing levels of psychosocial, emotional and cognitive distress due to the primary heart disease and the additional treatment for lethal arrhythmias. Although, the AICD implant is perceived subjectively and objectively as a lifesaving procedure; the increasing psychosocial and emotional distress and the impact of shocks on the quality of life of the patients definitely present a new challenge and responsibility for the concerned medical communities including the treating electrophysiologist, the referring cardiologist, medical specialist, psychologist, nurses, technicians and last but not least families. The lack of medical literature on the psychological, emotional, social and cognitive aspects that the ICD implies, not only for the recipient but for all the people involved in the process warrants us to study these aspects and their effects in order to suggest future perspectives.

Visionary Care for New Era Demands

Intelligent conceptualization of the emerging concerns, problems and complaints of ICD recipients is imperative. The accumulated experience with ICD subjects in the last two decades indicates a need for comprehensive care and management plans for those subjects taking-in consideration ICD implantation and at the same time warrants that serious considerations must be given to psychological, social and cognitive aspects secondary to defibrillator implant. The possibility to anticipate psychosocial and cognitive difficulties in ICD recipients, in addition to optimizing their rhythm control is the key toward successful comprehensive solutions for ICD patient management in the new era.

The Critical Decision in the Short Time: To Reject or Agree?

Decision research has detailed how cognitive, emotional, and social factors influence decision making [3, 4]. The ICD decision is unique because it is a major life decision that often must be made in a relatively short time period, and since implantation is not easily reversible, changing one's mind is not always a reasonable option. As the ICD decision may be challenging, patient involvement in medical decision making can vary considerably. When patients do take time to fully consider the pros and cons of a decision, this is labeled "systematic processing" [5]. When a patient is limited in his or her willingness or ability to process information, heuristic tendencies often influence decisions [4]. Optimizing patient decisions regarding device technologies remains a critical consideration for informed consent. Optimizing patient decisions regarding device technologies remains a critical consideration for informed consent. Decision making for new and improved technologies will increasingly become more difficult given the chasm between patient understanding and the advance of technology. Research suggests that assessing pros and cons of the ICD may predict their choice for the ICD. The ICD-DAS is an empirically based starting point for attempting to improve the ICD decision-making process and warrants more research.

Anthony Garrett Hazelton et al., studied decisional balance among potential implantable cardioverter defibrillator recipients. The purpose of this study was to create and evaluate a measure of patient valuated pros and cons of the ICD, and its relationship to patient decision regarding ICD implantation [6]. The quality and type of questions used by the authors are a new and practical step toward visionary consent which should serve to minimize personal and psychosocial aspects for ICD candidates in the post implant stage. The authors, examined the discriminant validity of the measure from existing psychological measures and tested the predictive validity of the proposed ICD measure on behavioral intention to receive the ICD. They discuss the potential clinical use of the ICD–decision analysis scale (ICD-DAS) on how the tool allows clinicians to explore why a patient has rated certain pros or cons in particular ways. If intervention can address patient concerns and provide meaningful knowledge, the quality of patient decisions is likely to improve (Fig. 2.1).

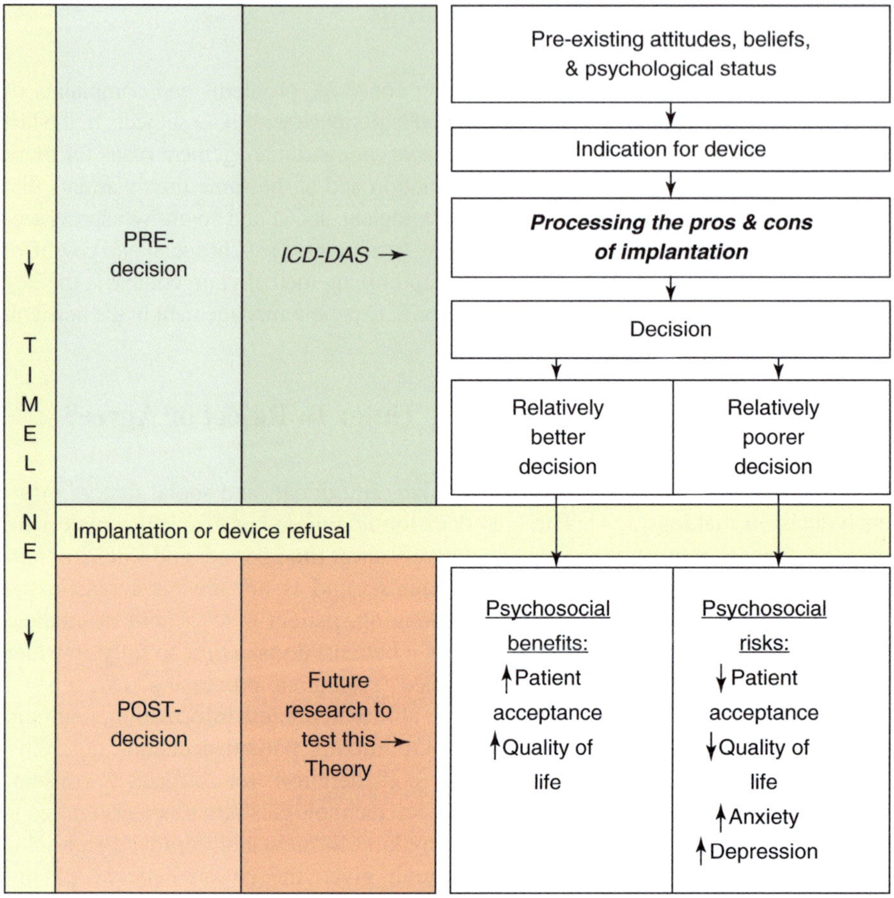

Fig. 2.1 Graphical representation of implantable cardioverter defibrillator (ICD) decision analysis scale. Notes: Timeline from before to after ICD decision from top to bottom. *Arrows* represent either [1] passage of time or [2] the potential impact of decision quality on a patient's psychosocial experience [6]

Cerebral Electrical Injury in ICD Patients

The defibrillation device provides high voltage therapy several seconds after the onset of ventricular fibrillation (VF). During this time, the cerebral nervous system is hypoperfused [7–10]. Electroencephalographic changes consistent with cerebral ischemia have been observed within 7.5–11 s of cardiac arrest [10, 11]. Older literature in the field based in electroencephalographic changes failed to document any correlation with neurologic outcome [10]. More recent publications investigated neuronal injury biomarkers to correlate between ICD shocks and associated cerebral hyoperfusion as evidence of neuronal injury. The release of neuron-specific enolase (NSE) and S100 has been reported after VF episodes aborted by implantable cardioverter-defibrillator (ICD) [12, 13]. Dworschak M et al., studied 45 patients undergoing implantable cardioverter/defibrillator insertion. Eleven patients with cardiac pacemaker implantation, which was performed in the same manner yet without the necessity to induce ventricular fibrillation, served as controls. They found that median neuron-specific enolase values climbed from a preoperative 9.9–12.3 and 14.4 μg/L at 2 and 24 h after surgery, respectively. This increase was associated with the number of shocks and the cumulative time in circulatory arrest. The highest median S100 level (0.075 μg/L) was reached 2 h after the procedure. Neuron-specific enolase and S100 were extremely elevated (13.7 and 0.970 μg/L, respectively) in one patient after an extended episode of ventricular fibrillation [12].

Disruption of the blood brain barrier occurs early in cerebral ischemia. Cytoplasmic proteins of cerebral origin can be detected in the blood. Elevated serum NSE could be detected as early as 1 h after cardiac arrest and levels of >33 ng/mL, predicted persistent coma. The specificity of serum NSE levels >80 ng/mL is sufficiently high that, when it is used with other clinical and electrophysiological data, it could be useful as a prognostic indicator of neurologic outcome after cardiac arrest [14]. Similarly, elevated serum S100, another cytosolic protein of mainly neuroglial origin, could be observed after cardiac arrest. Patients with S100 levels of 0.02 μg/L in the second day after cardiac arrest, all died within 2 weeks after the arrest. As compared with NSE, S100 seems to be more sensitive and specific as far as prognosis after global cerebral ischemia and cerebral damage is concerned. Furthermore, even slightly elevated NSE and S100 serum levels after stroke traumatic brain injury, hypothermic cardiac arrest and surgery correlated well with neurocognitive defects and neuropsychological outcome. Dworschak M et al. [12] concluded, even brief successive periods of global cerebral ischemia cause neuronal damage without obvious severe neurologic deficits, however, they may be related to subtle postoperative neurologic or cognitive dysfunctions that a number of implantable cardioverter defibrillator patients exhibit after implantation.

Prevalence and Impact of Psychosocial Distress in ICD Subjects

It is our belief that all figures estimating psychosocial distress and cognitive impairment in ICD subjects are underestimating the actual numbers. This is simply because the new experience of ICD implantation and the associated events must create emotional distress of some degree in all subjects who undergo the operation. In our experience patients tends to deny mild symptoms, as a way of self-protection, to maintain better self-image.

General or ICD-specific anxiety as a psychological morbidity has a point prevalence of 13–38% of ICD recipients in cross-sectional research [15]. Longitudinal assessment of anxiety has indicated that approximately 35% of patients at peri-implant met cutoff criteria for anxiety, whereas approximately 15% of patients remained above cutoff for anxiety at 6- and 12-month follow-ups [16]. Self-reported anxiety is also predictive of self-reported general health in ICD patients [17]. Significant depressive symptoms for ICD patients range from 10% to 41% [15]. Baseline depressive symptoms and the emotion of anger have also been associated with longitudinal increased risk of shock [18]. Finally, personality characteristics associated with negative emotional processes and social inhibition (type D personality) have also been established as prevalent (24%) in ICD patients and linked to increased risk of ventricular arrhythmia (hazard ratio, 1.89) and mortality (hazard ratio, 2:79) [19]. Taken together, sufficient evidence exists to warrant the inclusion of psychosocial factors in the routine treatment planning of ICD patients.

Post Traumatic Stress Disorder in ICD Patient, Fears and Available Facts

PTSD is a disorder that develops in some people who have seen or lived through a shocking, scary, or dangerous event, which tends to print a life stigma. In ICD patients, it is natural to feel afraid before, during, and after any shock experience. Fear triggers many split-secondary changes in the body to help the patient adapt with the shock. Nearly everyone will experience a spectrum of reactions after trauma, yet most people recover from the initial symptoms naturally. Those who continue to experience problems may be diagnosed with PTSD. People who have PTSD may feel stressed or frightened even when they are not in danger.

To be diagnosed with PTSD, an adult must have all of the following for at least 1 month:

1. At least one re-experiencing symptom.
2. At least one avoidance symptom.
3. At least two arousal and reactivity symptoms.
4. At least two cognition and mood symptoms.

Is there a Difference Between a Stressful Event and a Traumatic Event?

Most people with ICDs have faced stressful and potentially traumatic events at some point in their life. Reactions to traumatic events range from brief, normal, and healthy to long-term, pathological, and debilitating. The ICD patients are always at the risk of potentially traumatic events, the most serious are lethal arrhythmias and subsequent discharge of shock or multiple shocks. These stressful events are in addition to the inherent stressful cardiac condition, the ICD patient is suffering from, (see Fig. 2.2 for the time line of potentially stressful events in cardiac patient life).

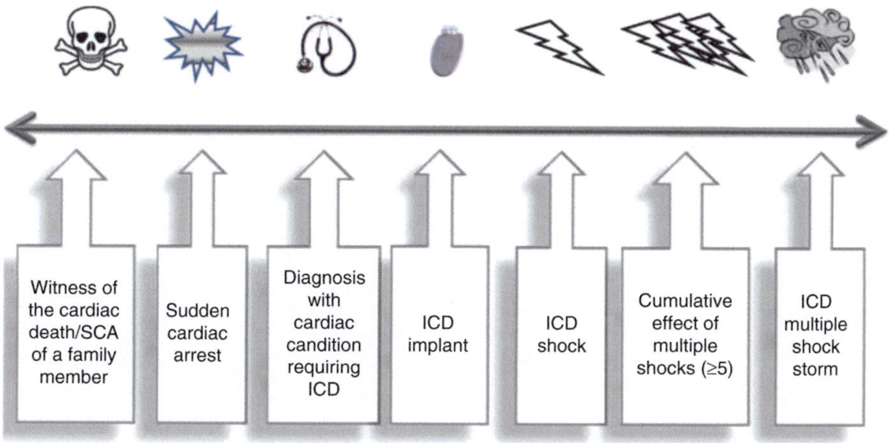

Fig. 2.2 Cardiac patient life potentially stressful and traumatic events

The difference between an event that is considered stressful and an event that is considered traumatic is primarily the personal perception and reaction to the event. If the reaction is one of *fear, helplessness, or horror*, it is typically considered traumatic by mental health specialists. Typical reactions of ICD patients to shock experience involves symptoms such as high anxiety, avoidance, and re-experiencing the event in the form of unwanted thoughts, dreams, or flashbacks. In the general public, approximately 8% of people meet the criteria for post-traumatic stress disorder [20], whereas 20% of ICD patients have significant symptoms of PTSD, meaning that one in five people with an ICD has PTSD [21]. Although many more than 20% of ICD patients experience ICD-related "traumatic experiences," not all develop trauma reactions such as PTSD. Risk factors for developing PTSD symptoms include lack of support from family or friends, a family or personal history of mental illness, a history of sexual or physical abuse as a child, or a cognitive or thought disorder [22]. Ultimately, the distinction between a stressful event and a traumatic event has more to do with a person's perception and reaction to the event than the event itself (see Fig. 2.3).

Post Traumatic Stress Disorder and ICD, Current Knowledge

The potential for PTSD in cardiac patients is increasingly recognized [21]. Rates of PTSD in the general public have been estimated at 7.8% [20]. PTSD rates in cardiac clinics range from 0% to 24% prevalence [23–29], and have recently been established in an ICD clinic to be approximately 20% [21]. It increases further in primary care settings to approximately 11–12% [30, 31]. Ladwig et al., [21] found that experience of sudden cardiac arrest outside of the hospital setting resulted in an even greater prevalence of PTSD (27–38%). Interestingly, these results did not differ,

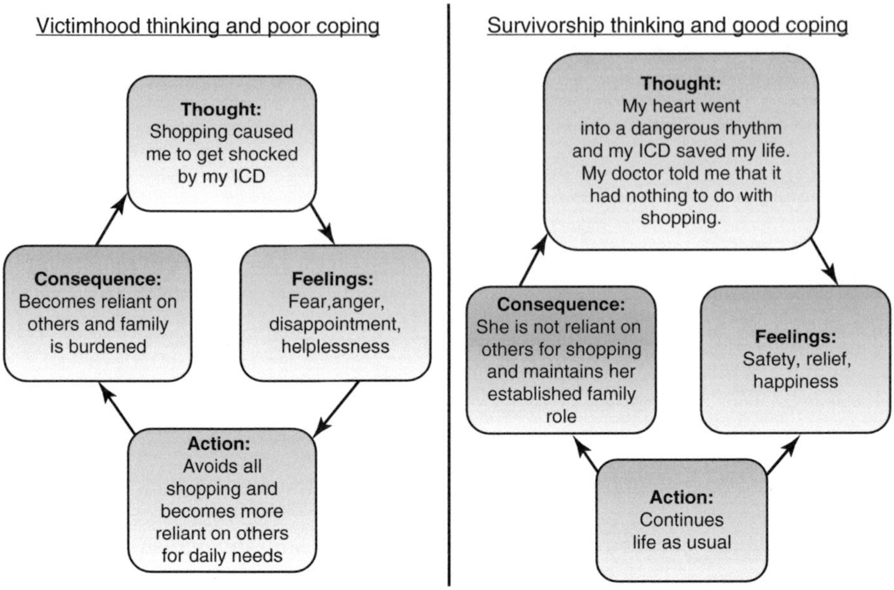

Fig. 2.3 Helpful and unhelpful thoughts and the effect of these thoughts on feelings, behaviors, and consequences. ICD indicates implantable cardioverter defibrillator

based on shock experience, suggesting that in this sample, the trauma associated with the cardiac condition was potentially more salient. In an another longitudinal assessment of PTSD symptoms in ICD patients, 21% were found to meet the cutoff for clinically significant PTSD symptoms at initial assessment. These rates dropped significantly in the first 6 months after implantation to 12% and remained stable at 13% at 1 year. Despite an initial reduction in the number of patients with PTSD, Von Kanel et al., found that 2 years after implant, there is a substantially greater prevalence of PTSD in ICD patients [32]. In fact, at 2 years after implant, 30.8% of patients had PTSD, and this increased to 36.4% at 4 years after implant. Nineteen percent of these patients had PTSD at both assessments, 12.1% remitted between times 1 and 2, and 17.8% had development of new PTSD between times 1 and 2. Altogether, 48.6% of the sample had clinically significant levels of PTSD during one of the time points. Moreover, ICD patients with elevated PTSD scores after device implantation were significantly more likely to have a shock storm [16]. Furthermore, elevated PTSD scores were associated with a 3.2 times greater likelihood of mortality within 5 years compared with ICD patients with moderate symptom levels of PTSD, even after controlling for disease and demographic parameters [21]. In addition to understanding the prevalence of psychosocial distress, possessing a working knowledge of the presentation of psychosocial distress in ICD patients is the most helpful method for facilitating appropriate intervention [33]. Figure 2.4 summarizes the key risk factors, prevalence, and presentation of psychosocial distress in ICD patients. A Venn diagram has been used to illustrate the likely overlap of symptoms and morbidities [34].

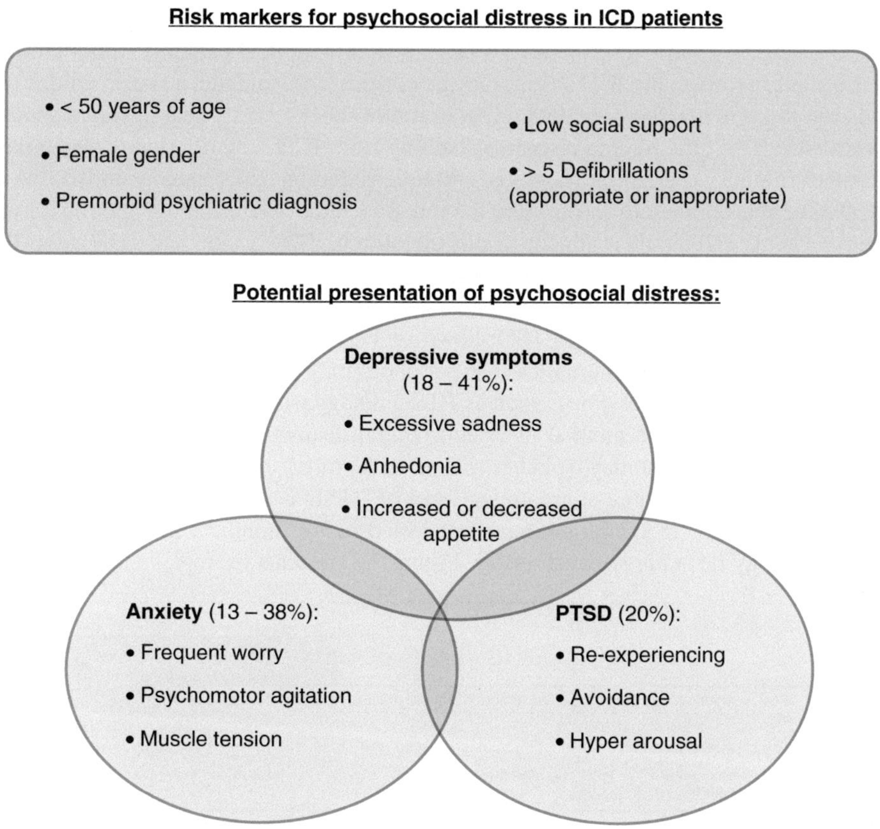

Fig. 2.4 Key risk factors, prevalence, and presentation of psychosocial distress in implantable cardioverter defibrillator (ICD) patients. PTSD indicates posttraumatic stress disorder [34]

Versteeg et al. [35], published a brief report that an ICD shock experience was the strongest determinant of PTSD at 3 months after implant. However, preimplantation anxiety and ICD concerns were the best predictors of PTSD at 6-month follow-up. Von Kanel et al., found that PTSD prevalence increases with time, 2 years after implant [32]. In their sample of patients surveyed, different PTSD predictors were found in 2 and 4 years after implantation. They found the significant predictors of PTSD at baseline (2 years after implantation) were: peritraumatic dissociation, feelings of helplessness, depression, female sex, history of being resuscitated, and greater number of cardiac symptoms. At 4 years after implantation predictors were: low education level, feelings of helplessness, alexithymia (sub-clinical inability to identify and describe emotions in the self and ineffective emotional responding), experience of >5 shocks, and previous history of PTSD.

Collectively, these results suggest that both preexisting psychological functioning and the eventual experience of ICD shocks relate to the presentation of PTSD symptoms in ICD patients. These preliminary results stimulate continual inclusion of both background (e.g., personality and trait variables) and experiential (e.g., shock and disease severity) variables in psychosocial research with ICD patients. Although the defibrillation (especially ICD storm) may be considered traumatic, it is also unique to other traumas in that the persistent threat of future shocks exists. Fear of future shock is realistic. Thus, the trauma response resulting from ICD defibrillation is dissimilar to other trauma experiences in which subsequent trauma experience is unlikely. An ICD patient is continually exposed to the threat of future defibrillation and must live with a visible and tactile reminder of this threat (e.g., ICD pocket and scar). In military trauma, when persons are continually exposed to war, a short-term and natural response to this stress is called "combat and operational stress reaction" [36]. These persons may go on to develop PTSD; however, because they are still exposed to the realistic threat of future trauma, their experiences may not warrant diagnosis with a potentially severe mental illness such as PTSD. Diagnosis with PTSD does not infer causality but is rather a method of categorizing a distinct presentation. The experience of the ICD patient may be better related to "combat and operational stress reaction" rather than the more stigmatizing label of PTSD because of the nature of the traumatic stressor. If symptoms have not lasted a full month, a more appropriate diagnosis may be *acute stress disorder*. Figure 2.5 presents examples of how PTSD

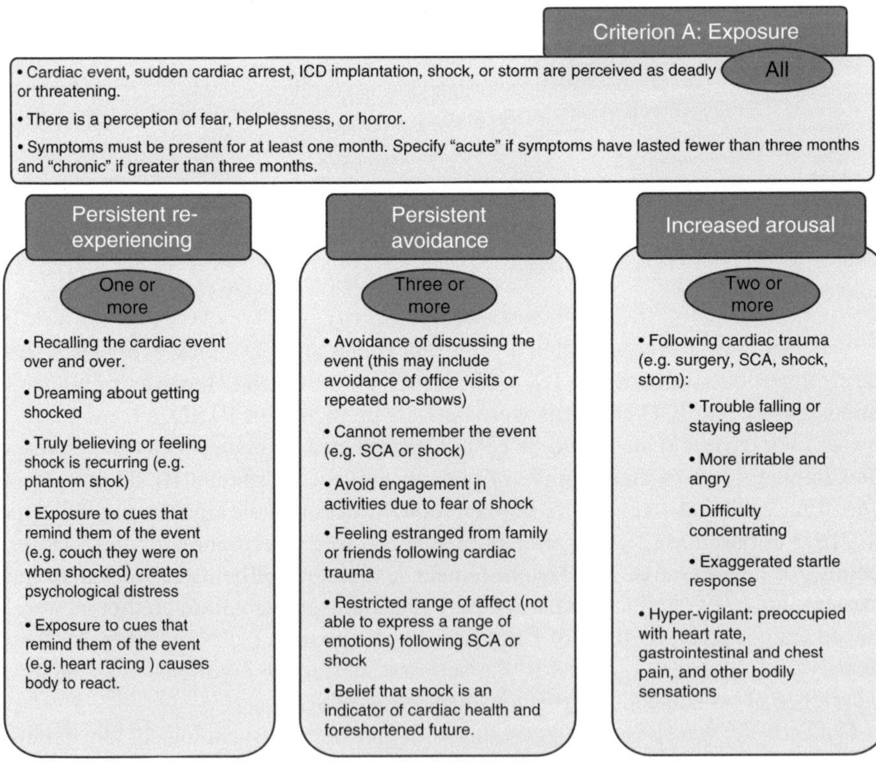

Fig. 2.5 Posttraumatic stress disorder symptom clusters and presentation in patients with implantable cardioverter-defibrillators (ICD). SCD indicated sudden cardiac death [34]

symptoms may be expressed in ICD patients. Formal diagnosis requires that the symptoms last >1 month and cause clinically significant impairment in occupational, social, or other important areas of functioning.

Quality of Life and the ICD

Quality of life is a generic term describing: *the health outcome of interdependent biological, psychological, occupational and social function*. Available evidence indicates that ICD recipients experience a brief decline in QOL from baseline but improve to pre-implant levels after 1 year of follow-up [37]. The largest clinical trial data published in final form is from the coronary artery bypass graft (CABG) Patch trial which randomized patients to ICD (n = 262) versus no ICD (n = 228) while undergoing CABG surgery [38]. In contrast to May and colleagues [37], data from this trial indicates that the QOL outcomes (mental and physical) for the ICD patients were significantly worse compared to patients with no ICD. Subanalyses revealed that there was no difference in QOL for non-shocked ICD patients versus patients with no ICD. These results indicate that the ICD group who had received shocks was responsible for the significantly worse mental and physical QOL outcome scores between the groups.

Collectively, this data suggest that the experience of shock may contribute to psychological distress and diminished QOL. Figure 2.6 details the psychological continuum a patient may experience secondary to shock.

Although detrimental, economic status is not considered in the current medical literature as a standing alone QOL indicator but is contemplated indirectly in

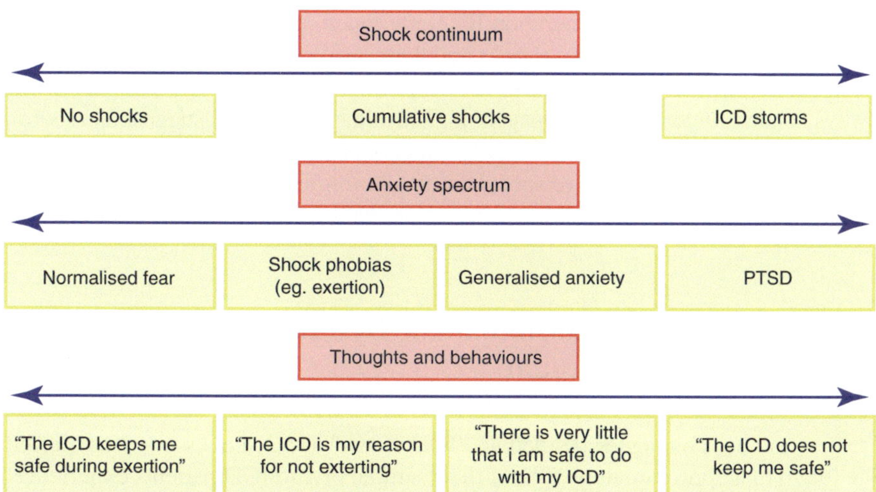

Fig. 2.6 Continuum of implantable cardioverter-defibrillator (ICD) shock response. PTSD, post-traumatic stress disorder [39]

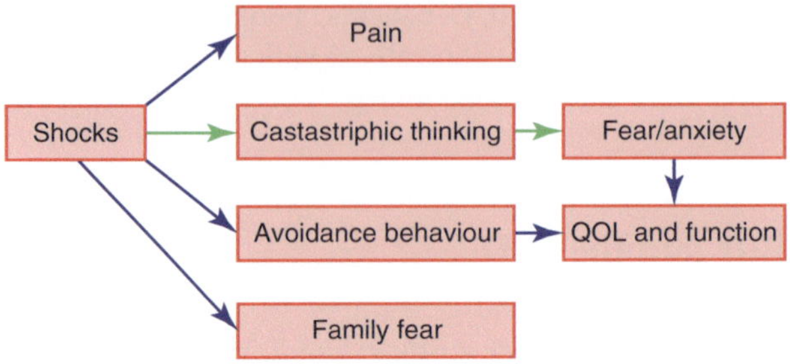

Fig. 2.7 Hypothesized interrelationship between shocks, psychological distress, and quality of life (QOL) [21]

discussions related to returning to work. In subset of patients it can dominate and directly affect psychological and social functions outcome and biological outcome indirectly. *Ability to return to work is accepted objective index of QOL.* ICD recipients have favorable return to work rates in currently available studies. The largest study (n = 101) indicated that 62% of patients had resumed employment [39]. Those who returned to work were more educated and less likely to have a history of myocardial infarction. Figure 2.7 illustrates shock consequences and its impact on QOL.

They concluded that The ICD is the treatment of choice for life threatening arrhythmias. All available data suggest that the ICD will achieve comparable if not better QOL than alternative treatments. Future research must place greater emphasis on ICD specific and arrhythmia specific measures that may be more sensitive to more changes in outcome. Measurement and interventions should focus on patient acceptance of the device. Interdisciplinary studies that include cardiology, psychology, nursing, and cardiac rehabilitation specialists are needed to guide best clinical practice. The reputation of the ICD as a "shock box" is a significant source of anxiety to potential patients. Today's generation ICDs are much improved in their sensing and tiered therapy options to reduce shocks and their resulting distress. Despite improvements in therapy such as anti-tachycardia pacing (ATP), ICD patients are likely always to need some attention to psychological adjustment. They suggest that routine consideration of psychosocial needs be integrated into the clinical care of ICD patients worldwide [40]. Future speculations to minimize the need for shock and its unfavorable consequences, will be discussed in the next sections of this chapter.

Anxiety, Depression and Autonomic Dysfunction: The Viscous Cycle for Shock Continuum

Credner and her colleagues defined an "ICD storm" as >3 shocks in a 24-h period. She found that approximately 10% of their sample of 136 ICD patients experienced an ICD storm during the first 2 years following ICD implantation [41]. Moreover, the mean (SD) number of shocks for this group of storm patients was 17 (range 3–50; median 8) [42]. The experience of an ICD storm may prompt catastrophic cognitions and feelings of increasing anxiety, depression and helplessness. These adverse psychological reactions have been linked in initial research as prospective predictors for the occurrence of subsequent arrhythmias and shocks at 1, 3, 6, and 9 month intervals. Although additional research focusing on a wide range of potentially identifiable "triggers" of arrhythmias is needed, the available evidence indicates that reducing negative emotions and psychological distress may also decrease the chances of receiving a shock. The evidence in this direction should alert electrophysiologists as well as psychologists and psychiatrists to focus their research and therapeutic measures in what we call: *Arrhythmogenicity of negative emotions.*

Anxiety and depression have been shown to be independent predictors of mortality in ischemic heart disease [43–49], raising the possibility that anxiety plays a contributing role in the high 1-year mortality rate observed after ICD implantation [50] despite the effectiveness of the ICD in preventing sudden death. Paradoxically, ICD patients might be at higher risk of having arrhythmias, and therefore of receiving shocks, because of their fear of receiving shocks. Although additional research focusing on a wide range of potentially identifiable "triggers" of arrhythmias is needed, the available evidence indicates that reducing negative emotions and psychological distress may also decrease the chances of receiving a shock. The role of anxiety and stress in inducing ventricular arrhythmias has been hypothesized since the 1970s [51, 52] and in the 1990s evidence indicated that strong emotions can precipitate cardiac events [53–55]. Emotional [56, 57] and mental stress [58] were shown to have a detrimental effect on both cardiac perfusion and function. This suggests that, at least in some settings, negative emotions may play a causal role in cardiac events, rather than being secondary phenomena. Anxiety may worsen cardiac outcomes by reducing heart rate variability (HRV) [59, 60] and baro-reflex control [61] or by inducing alterations in the coagulation system [62]. Conversely, conditions promoting psychological well-being such as social support, pet ownership [63, 64] or prayers may favorably influence variables such as HRV and survival.

Heart rate variability indicates psychological resiliency and behavioral flexibility, reflecting an individual's capacity to self-regulate and effectively adapt to changing social or environmental demands. Considerable evidence suggests evolution of the Autonomic Nervous System (ANS), specifically the vagus nerves, was central to development of emotional experience, the ability to self-regulate emotional processes and social behavior and that it underlies the social engagement system.

Jennifer L. et al. demonstrates that elevated levels of depression and anxiety are related to HRV based indices of autonomic nervous system dysfunction in patients with implantable cardioverter defibrillators [65]. A sympathovagal imbalance describing shift towards increased sympathetic and reduced parasympathetic nervous system activity may provide a pathophysiological mechanism accounting for the elevated arrhythmic risk in patients with psychological factors associated with elevated cardiovascular risk. Associations between depression and HRV tended to be stronger than associations between anxiety and HRV measures. Data analyses based on categorical data identifying relatively high levels of depression and anxiety versus low levels using previously published cut-off values revealed stronger associations with HRV than analyses examining depression and anxiety as continuous variables. These results suggest that psychosocial factors may adversely affect autonomic function only at levels above a certain critical threshold. Further research is needed to examine whether a formal clinical diagnosis of Major Depressive Disorder or specific anxiety disorders better identify cardiac patients at high risk of abnormal autonomic control.

Depression and anxiety often occur in the same patient and exploratory analyses indicate that the combination of high depression with high anxiety was associated with the most pronounced parasympathetic withdrawal as measured by the RMSSD and pNN50 indices. Reduced HRV in the group with elevated levels of both depression and anxiety levels was not merely a function of more severe depression symptoms because depression levels were not higher between the elevated depression subgroups with versus without elevated anxiety levels. These results raise the possibility that anxiety may exacerbate the relationship between depression and reduced HRV. Furthermore, some evidence suggests that high anxiety and not depression is associated with reduced vagal control among post myocardial infarction patients [61]. Symptomatic heterogeneity of HRV within depression [66] and evidence that worry episodes are associated with decreased HRV [67] indicates that attention to individual symptom profiles rather than diagnostic categories may be important. Additional research examining depression and anxiety symptoms is necessary to establish the neurobehavioral mechanisms that integrate central and autonomic nervous system activity.

Bekelman DB et al., documented strong inverse association between spiritual well-being and depression in 60 patients with heart failure, independent of gender, income, social support, physical symptoms, and health status [68].

Elena Salmoirago-Blotcher examined spiritual well-being in patients living with an implantable cardioverter defibrillator and investigated the possible impact of spiritual well-being on the self-reported psychological health of these patients [69]. They found that patients with higher spiritual well-being had significantly less psychological distress and a lower prevalence of concurrent psychiatric morbidity and psychotropic drug use compared with patients with lower spiritual wellbeing.

A new area of research is investigating the possibility to anticipate future cardiac events including sudden cardiac death. The natural variation in the geomagnetic field in and around the earth has been reportedly involved in relation to several human cardiovascular variables. These include blood pressure heart rate (HR), and heart rate variability (HRV) [70, 71]. Long term recordings of the earth magnetic field (MF) and heart rate variability (HRV) and the use of sophisticated mathematical methods indicate a strong correlation between earth MF and human heart, HRV [72]. The accumulated evidence of the sensitivity of the human autonomic nervous system (ANS) to geomagnetic changes should encourage us and other investigators to explore the possibility of establishing an international alarm system to anticipate cardiac events before they happen.

Management of Psychosocial Distress in ICD Patients

Awareness of the Magnitude of the Problem

Awareness of the significant proportion of psychophysiological distress in ICD patients is very important in their overall management, due to the detrimental effects it has on their psychosocial and physical health endpoints. Current available research suggests that approximately 20% of patients with ICDs have PTSD and a point prevalence of 13–38% for anxiety and 10–41% for depressive symptoms. This means that in every 10 ICD patients: up to *4 subject have depressive symptoms*, up to *4 subjects have anxiety* and *2 subjects have PTSD*. It is not wise to ignore this fact.

The presence of a mental health specialist or preferably, cardiac psychologist, as well as social specialist, is not only, fine addition in the comprehensive management of ICD patients but critical and integral to the usual device interrogation and overall care. It is the responsibility of the implanting electrophysiologist to plan for proper psychosocial care for both the short and long term. In our experience, employing specialists in psychosocial care could be difficult so a collaboration with the mental health provider to establish a screening and referral process in the neighborhood seems to be the practical solution.

The Intelligent Life Style and Therapies: The Intelligent Quality of Life

In recent years, advances in device technologies and optimal programming as well as the insight of using single and combined anti-arrhythmic medications has served to decrease the number of inappropriate shocks and shock-storms. Of particular importance, is the incorporation of anti-tachycardia pacing (ATP) and the increase of shocks for non-sustained tachycardia in the treatment algorithms [73].

Adjustments of anti-arrhythmic medication can also help reduce ventricular tachycardia/ventricular fibrillation episodes, thereby reducing shocks, in the first year, from as high as 38.5% (when β-blockers alone were given) to as low as 10.3%, (when β-blockers and amiodarone were administered) in the OPTIC study [74]. By use of these strategies, shock prevention can be tailored to the patient's unique cardiac profile [75]. An important publication in the field, Marcus GM et al., established that inappropriate shocks are the only reason why patients desire device deactivation [76]. Sears SF, one of the most important researchers of the psychosocial aspects of ICD patients, documented with his colleagues that cardiac rehabilitation efforts not only improve heart function, but that also the QOL benefits [77].

Berg SK et al., found that comprehensive cardiac rehabilitation combining exercise, training, and a psycho-educational intervention improves VO_2-uptake and general health. Furthermore, mental health seems improved [78].

Fitchet et al., compared the effects of a cardiac rehabilitation program with ICD patients that included exercise, education, and psychotherapy (12 weeks) with usual care. Exercise time improved 16%, with no ventricular tachycardia or shocks. In addition, anxiety and depression scores improved 25–30% [79].

It is wise to consider these important directives, interrupting the psychosocial distress and the shock continuum viscous cycle is paramount if we want to provide optimal comprehensive care to ICD patients and lead them towards an intelligent QOL.

Sparing Shock with Positive Emotion: The Cardiac Coherence

Increasing evidence is proving the impact of emotions on health and specifically, cardiovascular health. Research in the relatively new discipline of neurocardiology has confirmed that the heart is a sensory organ and acts as a sophisticated information encoding and processing center that enables it to learn, remember and make independent functional decisions that do not involve the cerebral cortex [80]. Spontaneous fluctuations of ongoing neural activity substantially affect sensory and cognitive performance. Because bodily signals are constantly relayed up to the neocortex, neural responses to bodily signals are likely to shape ongoing activity. Using magnetoencephalography which is a functional neuroimaging technique used for mapping brain activity by recording magnetic fields produced by electrical currents occurring in the brain, utilizing very sensitive magnetometers., Hyeong-Dong Park et al., showed that in humans, neural events locked to heartbeats before stimulus onset predict the detection of a faint visual grating in the posterior right inferior parietal lobule and the ventral anterior cingulate cortex, two regions that have multiple functional correlates and that belong to the same resting-state network [81] (Fig. 2.8).

Recent advances in neuroscience suggest the possibility of reprogramming and changing behavior patterns through modification techniques that go beyond the

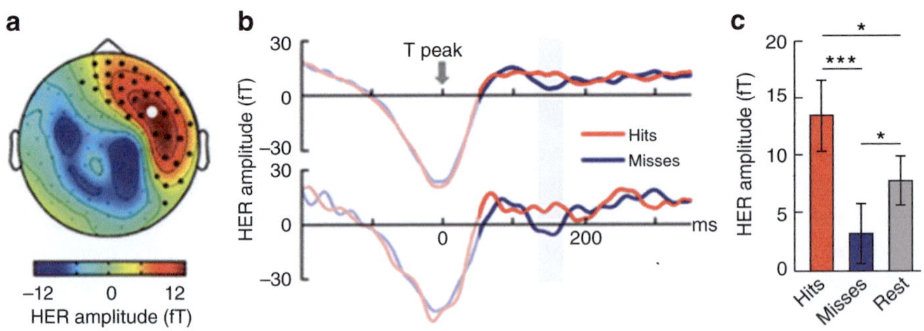

Fig. 2.8 Neural events locked to heartbeats before stimulus onset predict the detection of a faint visual grating in the posterior right inferior parietal lobule and the ventral anterior cingulate cortex [81]

paradigm of cognitive psychology. The modified patterns represent a new neuronal architecture, this technique was found to be successful in treating phobias, post-traumatic stress disorder, smoking addiction and even abnormal blood-pressure levels [82]. One of the most successful techniques in health and disease pattern modification is heart coherence, introduced to scientific committees in 1991 by HeartMath Institute (Ca, USA).

Negative emotions lead to an increased incidence of disorders in heart rhythms and in the autonomic nervous system, the positive psychophysiological state, called heart coherence, on the other hand is associated with high performance, stress reduction and greater emotional stability [83]. They developed a heart rhythm monitoring and feedback system that enables physiological coherence to be objectively monitored and quantified. Heart rhythm coherence feedback training has been successfully used in clinical settings by physicians, and mental health professionals to facilitate health improvements in patients with emotional instability.

ICD patients' efforts to self-regulate emotions can produce broad improvements in increasing or strengthening self-regulatory capacity, making them less vulnerable to depletions and fear of shock. Resilience is defined by the HeartMath researchers as the *capacity to prepare for, recover from and adapt in the face of stress, adversity, trauma or challenge*. Teaching how to improve self-resilience is especially important for highly potential subjects for PTSD like ICD patients. The ability to build and sustain resilience is related to self-management and efficient utilization of energy resources across four domains: *physical*, *emotional*, *mental* and *spiritual*. The integration and harmony between the four domains establish the coherent state [84] (Fig. 2.9). The patterns of afferent neural input to the brain affect emotional experience and modulate cortical function and self-regulatory capacity. Intentional activation of positive emotions plays an important role in

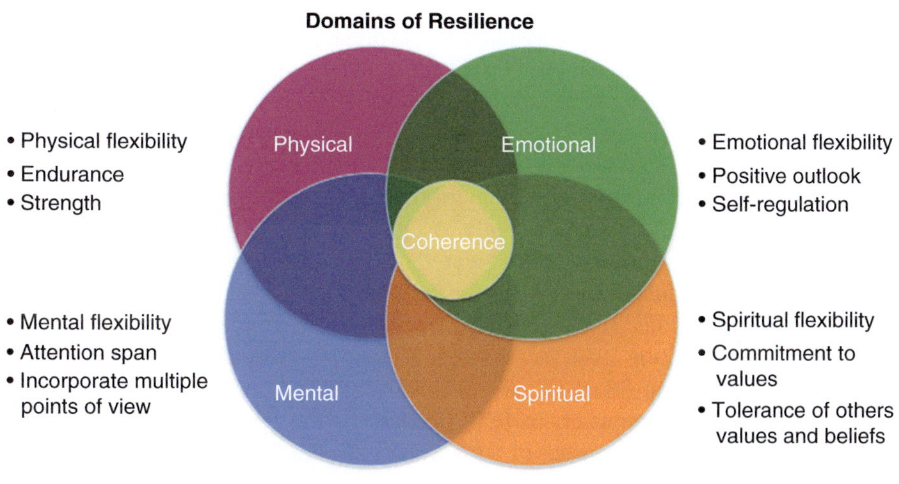

Fig. 2.9 Domains of resilience [84]

increasing cardiac coherence and thus self-regulatory capacity [85]. These findings expand on a large body of research into the ways positive emotional states can benefit physical, mental and emotional health [86–91].

In view of the role of the effects of negative emotions on induction of T Wave Alternans (TWA) and repolarization instability and its relation to future ventricular arrhythmias in patients with ICDs [92], we postulate that teaching the importance of positive emotional states and building a Heart Coherent pattern of life are promising non-pharmacological treatment options that can interrupt the negative emotion shock continuum for ICD patients.

The Psychotherapy: Cognitive Behavioral Therapy (CBT) for ICD Patients

A typical CBT programme would consist in face-to-face sessions between a patient and therapist but computerized cognitive behavioral therapy (CCBT) is now available. It was originally designed to treat depression, but is now used for a number of mental disorders. It works to solve current problems and change unhelpful thinking and behavior. Most therapists working with patients dealing with anxiety and depression use a blend of cognitive and behavioral therapy. This technique acknowledges that there may be behaviors that cannot be controlled through rational thought, but rather emerge based on prior conditioning from the environment and external or internal stimuli. CBT is problem-focused and action-oriented or directive in its therapeutic approach. It is different from the more traditional, psychoanalytical approach, where therapists look for the unconscious meaning behind the behaviors and then diagnose the patient. Instead, behaviorists believe that disorders, such as depression, have to do with the relationship between a feared stimulus and an avoidance response, resulting in a conditioned fear. The fear of shock in ICD patients is a typical example. Philippe Chevalier et al. found that by decreasing anxiety and possibly improving sympathovagal balance, cognitive behavior therapy may decrease the propensity for ventricular arrhythmias in ICD patients. However, these effects appear to be limited over time [93]. Lewin RJ, Coulton S et al., assessed the clinical and cost effectiveness of a brief home-based cognitive behavioral rehabilitation programme (the ICD plan) for patients undergoing implantation of a cardiac defibrillator [94]. They found the ICD plan improved health-related quality of life, reduced the incidence of clinically significant psychological distress and significantly reduced unplanned readmissions. It is a cost effective and easily implemented method for delivering rehabilitation and psychological care to patients undergoing ICD implantation. Pedersen SS et al., searched the PubMed and PsycInfo databases for psychological intervention in ICD patients in the period between January 1980 and April 2007, using a set of a priori determined keywords [95]. Based on the search and a hand search of the reference lists of the included articles, they identified nine studies that fulfilled the inclusion criteria. They concluded that small-scale intervention trials suggest that psychological intervention is worthwhile in ICD patients. Nevertheless, large-scale, well-designed trials are warranted to substantiate these findings. A multifactorial approach using a cognitive behavioral component paired with exercise training is likely to be the most successful. Sears S et al., investigated an ICD stress and shock management program delivered in either a 6-week format or a 1-day workshop format. The intervention was aimed at reducing psychological (anxiety) and physiological (salivary cortisol) markers of distress in ICD patients. Secondary endpoints included measures of quality of life (QOL) and patient acceptance of device therapy, as well as biological mediators of inflammation (TNFalpha and IL-6) [96]. Their results suggest that structured interventions for shocked ICD patients involving ICD education and cognitive-behavioral strategies can reduce psychological distress and improve quality of life, regardless of format. *As a matter of fact, there is a substantial amount of evidence suggesting that CBT for anxiety disorders tends to result in greater decrement of symptoms than either medication or combined medication and CBT* [97]. Reviews specifically examining these studies in the context of the anxiety disorder treatment literature suggest that the use of medication during initial stages of CBT, followed by tapering of medication and continuation of CBT, may be optimal [97]. Bradley R et al., present a multidimensional meta-analysis of studies published between 1980 and 2003 on psychotherapy for PTSD [98]. *They found the psychotherapy research literature has focused primarily on cognitive behavior therapy approaches* (particularly exposure and cognitive restructuring) and eye movement desensitization and reprocessing. Exposure therapy includes confrontation of memories of the trauma or cues ("triggers") related to the traumatic event. Other cognitive behavior therapy approaches focus on developing skills for anxiety management or challenging distorted cognitions. Another treatment approach is eye movement desensitization and reprocessing in which the patient is asked to develop a mental image of a traumatic event and related negative cognitions while tracking a bilateral stimulus. The mechanisms of action are largely unknown. Psychodynamic psychotherapy reviews and meta-analyses have supported the efficacy of psychotherapy for PTSD, particularly cognitive behavior therapy and, more recently, eye movement desensitization and reprocessing. Although, case studies have suggested the potential utility of other therapeutic approaches, such as psychodynamic and humanistic/experiential psychotherapy, research is not available to draw strong conclusions. *They concluded that the majority of patients treated with psychotherapy for PTSD in randomized trials recover or improve, rendering these approaches some of the most effective psychosocial treatments devised to the date of their study.*

Despite the encouraging results that psychotherapy has given in the treatment for PTSD, we recommended that large scale ICD patient targeted PTSD psychotherapy projects conceptualize clear treatment outlines for this unique subset of PTSD individuals.

Pharmacological Treatment of PTSD

Acute Treatment

The findings of randomized placebo-controlled treatment studies indicate that there is evidence for the efficacy of a range of antidepressants including some SSRIs (fluoxetine, paroxetine, sertraline), amitriptyline, imipramine, mirtazapine, nefazodone, phenelzine and venlafaxine [99]. There is also evidence for the efficacy of the antipsychotics risperidone [100], olanzapine [101] and the anticonvulsant topiramate [102]. Medications which have not been found efficacious in placebo-controlled trials include citalopram, alprazolam, and the anticonvulsants tiagabine and divalproex.

Longer Term Treatment

Although many patients with post-traumatic stress disorder experience a prolonged illness, there is some uncertainty about the course of the condition, as most longitudinal studies in post-traumatic stress disorder are retrospective in design. Few prospective studies have been published, although the findings of a prospective study in adolescents and young adults with post-traumatic stress disorder or sub-threshold post-traumatic stress disorder indicate that around 50% will experience a chronic course of illness [103]. The findings of acute and continuation treatment studies indicate that the proportion of responding patients increases steadily over time [104, 105]. A small number of randomized double-blind placebo-controlled relapse prevention studies found evidence of the efficacy of longer-term treatment, for fluoxetine [106] and sertraline [107], but not tiagabine [108].

The Future of Care

System NeuroPsychoBiological Approach

It is constantly underlined that the "modern" physician has lost the human touch and has become too mechanical or too scientific in his approach. The negligence of psychosocial and subtle cognitive issues in cardiac disease evaluation is evident by the total absence of psychosocial and cognitive indicators in the most important prognostic marker known for heart failure, namely the New York Heart Association (NYHA) Functional Classification. The biomedical model is disease-oriented, not patient-oriented. To be patient-oriented, the model must include psychosocial dimensions. But even the term, psychosocial has a strange and esoteric ring for biomedically-trained physicians. For most, "psychosocial" means problems that are primarily of concern to the psychiatrist or the social worker. The number of ICD patients constantly increases, creating a distinct group of human beings with their own demands and complaints: a specific total solution of care should emerge which must take into consideration biological as well as psychosocial and cognitive aspects of ICD patients.

Technical Aspects of the Device

In February 1980 at Johns Hopkins Hospital, Dr. Levi Watkins performed the first ICD implant which had the simple task of recognizing and correcting by defibrillation an abnormal heart rhythm. In the last 36 years, ICD underwent a tremendous and sophisticated programming upgrade, ultimately aiming at more accurate diagnoses and intelligent tiered therapy. We mention biomedical and technical issues in the current and future psychosocial functioning management of ICD patients to emphasize its importance and at the same time, because minimizing the number of shocks has important psychosocial implications and consequences for ICD patients. The details of these advances are not the scope of this chapter.

The New NeuroPsychoBiological Perspective: From Genes to Galaxies

Every cell in our body is immersed in an environment of both external and internal fluctuating magnetic fields that can affect virtually every cell and circuit in biological systems to a certain degree. Numerous studies have shown that various physiological rhythms and global collective behaviors can be synchronized with the solar and geomagnetic activity; and that disruptions in these fields may have adverse effects on human health and behavior [109, 110].

The natural variation in the geomagnetic field in and around earth has been reportedly involved in relation to several human cardiovascular variables. These include blood pressure [111], heart rate (HR), and heart rate variability (HRV) [70, 71]. A growing body of evidence suggests that an energetic field is formed between individuals in groups through which communication among all the group members occurs simultaneously. In other words, there is a literal group "field" that connects all the members. Sociologist Raymond Bradley in collaboration with neuroscientist Karl Pribram, developed a general theory of social communication to explain the patterns of social organization common to most groups, independent of size, culture, degree of formal organization, length of existence, or member characteristics. Energetic influxes from solar and geomagnetic fields have been associated with numerous aspects of human health and wellness, both positively and negatively. From a social perspective, humans are embedded within social networks that exist on the earth, which is part of the solar system. Therefore, it should not be surprising that human physiological rhythms and global behaviors are synchronized with solar and geomagnetic activity [112, 113].

Magnetic storms have been associated with a decrease in heart rate variability [114–116]. Magnetic storms have also been associated with an increase in myocardial infarctions and strokes [117]. In a prospective study, Wolpert et al. [118], evaluated the daily and weekly distributions of malignant ventricular tachyarrhythmia in different patient populations. These authors report a higher incidence of malignant ventricular tachyarrhythmia on Saturdays in patients with coronary heart disease, but on Mondays and Wednesdays for patients with dilated cardiomyopathy or non-ischemic heart disease. This result was interpreted as indicating the operation of different triggers in coronary heart disease that do not operate in dilated cardiomyopathy.

These critical observations indicate that understanding the complex field of energetic networks and sophisticated cosmo biological interactions, is imperative for the comprehensive management of rhythm as well as psychosocial care of ICD patients.

Although PTSD is still largely regarded as a psychological phenomenon, over the past three decades the growth of the biological PTSD literature has been explosive and thousands of references now exist. Ultimately, the impact of an environmental event such as a psychological trauma must be understood at organic, cellular, and molecular levels. Shalev I et al., tested the association between the persistence of internalizing disorders (depression, generalized anxiety disorder, and post-traumatic stress disorder) and leukocyte telomere length (LTL) [119]. Their findings point to a potential mechanism linking internalizing disorders to accelerated biological aging in the first half of the life course, particularly in men. Because internalizing disorders are treatable, the findings suggest the hypothesis that treating psychiatric disorders in the first half of the life course may reduce the population burden of age-related disease and extend health expectancy for internalizing disorders patients in general and PTDS in ICD patients in specific.

Logue MW et al., describe the results of the first genome-wide association study (GWAS) of post-traumatic stress disorder (PTSD) performed using trauma-exposed white non-Hispanic participants. *RORA* gene has been implicated in prior GWAS studies of psychiatric disorders and is known to have an important role in neuroprotection and other behaviorally relevant processes. In association with PTSD, the RORA gene was found to be a significant risk locus. This study represents an important step toward identifying the genetic underpinnings of PTSD [120]. Liboff AR et al., investigated time-varying magnetic fields effect on DNA synthesis [121]. The range of magnetic field amplitudes they tested encompass the geomagnetic field, suggesting the possibility of mutagenic interactions directly arising from short-term changes in the earth's field.

Recently, Yang R et al., have developed computational tools for identifying PTSD biomarkers from "multi-omic" data. Specifically, they integrate genome-wide blood measurements of messenger RNA levels, microRNA levels and DNA methylation levels from both PTSD patients and controls to identify multi-modal disease biomarkers.

These biomarkers provide both a *means for diagnosing new patients as well as a molecular network-level description of the PTSD phenotype* (Fig. 2.10a, b) [122].

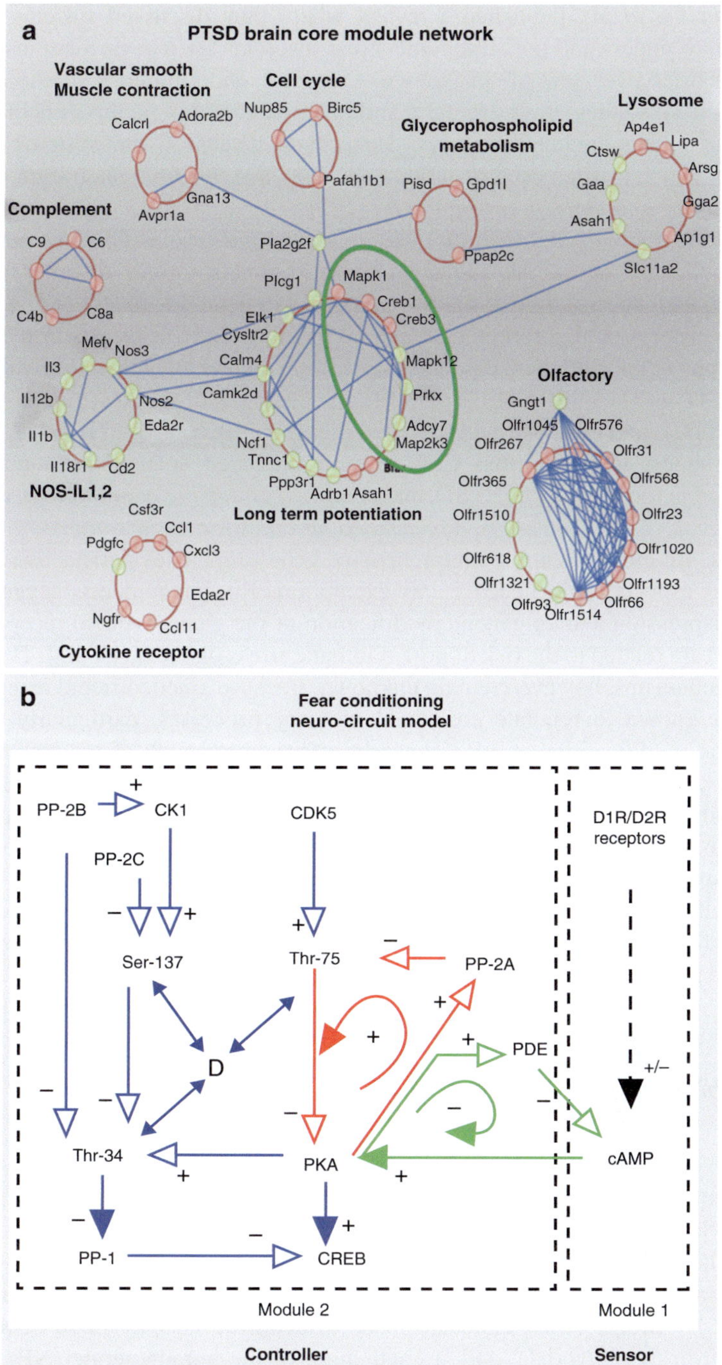

Fig. 2.10 (**a**, **b**) Computational tools for identifying PTSD biomarkers from "multiomic" data, illustrated biomarkers provide both a means for diagnosing new patients as well as a molecular network-level description of the PTSD phenotype. (**a**) Reproduced with permission of the Regents of The University of California (**b**) IEEE grants to Prof. Abdullah Alabdulgader, License Number 4177010395849, a non-exclusive, non-transferable worldwide license to use this image in accordance with the terms and conditions of the agreement [122]

Thakur GS et al., published a review where they discussed systems biology approach to understand post-traumatic stress disorder. Their review begins by providing a brief overview of the known biological underpinnings of the disorder resulting from studies using structural and functional neuroimaging, endocrinology, and genetic and epigenetic assays. Next, they discussed the systems biology approach which is often used *to gain mechanistic insights from the wealth of available high-through put experimental data* [123].

Endocannabinoids and their attending cannabinoid type 1 (CB1) receptor have been implicated in animal models of post-traumatic stress disorder (PTSD). However, their specific role has not been studied in people with PTSD.

Neumeister A et al., presented an in vivo imaging study using positron emission tomography (PET) and the CB1-selective radiolig and [(11)C]OMAR in individuals with PTSD, and healthy controls with lifetime histories of trauma (trauma-exposed controls (TC)) and those without such histories (healthy controls (HC)) [124]. Their results suggest that abnormal CB1 receptor-mediated anandamide signaling is implicated in the etiology of PTSD, and *provide a promising neurobiological model to develop novel, evidence-based pharmacotherapies for this disorder.*

As we are emphasizing a comprehensive gene to galaxies perspective for psychosocial aspects, epigenetics is no exemption. Recent evidence suggests that altered expression and epigenetic modification of the glucocorticoid receptor gene (NR3C1) are related to the risk of post-traumatic stress disorder (PTSD). The underlying mechanisms, however, remain unknown. Because glucocorticoid receptor signaling is known to regulate emotional memory processes, particularly in men, epigenetic modifications of NR3C1 might affect the strength of traumatic memories. They found that increased DNA methylation at the NGFI-A (nerve growth factor-induced protein A) binding site of the NR3C1 promoter was associated with less intrusive memory of the traumatic event and reduced PTSD risk in male, but not female survivors of the Rwandan genocide (Fig. 2.11). Together, these findings indicate that an epigenetic modification of the glucocorticoid receptor gene promoter is linked to interindividual and gender-specific differences in memory functions and PTSD risk [125].

Neurobiology and PTSD

Research on the neurobiology of the stress response in animals has led to successful new treatments for Post-Traumatic Stress Disorder (PTSD) in humans [126]. Basic research has found that high levels of catecholamine release during stress rapidly impair the top-down cognitive functions of the prefrontal cortex (PFC), while strengthening the emotional and habitual responses of the amygdala and basal ganglia [126]. Chronic stress exposure leads to dendritic atrophy in PFC, dendritic extension in the amygdala, and strengthening of the noradrenergic (NE) system. High levels of NE release during stress engage low affinity alpha-1 adrenoceptors, (and likely beta-1 adrenoceptors), which rapidly reduce the firing of PFC neurons,

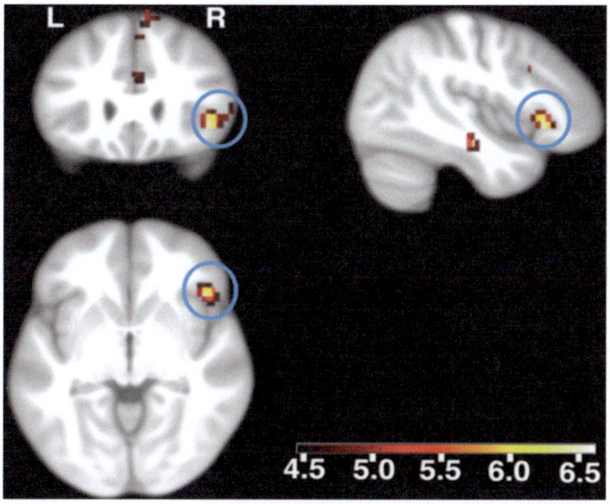

Fig. 2.11 Methylation-dependent differences in brain activity related to successful recognition of previously seen pictures in healthy men. Displayed are voxels with a positive correlation between methylation values (at NR3C1_CpG3) and activity, using color-coded t values. The *blue circles* show the activation in the pars triangularis and pars orbitalis of the inferior frontal gyrus [125]

but strengthen amygdala function. In contrast, moderate levels of NE release during nonstress conditions engage higher affinity alpha-2A receptors, which strengthen PFC, weaken amygdala, and regulate NE cell firing. Thus, either alpha-1 receptor blockade or alpha-2A receptor stimulation can protect PFC function during stress. Patients with PTSD have signs of PFC dysfunction (see Fig. 2.12). Clinical studies have found that blocking alpha-1 receptors with prazosin, or stimulating alpha-2A receptors with guanfacine or clonidine can be useful in reducing the symptoms of PTSD. Placebo-controlled trials have shown that prazosin is helpful in veterans, active duty soldiers and civilians with PTSD, including improvement of PFC symptoms such as impaired concentration and impulse control. Open label studies suggest that guanfacine may be especially helpful in treating children and adolescents who have experienced trauma. Knowledge of PTSD neurological pathways should open new era for successful therapies for ICD with PTSD patients and others.

The Electromagnetic Therapy: Transcranial Magnetic Stimulation in Post-traumatic Stress Disorder

Transcranial Magnetic Stimulation (TMS) is a term used to describe a technology that uses magnetic currents applied to a conscious individual through the scalp to alter the electrical charge of his/her brain's cortex and therefore cause neuronal excitability or brain stimulation without the need of medication or invasive surgery. TMS has been researched for the last 36 years when Tofts [127] suggested

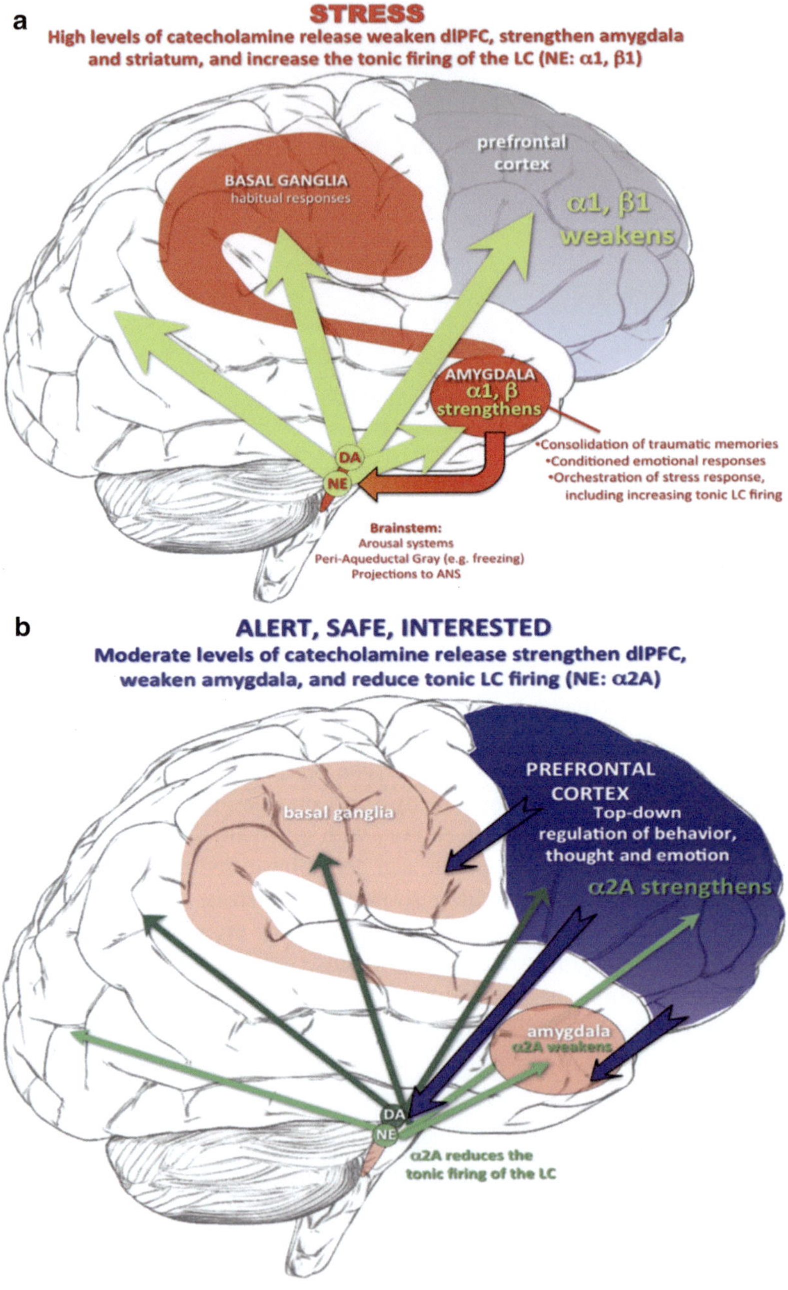

Fig. 2.12 (**a**) During nonstressed arousal conditions when the subject is alert, safe and interested, the highly evolved prefrontal cortex (highlight in *blue*) provides top-down regulation of behavior, thought and emotion. (**b**) Under conditions of uncontrollable stress, there are high levels of catecholamine release in brain, which weaken PFC function but strengthen the affective responses of the amygdala and the habitual responses of the basal ganglia [129]

parameters for the safe use among humans. There are various forms of this procedure: single-pulse TMS, paired-pulse TMS, repetitive TMS, synchronized TMS, and deep TMS. These different TMS versions have been developed to address different assessment and treatment needs. To date, PTSD psychotherapy and drug treatment achieve only partial success, indicating need for further development of treatment strategies. Recent research has found that impaired acquired fear extinction capability serves as an important factor at the pathogenesis of the disorder. Medial prefrontal cortex hypo-activity has been implicated in this extinction impairment, providing insight as to why some trauma exposed individuals will develop PTSD. Isserles M et al., test whether fear extinction can be facilitated and therapeutic effect achieved by repeated medial prefrontal cortex deep transcranial magnetic stimulation (DTMS) of PTSD patients resistant to standard treatment. They concluded that combining brief script-driven exposure with DTMS can induce therapeutic effects in PTSD patients [128]. Karsen E et al., performed literature review with descriptions of primary studies as well as meta analysis of studies with a control group. They found eight primary studies were identified and three studies met criteria for meta-analysis. *All studies suggest effectiveness of TMS for PTSD. Additionally, right-sided may be more effective than left-sided treatment.* There is no clear advantage in high versus low frequency, and the treatment is generally well tolerated. Meta-analysis shows significant effect size on PTSD symptoms that may be correlated with total number of stimulations. They concluded that TMS for PTSD appears to be an effective and well-tolerated treatment [129]. TMS in our perspective is very promising non invasive treatment for PTSD in ICD patients and others.

References

1. Bardy GH, Lee KL, Mark DB, Poole JE, Packer DL, Boineau R, Domanski M, Troutman C, Anderson J, Johnson G, McNulty SE, Clapp-Channing N, Davidson-Ray LD, Fraulo ES, Fishbein DP, Luceri RM, Ip JH. Amiodarone or an implantable cardioverter-defibrillator for congestive heart failure. N Engl J Med. 2005;352:225–37.
2. Daubert JP, Zareba W, Cannom DS, McNitt S, Rosero SZ, Wang P, Schuger C, Steinberg JS, Higgins SL, Wilber DJ, Klein H, Andrews ML, Hall J, Moss AJ. Inappropriate implantable cardioverter-defibrillator shocks in MADIT II: frequency, mechanisms, predictors, and survival impact. J Am Coll Cardiol. 2008;51:1357–65.
3. Patel VL, Kaufman DR, Arocha JF. Emerging paradigms of cognition in medical decision making. J Biomed Inform. 2002;5:52–75.
4. Tversky A, Kahneman D. Judgment under uncertainty: heuristics and biases. Science. 1974;185:1124–31.
5. Chaiken S, Maheswaran D. Heuristic processing can bias systematic processing: effects of source credibility, argument ambiguity, and task importance on attitude judgment. J Pers Soc Psychol. 1994;66:460–73.
6. Garrett Hazelton A, Sears SF, Ford J, Cahill J, Nekkanti R, Deantonio H, Ottoboni L, Norton L, Wang P. Decisional balance among potential implantable cardioverter defibrillator recipients: development of the ICD-decision analysis scale (ICD-DAS). PACE. 2014;37:63–72.
7. Aminoff MJ, Scheinman MM, Griffin JC, Herre JM. Electrocerebral accompaniments of syncope associated with malignant ventricular arrhythmias. Ann Intern Med. 1988;108:791–6.

8. Clute HL, Levy WJ. Electroencephalographic changes during brief cardiac arrest in humans. Anesthesiology. 1990;73:821–5.
9. Skhirtladze K, Birkenberg B, Mora B, et al. Cerebral desaturation during cardiac arrest: its relation to arrest duration and left ventricular pump function. Crit Care Med. 2009;37:471–5.
10. De Vries JW, Bakker PFA, Visser GH, et al. Changes in cerebral oxygen uptake and cerebral electrical activity during defibrillation threshold testing. Anesth Analg. 1998;87:16–20.
11. Adams DC, Heyer EJ, Emerson RG, et al. Evaluation of clinical neurologic outcome and electroencephalographic changes during implantation. J Thorac Cardiovasc Surg. 1995;109:565–73.
12. Dworschak M, Franz M, Czerny M, Gorlitzer M, Blaschek M, Grubhofer G, Haider W. Release of neuron-specific enolase and S100 after implantation of cardioverters/defibrillators. Crit Care Med. 2003;31(8):2085–9.
13. Weigl M, Moritz A, Steinlechner B, et al. Neuronal injury after repeated brief cardiac arrests during internal cardioverter defibrillator implantation is associated with deterioration of cognitive function. Anesth Analg. 2006;103:403–9.
14. Almaraz AC, Bobrow BJ, Wingerchuk DM, Wellik KE, Demaerschalk BM. Serum neuron specific enolase to predict neurological outcome after cardiopulmonary resuscitation: a critically appraised topic. Neurologist. 2009;15(1):44–8.
15. Sears S, Matchett M, Conti J. Effective management of ICD patient psychosocia lissues and patient critical events. J Cardiovasc Electrophysiol. 2009;20:1297–304.
16. Kapa S, Rotondi-Trevisan D, Mariano Z, Aves T, Irvine J, Dorian P, Hayes DL. Psychopathology in patients with ICDs over time: results of a prospective study. Pacing Clin Electrophysiol. 2010;33:198–208.
17. Broek K, Nyklícek I, Denollet J. Anxiety predicts poor perceived health in patients with an implantable defibrillator. Psychosomatics. 2009;50:483–92.
18. Whang W, Albert C, Sears S, Lampert R, Conti JB, Wang PJ, Singh JP, Ruskin JN, Muller JE, Mittleman MA. Depression as a predictor for appropriate shocks among patients with implantable cardioverter defibrillators: results from the triggers of ventricular arrhythmias (TOVA) study. J Am Coll Cardiol. 2005;45:1090–5.
19. Pedersen S, Broek K, Berg M, Theuns DAMJ. Shock as a determinant of poor patient-centered outcomes in implantable cardioverter defibrillator patients: is there more to it than meets the eye? Pacing Clin Electrophysiol. 2010;33:1430–6.
20. Kessler RC, Sonnega A, Bromet E, Hughes M, Nelson CB. Posttraumatic stress disorder in the National Comorbidity Survey. Arch Gen Psychiatry. 1995;52:1048–60.
21. Ladwig KH, Baumert J, Marten-Mittag B, Kolb C, Zrenner B, Schmitt C. Posttraumatic stress symptoms and predicted mortality in patients with implantable cardioverter defibrillators: results from the prospective living with an implanted cardioverter-defibrillator study. Arch Gen Psychiatry. 2008;65:1324–30.
22. Ozer EJ, Best SR, Lipsey TL, Weiss DS. Predictors of posttraumatic stress disorder and symptoms in adults: a meta-analysis. Psychol Bull. 2003;129:52–73.
23. Kutz I, Shabata H, Solomon Z, Neumann M, David D. Post-traumatic stress disorder in myocardial infarction patients: prevalence study. Isr J Psychiatry Relat Sci. 1994;31:48–56.
24. Bennett P, Brooke S. Intrusive memories, post-traumatic stress disorder and myocardial infarction. Br J Clin Psychol. 1999;38:411–6.
25. Bennett P, Conway M, Clatworthy J, Brooke S, Owen R. Predicting post-traumatic symptoms in cardiac patients. Heart Lung J Acute Crit Care. 2001;30:458–65.
26. Bennett P, Owen RL, Koutsakis S, Bisson J. Personality, social context and cognitive predictors of post-traumatic stress disorder in myocardial infarction patients. Psychol Health. 2002;17:489–500.
27. Pedersen S, Domburg R, Theuns D, Jordaens L, Erdman RAM. Type D personality is associated with increased anxiety and depressive symptoms in patients with an implantable cardioverter defibrillator and their partners. Psychosom Med. 2004;66:714–9.

28. Cotter G, Milo-Cotter O, Rubinstein D, Shemesh E. Posttraumatic stress disorder: a missed link between psychiatric and cardiovascular morbidity? CNS Spectr. 2006;11:129–36.
29. Shemesh E, Koren-Michowitz M, Yehuda R, Milo-Cotter O, Murdock E, Vered Z, Shneider BL, Gorman JM, Cotter G. Symptoms of posttraumatic stress disorder in patients who have had a myocardial infarction. Psychosomatics. 2006;47:231–9.
30. Magruder KM, Frueh BC, Knapp RG, Davis L, Hamner MB, Martin RH, Gold PB, Arana GW. Prevalence of posttraumatic stress disorder in veterans affairs primary care clinics. Gen Hosp Psychiatry. 2005;27:169–79.
31. Stein MB, McQuaid JR, Pedrelli P, Lenox R, Cahill ME. Posttraumatic stress disorder in the primary care medical setting. Gen Hosp Psychiatry. 2000;22:261–9.
32. Von Kanel R, Baumert J, Kolb C, Cho EN, Ladwig KH. Chronic posttraumatic stress and its predictors in patients living with an implantable cardioverter defibrillator. J Affect Disord. 2010;131(1–3):344–52.
33. Sears S, Hauf J, Kirian K, Hazelton G, Conti J. Posttraumatic stress and the implantable cardioverter-defibrillator patient: what the electrophysiologist needs to know. Circ Arrhythm Electrophysiol. 2011;4(2):242–50.
34. Sears S, Conti J. Understanding implantable cardioverter defibrillator shocks and storms: medical and psychosocial considerations for research and clinical care. Clin Cardiol. 2003;26:107–11.
35. Versteeg H, Theuns DAMJ, Erdman RAM, Jordaens L, Pedersen SS. Posttraumatic stress in implantable cardioverter defibrillator patients: the role of preimplantation distress and shocks. Int J Cardiol. 2011;3:438–9.
36. Figley CR, Nash WP, editors. Combat stress injury theory, research, and management. New York: Routledge; 2007.
37. May CD, Smith PR, Murdock CJ, et al. The impact of the implantable cardioverter defibrillator on quality of life. Pacing Clin Electrophysiol. 1995;18:1411–8.
38. Namerow PB, Firth BR, Heywood GM, et al. Quality of life six months after CABG surgery in patients randomized to ICD versus no ICD therapy: findings from the CABG patch trial. Pacing Clin Electrophysiol. 1999;22:1305–13.
39. Kalbfleisch KR, Lehmann MH, Steinman RT, et al. Reemployment following implantation of the automatic cardioverter defibrillator. Am J Cardiol. 1989;64:199–202.
40. Sears SF Jr, Conti J. Quality of life and psychological functioning of ICD patients. Heart. 2002;87:488–93.
41. Credner SC, Klingenheben T, Mauss O, et al. Electrical storm in patients with transvenous implantable cardioverter defibrillators. J Am Coll Cardiol. 1998;32:1909–15.
42. Sears SF Jr, Burns JL, Handberg E, et al. Young at heart: understanding the unique psychosocial adjustment of young implantable cardioverter defibrillator recipients. Pacing Clin Electrophysiol. 2001;24:1113.
43. Kawachi I, Sparrow D, Vokonas PS, Weiss ST. Symptoms of anxiety and risk of coronary heart disease. The normative aging study. Circulation. 1994;90(5):2225–9.
44. Barefoot JC, Helms MJ, Mark DB, Blumenthal JA, Califf RM, Haney TL, O'Connor CM, Siegler IC, Williams RB. Depression and long-term mortality risk in patients with coronary artery disease. Am J Cardiol. 1996;78(6):613. doi:10.1016/S0002-9149(96)00380-3.
45. Thomas SAFE, Wimbush F, Schron E. Psychological factors and survival in the cardiac arrhythmia suppression trial (CAST): a reexamination. Am J Crit Care. 1997;6(2):116–26.
46. Carney RM, Freedland KE, Jaffe AS, Frasure-Smith N, Lesperance F, Sheps DS, Glassman AH, O'Connor CM, Blumenthal JA, Kaufmann PG, et al. Depression as a risk factor for post-MI mortality. J Am Coll Cardiol. 2004;44(2):472. doi:10.1016/j.jacc.2004.04.030.
47. Lesperance F, Frasure-Smith N, Talajic M, Bourassa MG. Five-year risk of cardiac mortality in relation to initial severity and one-year changes in depression symptoms after myocardial infarction. Circulation. 2002;105(9):1049–53. doi:10.1161/hc0902.104707.
48. Grace S, Abbey S, Irvine J, Zachary M, Stewart D. Prospective examination of anxiety persistence and its relationship to cardiac symptoms and recurrent cardiac events. Psychother Psychosom. 2004;73:344–52. doi:10.1159/000080387.

49. Moser D, Dracup K. Is anxiety early after myocardial infarction associated with subsequent ischemic and arrhythmic events? Psychosom Med. 1996;58:395–401.
50. Moss AJ, Greenberg H, Case RB, Zareba W, Hall WJ, Brown MW, Daubert JP, McNitt S, Andrews ML, Elkin AD, et al. Long-term clinical course of patients after termination of ventricular tachyarrhythmia by an implanted defibrillator. Circulation. 2004;110(25):3760–5. doi:10.1161/01.CIR.0000150390.04704.B7.
51. Lown B, Temte JV, Reich P, Gaughan C, Regestein Q, Hal H. Basis for recurring ventricular fibrillation in the absence of coronary heart disease and its management. N Engl J Med. 1976;294(12):623–9. doi:10.1056/NEJM197603182941201.
52. Lown B, DeSilva R, Reich P, Murawski B. Psychophysiologic factors in sudden cardiac death. Am J Psychiatry. 1980;137(11):1325–35.
53. Leor J, Poole WK, Kloner RA. Sudden cardiac death triggered by an earthquake. N Engl J Med. 1996;334(7):413–9. doi:10.1056/NEJM199602153340701.
54. Kloner RA, Leor J, Poole WK, Perritt R. Population-based analysis of the effect of the northridge earthquake on cardiac death in Los Angeles County, California. J Am Coll Cardiol. 1997;30(5):1174. doi:10.1016/S0735-1097(97)00281-7.
55. Meisel S, Kutz I. Effect of Iraqi missile war on incidence of acute myocardial infarction and sudden death in Israeli civilians. Lancet. 1991;338(8768):660–1. doi:10.1016/0140-6736(91)91234-L.
56. Ironson GTC, Boltwood M, Bartzokis T, et al. Effects of anger on left ventricular ejection fraction in coronary artery disease. Am J Cardiol. 1993;70(3):281–5. doi:10.1016/0002-9149(92)90605-X.
57. Wittstein IS, Thiemann DR, Lima JAC, Baughman KL, Schulman SP, Gerstenblith G, Wu KC, Rade JJ, Bivalacqua TJ, Champion HC. Neurohumoral features of myocardial stunning due to sudden emotional stress. N Engl J Med. 2005;352(6):539–48. doi:10.1056/NEJMoa043046.
58. Rozanski A, Bairey C, Krantz D, Friedman J. Mental stress and the induction of silent myocardial ischemia in patients with coronary artery disease. N Engl J Med. 1988;318(16):1005–12. doi:10.1056/NEJM198804213181601.
59. Kawachi I, Sparrow D, Vokonas PS, Weiss ST. Decreased heart rate variability in men with phobic anxiety (data from the normative aging study). Am J Cardiol. 1995;75(14):882. doi:10.1016/S0002-9149(99)80680-8.
60. Thayer JF, Friedman BH, Borkovec TD. Autonomic characteristics of generalized anxiety disorder and worry. Biol Psychiatry. 1996;39(4):255–66. doi:10.1016/0006-3223(95)00136-0.
61. Watkins LL, Blumenthal JA, Carney RM. Association of anxiety with reduced baroreflex cardiac control in patients after acute myocardial infarction. Am Heart J. 2002;143:460–6. doi:10.1067/mhj.2002.120404.
62. von Kanel R, Mills PJ, Fainman C, Dimsdale JE. Effects of psychological stress and psychiatric disorders on blood coagulation and fibrinolysis: a biobehavioral pathway to coronary artery disease? Psychosom Med. 2001;63(4):531–44.
63. Friedmann E, Thomas S. Pet ownership, social support, and one-year survival after acute myocardial infarction in the cardiac arrhythmia suppression trial (CAST). Am J Cardiol. 1995;76:1213–7. doi:10.1016/S0002-9149(99)80343-9.
64. Friedmann E, Thomas SA, Stein PK, Kleiger RE. Relation between pet ownership and heart rate variability in patients with healed myocardial infarcts. Am J Cardiol. 2003;91(6):718. doi:10.1016/S0002-9149(02)03412-4.
65. Francis J, Weinstein A, Krantz D, Haigney M, Stein P, Stone P, Gottdiener J, Kop W. Association between symptoms of depression and anxiety with heart rate variability in patients with implantable cardioverter defibrillators. Psychosom Med. 2009;71(8):821–7. doi:10.1097/PSY.0b013e3181b39aa1.
66. Rottenberg J, Chambers AS, Allen JJ, Manber R. Cardiac vagal control in the severity and course ofdepression: the importance of symptomatic heterogeneity. J Affect Disord. 2007;103(1–3):173–9.

67. Pieper S, Brosschot JF, van der Leeden R, Thayer JF. Cardiac effects of momentary assessed worry episodes and stressful events. Psychosom Med. 2007;69(9):901–9.
68. Bekelman DB, Dy SM, Becker DM, et al. Spiritual well-being and depression in patients with heart failure. J Gen Intern Med. 2007;22(4):470–7.
69. Salmoirago-Blotcher E, Crawford S, Tran C, Goldberg R, Rosenthal L, Ockene I. Spiritual well-being may buffer psychological distress in patients with implantable cardioverter defibrillators (ICD). J Evid Based Complementary Altern Med. 2012;17(3):148–54.
70. Baevsky RM, Petrov VM, Chernikova AG. Regulation of autonomic nervous system in space and magnetic storms. Adv Space Res. 1998;22(2):227–34.
71. Cornelissen G, McCraty R, Atkinson M, Halberg F. Gender differences in circadian and extra-circadian aspects of heart rate variability (HRV). 1st International Workshop of the Tsim Tsoum Institute. Krakow, Poland; 2010.
72. Alabdulgader A, McCraty R, Atkinson M, Vainoras A, Berškienė K, Mauricienė V, Daunoravičienė A, Navickas Z, Šmidtaitė R, Landauskas M. Human heart rhythm sensitivity to earth local magnetic field fluctuations. J Vibroeng. 2015;17(6):3271–8.
73. Wilkoff BL, Williamson BD, Stern RS, Moore SL, Lee SW, Birgersdotter-Green UM, Wathen MS, VanGelden IC, Heubner BM, Brown ML, Holloman KK. Strategic programming of detection and therapy parameters in implantable cardioverter-defibrillators reduces shock in primary prevention patients. J Am Coll Cardiol. 2008;52:541–51.
74. Connolly SJ, Dorian P, Roberts RS, Gent M, Bailin S, Fain ES, Thorpe K, Champagne J, Talajic M, Coutu B, Gronefeld GC, Hohnloser SA. Comparison of beta-blockers, amiodarone plus beta-blockers, or sotalol for prevention of shocks from implantable cardioverter defibrillators: the OPTIC study: a randomized trial. JAMA. 2006;295:165–71.
75. Mishkin J, Saxonhouse S, Woo G, Burkart TA, Miles WM, Conti JB, Shofield KS, Sears SF, Aranda JM. Appropriate evaluation and treatment of heart failure patients after implantable cardioverter-defibrillator discharge: time to go beyond the initial shock. J Am Coll Cardiol. 2009;54:1993–2000.
76. Marcus GM, Chan DW, Redberg RF. Recollection of pain due to inappropriate versus appropriate implantable cardioverter-defibrillator shocks. Pacing Clin Electrophysiol. 2010;34: 348–53.
77. Sears SF, Kovacs AH, Conti JB, Handberg E. Expanding the scope of practice for cardiac rehabilitation: managing patients with implantable cardioverter defibrillators. J Cardiol Rehab. 2004;24:209–15.
78. Berg SK, Pedersen PU, Zwisler AD, Winkel P, Gluud C, Pedersen BD, Svendsen JH. Comprehensive cardiac rehabilitation improves outcome for patients with implantable cardioverter defibrillator. Findings from the COPE-ICD randomised clinical trial. Eur J Cardiovasc Nurs. 2015;14(1):34–44. doi:10.1177/1474515114521920. Epub 2014 Feb 5.
79. Fitchet A, Doherty P, Bundy C, Bell W, Fitzpatrick AP, Garratt CJ. Comprehensivecardiac rehabilitation programme for implantable cardioverter-defibrillator patients: a randomised controlled trial. Heart. 2003;89:155–60.
80. McCraty R, Zayas MA. Cardiac coherence, self-regulation, autonomic stability, and psychosocial well-being. Front Psychol. 2014;5:1090.
81. Park HD, Correia S, Ducorps A, TallonBaudry C. Spontaneous fluctuations in neural responses to heartbeats predict visual detection. Nat Neurosci. 2014;17:612–8.
82. Alabdulgader A. Coherence: a novel nonpharmacological modality for lowering blood pressure in hypertensive patients. Glob Adv Health Med. 2012;1:54–62.
83. Sarabia-Cobo CM. Heart coherence: a new tool in the management of stress on professionals and family caregivers of patients with dementia. Appl Psychophysiol Biofeedback. 2015;40(2):75–83. doi:10.1007/s10484-015-9276-y.
84. HeartMathInstitute. Chapter 2: Resilience and stress and emotion. In: Science of the heart, exploring the role of the heart in human performance. Boulder Creek: HeartMathInstitute; 2016.

85. McCraty R, Atkinson M, Tomasino D, Bradley RT. The coherent heart: heart-brain interactions, psychophysiological coherence, and the emergence of system-wide order. Integral Rev. 2009;5(2):10–115.
86. Fredrickson BL. Positive emotions. In: Snyder CR, Lopez SJ, editors. Handbook of positive psychology. New York: Oxford University Press; 2002. p. 120–34.
87. Isen AM. Positive affect. In: Dalgleish T, Power M, editors. Handbook of cognition and emotion. New York: Wiley; 1999. p. 522–39.
88. Wichers MC, et al. Evidence that moment-to-moment variation in positive emotions buffer genetic risk for depression: a momentary assessment twin study. Acta Psychiatr Scand. 2007;115(6):451–7.
89. Fredrickson BL. The role of positive emotions in positive psychology. The broaden-and-build theory of positive emotions. Am Psychol. 2001;56(3):218–26.
90. Fredrickson BL, Joiner T. Positive emotions trigger upward spirals toward emotional well-being. Psychol Sci. 2002;13(2):172–5.
91. Fredrickson BL, et al. What good are positive emotions in crises? A prospective study of resilience and emotions following the terrorist attacks on the United States on September 11th, 2001. J Pers Soc Psychol. 2003;84(2):365–76.
92. Lampert R, Shusterman V, Burg M, McPherson C, Batsford W, Goldberg A, Soufer R. Anger-induced T-wave alternans predicts future ventricular arrhythmias in patients with implantable cardioverter-defibrillators. J Am Coll Cardiol. 2009;53(9):774–8. doi:10.1016/j.jacc.2008.10.053.
93. Chevalier P, Cottraux J, Mollard E, Sai NY, Brun S, Burri H, Restier L, Adeleine P. Prevention of implantable defibrillator shocks by cognitive behavioral therapy. Am Heart J. 2006; 151(1):191.e1–6.
94. Lewin RJ, Coulton S, Frizelle DJ, Kaye G, Cox H. A brief cognitive behavioural pre-implantation and rehabilitation programme for patients receiving an implantable cardioverter-defibrillator improves physical health and reduces psychological morbidity and unplanned readmissions. Heart. 2009;95:63–9. doi:10.1136/hrt.2007.129890.
95. Pedersen SS, Broek KC, Sears SF. Psychological intervention following implantation of an implantable defibrillator: a review and future recommendations. Pacing Clin Electrophysiol. 2007;30:1546–54.
96. Sears S, Sowell L, Kuhl E, Kovacs AH, Serber ER, Handberg E, Kneipp SM, Zineh I, Conti JB. The ICD shock and stress management program: a randomized trial of psychosocial treatment to optimize quality of life in ICD patients. Pacing Clin Electrophysiol. 2007; 30:858–64.
97. Otto MW, Smits JAJ, Reese HE. Cognitive-behavioral therapy for thetreatment of anxiety disorders. J Clin Psychiatry. 2004;65(5):34–41.
98. Bradly R, Greene J, Russ E, Dutra L, Westen D. A multidimensional meta-analysis of psychotherapy for PTSD. Am J Psychiatry. 2005;162:214–27.
99. Ipser JC, Stein DJ, Hawkridge S, et al. Pharmacotherapy for anxiety disorders in children and adolescents (review). Cochrane Database Syst Rev. 2009;3:CD005170. doi:10.1002/14651858.CD005170.pub2.
100. Padala PR, Madison J, Monnahan M, et al. Risperidone monotherapy for post-traumatic stress disorder related to sexual assault and domestic abuse in women. Int Clin Psychopharmacol. 2006;21:275–80.
101. Carey P, Suliman S, Ganesan K, et al. Olanzapine monotherapy in posttraumatic stress disorder: efficacy in a randomized, double-blind, placebo-controlled study. Hum Psychopharmacol. 2012;27:386–91.
102. Yeh MSL, Mari JJ, Pupo Costa MC, et al. A double-blind randomized controlled trial to study the efficacy of topiramate in a civilian sample of PTSD. CNS Neurosci Ther. 2011;17: 305–10.
103. Perkonigg A, Pfister H, Stein MB, et al. Longitudinal course of posttraumatic stress disorder and posttraumatic stress disorder symptoms in a community sample of adolescents and young adults. Am J Psychiatry. 2005;162:1320–7.

104. Davidson J, Baldwin D, Stein DJ, et al. Treatment of posttraumatic stress disorder with venlafaxine extended release—a 6-month randomized controlled trial. Arch Gen Psychiatry. 2006;63:1158–65.
105. Londborg PD, Hegel MT, Goldstein S, et al. Sertraline treatment of posttraumatic stress disorder: results of 24 weeks of open-label continuation treatment. J Clin Psychiatry. 2001; 62:325–31.
106. Martenyi F, Brown EB, Zhang H, et al. Fluoxetine v. Placebo in prevention of relapse in posttraumatic stress disorder. Br J Psychiatry. 2002;181:315–20.
107. Davidson JRT, Connor KM, Hertzberg MA, et al. Maintenance therapy with fluoxetine in posttraumatic stress disorder: a placebo-controlled discontinuation study. J Clin Psychopharmacol. 2005;25:166–9.
108. Connor KM, Davidson JRT, Weisler RH, et al. Tiagabine for posttraumatic stress disorder: effects of open-label and double-blind discontinuation treatment. Psychopharmacology. 2006;184:21–5.
109. Stoupel EG, Tamoshiunas A, Radishauskas R, Bernotiene G, Abramson E, et al. Neutrons and the plaque: AMI (n-8920) at days of zero GMA/high neutron activity (n-36) and the following days and week. Kaunas, Lithuania, 2000-2007. J Clin Exp Cardiol. 2011; 2(1):121.
110. Stoupel EG, Tamoshiunas A, Radishauskas R, Bernotiene G, Abramson E, et al. Acute myocardial infarction (AMI) and intermediate coronary syndrome (ICS). Health. 2010;2(2):131–6.
111. Stoupel EG, Wittenberg C, Zabludowski J, Boner G. Ambulatory blood pressure monitoring inpatients with hypertension on days of high and low geomagnetic activity. J Hum Hypertens. 1995;9(4):293–4.
112. McCraty R, Childre D. Coherence: bridging personal, social and global health. Altern Ther Health Med. 2010;16(4):10–24.
113. Halberg F, Cornelissen G, McCraty R, Al-Abdulgader A. Time structures (chronomes) of the blood circulation, populations' health, human affairs and space weather. World Heart J. 2011;3(1):1–40.
114. Cornélissen G, Halberg F, Schwartzkopff O, et al. Chronomes, time structures, for chronobioengineering for a full life. Biomed Instrum Technol. 1999;33:152–87.
115. Otsuka K, Cornélissen G, Weydahl A, et al. Geomagnetic disturbance associated with decrease in heart rate variability in a subarctic area. Biomed Pharmacother. 2001;55(Suppl 1):51–6.
116. Baevsky RM, Petrov VM, Cornélissen G, et al. Meta-analyzed heart rate variability, exposure to geomagnetic storms, and the risk of ischemic heart disease. Scr Med. 1997;70:199–204.
117. Cornélissen G, Halberg F, Breus T, et al. Non-photic solar associations of heart rate variability and myocardial infarction. J Atmos Sol Terr Phys. 2002;64:707–20.
118. Wolpert C, Jung W, Spehl S, et al. Zirkadiane und wochentliche verteilung maligner ventrikularer tachyarrhythmienbei patientenmitkoronarer herzkrankheitoderdilatativer kardiomyopathiemit implantiertem kardioverter-defibrillator. Dtsch Med Wochenschr. 1998;123: 140–5.
119. Shalev I, Moffitt TE, Braithwaite AW, Danese A, Fleming NI, Goldman-Mellor S, Harrington HL, Houts RM, Israel S, Poulton R, Robertson SP, Sugden K, Williams B, Caspi A. Internalizing disorders and leukocyte telomere erosion: a prospective study of depression, generalized anxiety disorder and post-traumatic stress disorder. Mol Psychiatry. 2014;19:1163–70. doi:10.1038/mp.2013.183.
120. Logue W, Baldwin C, Guffanti G, Melista E, Wolf EJ, Reardon AF, Uddin M, Wildman D, Galea S, Koenen KC, Miller MW. A genome-wide association study of post-traumatic stress disorder identifies the retinoid-related orphan receptor alpha (*RORA*) gene as a significant risk locus. Mol Psychiatry. 2013;18:937–42. doi:10.1038/mp.2012.113.
121. Liboff AR, Williams T Jr, Strong DM, Wistar R Jr. Time-varying magnetic fields: effect on DNA synthesis. Science. 1984;223(4638):818–20.

122. Yang R, Daigle JBJ, Muhie SY, Hammamieh R, Jett M, Petzold LR, Doyle IIIFJ. Core modular blood and brain biomarkers in social defeat mouse model for post traumatic stress disorder. BMC Syst Biol. 2013;7:80. doi:10.1186/1752-0509-7-80.
123. Thakur GS, Daigle BJ Jr, Dean KR, Zhang Y, Rodriguez-Fernandez M, Hammamieh R, Yang R, Jett M, Palma J, Petzold LR, Doyle FJ III. Systems biology approach to understanding post-traumatic stress disorder. Mol Biosyst. 2015;11(4):980–93. doi:10.1039/c4mb00404c.
124. Neumeister A, Normandin MD, Pietrzak RH, Piomelli D, Zheng MQ, Gujarro-Anton A, Potenza MN, Bailey CR, Lin SF, Najafzadeh S, Ropchan J, Henry S, Corsi-Travali S, Carson RE, Huang Y. Elevated brain cannabinoid CB1 receptor availability in post-traumatic stress disorder: a positron emission tomography study. Mol Psychiatry. 2013;18(9):1034–40. doi:10.1038/mp.2013.61. Epub 2013 May 14.
125. Vukojevic V, Kolassa IT, Fastenrath M, Gschwind L, Spalek K, Milnik A, Heck A, Vogler C, Wilker S, Demougin P, Peter F, Atucha E, Stetak A, Roozendaal B, Elbert T, Papassotiropoulos A, de Quervain DJ. Epigenetic modification of the glucocorticoid receptor gene is linked to traumatic memory and post-traumatic stress disorder risk in genocide survivors. J Neurosci. 2014;34(31):10274–84. doi:10.1523/JNEUROSCI.1526-14.2014.
126. Arnsten AFT, Raskind MA, Taylor FB, Connor DF. The effects of stress exposure on prefrontal cortex: translating basic research into successful treatments for post-traumatic stress disorder. Neurobiol Stress. 2015;1:89–99.
127. Tofts PS. The distribution of induced currents in magnetic stimulation of the nervous system. Phys Med Biol. 1990;35:1119–28.
128. Isserles M, Shalev AY, Roth Y, Peri T, Kutz I, Zlotnick E, Zangen A. Effectiveness of deep transcranial magnetic stimulation combined with a brief exposure procedure in post-traumatic stress disorder—a pilot study. Brain Stimul. 2013;6(3):377–83.
129. Karsen EF, Watts BV, Holtzheimer PE. Review of the effectiveness of transcranial magnetic stimulation for post-traumatic stress disorder. Brain Stimul. 2014;7(2):151–7.

Chapter 3
Psychosocial Concerns in Patients Living with an Implantable Cardioverter Defibrillator

Ingela Thylén

Abstract Despite the unquestionable mortality advantages of implantable cardioverter defibrillators [ICDs], some patients with ICDs will experience psychosocial concerns after implantation, including symptoms of anxiety, depression, and post traumatic stress disorder, as well as ICD-related distress. Factors that can influence the impact of these psychological disorders include socio-demographic variables, variables related to the ICD and psychosocial variables. Unfortunately, it is uncommon for patients to seek help for their anxiety and depression. It is therefore of paramount importance that the healthcare professionals actively ask their patients about their psychological state during follow-up of the device. By discussing concerns and common reactions to the ICD, potential anxiety or depression can be prevented or alleviated.

Keywords Age • Anxiety • Depression • Gender • ICD shock • ICD-related concerns • Patient outcomes • Personality traits • Posttraumatic stress disorder • Psychological distress • Type-D personality

Based on the results of primary and secondary prevention trials, implantable cardioverter defibrillators [ICDs] are currently first line therapy for patients at risk of sudden cardiac death. The ICD is generally well accepted by the majority of patients and is perceived as a lifesaving and life transforming device. Existing literature describes the ICD as a device that gives the recipient a sense of security and trust in

---

I. Thylén, R.N., Ph.D.
Department of Cardiology and Department of Medical and Health Sciences, Linköping University, Linköping, Sweden
e-mail: ingela.thylen@regionostergotland.se

© Springer International Publishing AG 2017
R. Proietti et al. (eds.), *Psychological, Emotional, Social and Cognitive Aspects of Implantable Cardiac Devices*, DOI 10.1007/978-3-319-55721-2_3

its capabilities to save their life in the event of dysrhythmia. Patients report that after ICD implantation they strive to resume command over their life again and experience both positive feelings, such as acceptance of the device, gratitude, re-evaluation of life, and negative feelings related to restriction of physical activities and fear of being alone. Despite the positive attributes of the ICD, living with an ICD has been found to cause varying levels of psychological distress, which consist in fear of device malfunction, fear of having shocks in public, or the embarrassment of becoming unconscious, but also thoughts about death, all contributing to different psychosocial responses. Some patients with ICDs become concerned with body image because the device's silhouette may be visible under the skin, and it is common to have problems with stiffness in the shoulder in the immediate postoperative period. A close relationship between ICD satisfaction and the prevalence of psychological problems has also been demonstrated. Moreover, undergoing the implantation of an ICD may cause patients to feel a loss of personal, social, and material resources. The higher the patient's sense of loss of emotional or physical well-being, the higher the risk of symptoms of depression and anxiety. The ICD patients' relationships may also become strained because of changes in their ability to maintain previous physical, social, and sexual activity. Depression or anxiety can in turn cause patients to be withdrawn or become irritable. Factors that can influence the impact of psychosocial distress include particularly (1) socio-demographic variables (age, gender, and multi-morbidity), (2) variables related to the ICD (number of ICD shocks, generator size, time from ICD implant, and device indication), and (3) psychosocial variables (negative coping strategies, lack of social support, poor knowledge of the heart condition, and personality traits).

Magyar-Russell et al. [1] presented a review of 45 studies regarding the prevalence of anxiety and depression in adult patients with ICDs. Of the 45 studies, 31 measured depression and anxiety 12 months or more following implant with a range of 12–645 participants. This review found the prevalence of psychosocial distress to be higher in patients with ICDs than in the general population; in particular, prevalences of an anxiety disorder ranged between 11 and 26% and prevalences of a depressive disorder between 11 and 28% when validated diagnostic interviews were used [1]. Similar rates of a depressive disorder were found in other cardiac populations [2, 3]. However, the rates of elevated symptoms of anxiety (8–63%) and depression (5–41%) ranged widely across studies and times of assessment when validated self-report questionnaires were used [1]. The psychological distress usually decreases during the first year after implantation [4, 5], but approximately 25% of patients have difficulty adjusting and continue to experience high levels of anxiety and depression throughout life [4]. The experience of a shock—or simple awareness of this function—may indeed result in a significantly increased and distressing concern about future shocks, which in turn may lead to avoidance behaviours, e.g., refraining from engaging in physical exercise due to fear of shocks [4]. Ultimately, shock anxiety may develop into a clinically significant generalised anxiety disorder or in avoidance of behaviours associated with a previous ICD shock experience.

Definitions and Measurements

Generalised anxiety disorder is defined through cognitive and somatic symptomatology that primarily consist in excessive chronic worry and anticipatory anxiety without a specific cause [6], in addition to sleep disturbances, restlessness, irritability, fatigue, concentration difficulties, and muscular tension [7]. Individuals with generalised anxiety disorder may worry about minor things, daily events, or the future. In ICD studies it is common to measure both general as well as disease-related anxiety. Worries about the illness trajectory or future ICD shocks overlap with general anxiety [8], nevertheless they can impact patients differently. For example, disease-related anxiety in patients with an ICD is more strongly related to Quality of Life (QoL) than general anxiety is [9]. Fortunately, both conditions and their symptoms can be prevented, treated, and managed if effectively recognized using reliable and valid assessment instruments designed specifically for patients with ICDs. Several self-report questionnaires have been developed for this purpose; the most frequently used are the 10-item Florida Shock Anxiety Scale [FSAS] [10] and the 20-item ICD Patient Concerns Questionnaire [ICDC] [11] or the shorter 8-item version [8]. Statements listed in these questionnaires are for example "I am scared to exercise because I am scared that it will increase my heart rate and cause my device to fire" [10] and "I am worried about symptoms/pain associated with my ICD firing" [8].

Even if some patients' psychosocial distress is limited to their ICDs, more general measures could be used when screening for symptoms of anxiety and depression, for example the Patient Health Questionnaire [PHQ]. This self-report instrument starts with two simple questions: "over the last 2 weeks, has the patient been bothered by any of the following problems: (1) little interest or pleasure in doing things, and (2) feeling down, depressed, or hopeless", and then progresses to the full 9-item questionnaire if the answer to one of these two questions is positive [12]. Other frequently used screening instruments for anxiety and depression in patients with ICDs are the Hospital Anxiety and Depression Scale [HADS] [13], the Beck Depression Inventory [BDI] [14], the Beck Anxiety Inventory [BAI] [15], and the Brief Symptom Inventory-18 Item [BSI-18] [16].

Having experienced a sudden aborted cardiac arrest, multiple shocks or other near-death situations can also bring about post-traumatic stress disorder [PTSD] and may affect the amount and severity of anxiety and/or depressive symptoms [17]. In addition to having faced a life-threatening event, the diagnosis of PTSD requires the patient's response to be associated with severe panic and the presence of dissociative symptoms (e.g., flashbacks) in which the individual feels or acts as if the traumatic event(s) was recurring [7]. Psychosocial research has recently began studying the incidence of PTSD in the ICD population. One of the most commonly used instruments to measure PTSD in patients with ICD is the Impact of Event Scale Revised [IES-R] [18]. Current available research suggests that approximately 20% of patients with an ICD have PTSD [19], the percentage is higher in the female population [20]. When von Känel et al. [17] followed 107 patients with an ICD, they found that rates of PTSD increased from baseline to follow-up; in particular, 19% of patients were diagnosed with PTSD at both assessments, 12% at baseline only and 18% at follow-up only. Female gender, feelings of helplessness, and a history of depression predicted greater PTSD at baseline, while low education, greater baseline PTSD, feelings of helplessness and ≥5 shocks during follow-up predicted greater PTSD between 2 and 5.5 years post-ICD implantation [17].

The psychological response and adjustment to ICD implant is complex and multifactorial, and it has been suggested that psychological distress seems to emerge more from the psychological profile of the patient [5] and to a lesser extent from ICD shocks [21]. Patients, particularly women, with substantial ICD-related concerns and a type-D personality have been identified in literature at a higher risk of psychological distress post implantation [5]. Individuals with a type-D personality tend to experience a wide range of negative emotions (e.g., feel unhappy, worry, and feel down in the dumps), however they tend not to express these emotions due to fear of rejection by others [22]. Type-D personality is considered a distressed personality characterized by two relatively stable traits: negative affectivity (e.g., "I often feel unhappy"), and social inhibition (e.g., "I am a closed kind of person"). This personality can be assessed with the 14-item Type-D Scale [DS14] [22].

Driving Restrictions and Its Impact on Psychosocial Distress

Individuals with an ICD are prohibited from driving a motor vehicle for a restricted period after the implantation and/or shock, this is likely to influence their everyday living in different ways. The willingness to accept the restriction differs between individuals. Some patients change their driving behaviour because of uncertainty of their driving abilities or fear of having arrhythmias/shocks while driving. In qualitative research it has been found that driving restrictions may lead to decreased self-esteem, relationship problems, loss of independence, and social isolation [23, 24]. Similarly, Schuster et al. [25] found that driving restrictions correlated significantly to decreased self-efficacy and anxiety. Handling driving restrictions and shocks after ICD implantation is a complex issue that clinicians need to address through direct communication with the patient. More individualized and structured information, that respects the patients' experiences and needs [24] may help to handle the driving restrictions in a less distressful way, as the literature suggests [26–28]. Many ICD patients experience a loss of independence during the period of driving restrictions. They feel limited in their ability to visit friends and family, and to participate in social activities; they are also forced to change their everyday life during the driving restriction [24, 29, 30]. Patients living with an ICD have expressed anxiety about the future, with worries about having new driving restrictions if any arrhythmias should be detected when going to the regular ICD follow-up visits [24, 31]. Hence, patients must be instructed at discharge from the hospital about the risks of possible arrhythmias in the future in order to have realistic expectations about the driving restrictions. Patients also describe how they become more attentive to warning signs from their body and use this as a tool for determining whether they should continue driving [24]. This so-called sickness scoreboard, when patients use ICD shocks and/or other physical symptoms to predict future cardiac health, may give the patient a greater perceived sense of control, particularly regarding readiness to drive [32].

Psychosocial Distress in the Partner

Also partners have to cope with the possibility that the ICD can unexpectedly shock the patient which in turn may lead to fear, anxiety and overprotectiveness, and may have a particularly profound impact if the partner has witnessed the patient having a previous cardiac arrest [33]. Van den Broek and colleagues [34] presented a review of 22 studies on emotional distress in partners of patients with an ICD and found that partners' levels of distress were at least equal, and sometimes higher, compared to patients' levels. The majority of large-scale studies suggested that partners' distress levels decrease in the first year post implantation [34]. Domains of concern emerging from qualitative studies were related to patient care, helplessness and uncertainties related to shocks, role changes, sexual activities, overprotectiveness, and driving [34]. Since partners serve as important sources of support for patients with ICDs, this role may be hampered if they experience increased distress. It is therefore of paramount importance that also the partners are involved in the follow-ups of the ICD.

Age and Multi-morbidities

A review of descriptive studies with symptoms of general anxiety and depression as outcomes demonstrated that age has mixed effects on the psychosocial responses of patients with an ICD [35]. Several studies have identified that young adult patients are at greater risk of intensified anxiety [36–40], depression [39] and ICD-related concerns compared to older patients [39], while other studies have not found that age affects the level of general anxiety [41–43]. In a recent cross-sectional study describing 229 octo-nonagenerians' levels of distress, it was found that 11% reported symptoms of depression, 15% experienced anxiety and 26% had ICD-related concerns with worries of future ICD shocks [44]; these rates of psychological distress were not higher than those found in younger patients. The discrepancies related to age may be caused by the heterogeneity of the studies in terms of age ranges of participants, disease causes and device indications, confounded by age, sensitivity of the measures of psychological responses, and analysis approaches. Nevertheless, the trend is for younger adults to experience greater concerns and negative psychosocial responses to the ICD, particularly women and patients with a shock experience. For example, in order to prevent ICD shocks, half of the younger patients have been found to decrease their activity [40, 45]. In qualitative studies, the lived experiences of young patients with an ICD often mirror that of older adults. The challenges of living with an ICD include insecurity about physical appearance, device compliance, bodily sensations of the device, body image concerns, future uncertainty, financial security, and limited support. The overall lived experience consists in appreciation for device benefits, fear of device malfunction, and attracting attention [46].

Multi-morbidity is defined in literature as two, three or more co-occurring conditions not related to the index condition [47]. The prevalence of multiple chronic illnesses in the ICD population is reported to be approximately 25% [48], but its impact on psychosocial distress has not really been studied. However, multiple co-morbidities have been found to be linked with poor outcomes in this population [49, 50], and this association between illness burden and poor survival may affect the patients' quality-of-life and psychological responses [48, 51, 52].

Gender

Approximately 20–30% of patients with ICD are women and there are a number of well-documented gender differences within the ICD population [53, 54]. Although mortality outcomes appear to be similar between males and females, women receive appropriate ICD shocks less often than men, have worse functional status at ICD implantation and have higher rates of adverse events in the hospital after ICD implantation [54–57]. Most patients with ICDs report a good quality-of-life, without emotional distress, but among those who experience distress, women are the more strongly affected. [58]. Potential explanations of increased anxiety in female patients with ICDs include receipt of shock, fear of death, body image change and specific anxieties related to role loss [59, 60]. Still, some studies report no gender differences in symptoms of depression [61–63] or anxiety [20, 61, 64] among patients with ICDs. These results, however, are contradicted by studies that do report an increase of depression [20, 41] and anxiety [41, 58, 62, 63] in female patients, independently of other variables. Furthermore, younger women under the age of 50 appear to be at greater risk to develop psychosocial distress associated with ICD-related concerns, shock anxiety, death anxiety and body image concerns than middle- and older-aged women [38]. However, the numbers of women represented in these studies are low, making the comparison of outcomes related to gender differences difficult. A most recent adequately powered study with >3000 patients with ICD and focusing on gender differences found that a higher proportion of women (20%) than men (15%) had anxiety symptoms, while there were no differences in the proportion of men (8%) and women (9%) with depressive symptoms [58]. Additionally, women had poorer quality-of-life, lower perceived control in life and lower levels of social support than men [58]. Specifically, lower perceived control, symptoms of depression and a type-D personality were predictors of symptoms of anxiety in women. Among men, younger age, primary prevention indication, previous shock experience, higher comorbidity burden, poor social support, low perceived control, depressive symptoms and type-D personality predicted presence of anxiety. With regard to symptoms of depression, older age, lower education level, longer time since ICD implantation, ICD implanted for secondary prevention, higher comorbidity burden, lower levels of social support, low perceived control, higher anxiety and higher type-D personality scores were independently associated with higher depression scores in men. Among women, the only significant independent predictors of depressive symptoms were higher comorbidity burden, poor social support, symptoms of anxiety and a type-D personality [58].

ICD Shock Therapy

Appropriate adjustment to device implant and freedom from psychosocial distress following the implant of an ICD may depend in part upon whether or not shocks have been delivered by the device. During the first years after implantation, the chances of receiving at least one ICD shock can range from one third in primary preventive patients [65, 66] to up to 50% in patients with a secondary indication [67, 68]. Even among those without shocks during first battery life, the incidence of shocks at 5 years following generator exchange is >25% [65]. Today, the majority of new ICD implants are performed for primary prevention and long-term follow-up from clinical trials suggests that the annual rate of appropriate ICD shock therapy in these patients ranges between 5 and 12% per year [69–73]. Men and younger patients are at greater risk of experiencing ICD shocks [65].

Shocks have been described by patients as unpleasant, painful and unpredictable [74, 75], "like a blow to the body, a punch in the chest, like being hit by a truck, kicked by a mule, or putting a finger in a light socket" [76]. The ICD shock experience has also been described as moderate (i.e. 5) when rated on a visual analogue scale (where 0 means no pain and 10 the worst possible pain imaginable) [77]. Although most people are able to tolerate a shock to some extent, the shock experience is discomforting and can prompt feelings like anxiety, depression, helplessness, anger or fear of future shocks [41, 78–80]. The patient's cardiac status, history of psychiatric illness and other factors increase the risk of experiencing these symptoms. ICD shocks may also affect relationships and sexual relations [81] with fear of receiving a shock during intercourse. Nevertheless, studies have been inconsistent about how, and if, receipt of ICD shocks and psychosocial distress are associated [41, 82–86]. Some of the studies have found a relationship between ICD shocks and anxiety [5, 75], while others [83, 85] did not find evidence of such a relationship and suggest that anxiety is stable over time. Instead, it has been suggested that ICD-related concerns, patients' perceptions of their personal control over shocks and their attributions regarding the predictability of shocks have a bigger impact on psychological distress than receipt of an actual shock and are an important indicator of psychosocial adjustment [8, 79, 87]. A shock from an ICD can be lifesaving but it can also affect a person's psychological state leading them to being constantly afraid that the device is about to deliver a new or recurrent shock. Moreover, disease-specific anxiety and avoidance of behaviours that patients believe elicit cardiac symptoms [88] or triggers shocks can limit the frequency and intensity of activities of daily life [32]. ICD-related concerns, with worries about the ICD firing, doing activities that may cause shocks, pain associated with the ICD firing and not being able to prevent shocks in the future has been identified as a major determinant of psychological distress and impaired QoL [79, 89]. This concern is substantially higher in those who are younger, female, have experienced more than one ICD shock and are anxious or depressed [79].

After receiving a shock feeling a "loss of control" is common among patients with an ICD and might lead them to continually avoid the activity they were doing when the discharge occurred. This avoidance behaviour may reduce anxiety but is negatively reinforcing. Patients are typically troubled by the ICDs' uncontrollable and unpredictable nature, and feel compelled to try to predict when the device will shock. Often patients become attuned to minor bodily sensations and incorrectly interpret normal sympathetic responses as precursors of an up-coming ICD shock. Fearful assessment of these symptoms can activate anxiety-related sympathetic arousal, creating a "fear of fear" cycle that mimics the catastrophic interpretation of patients with panic disorder. "Overgeneralizing" occurs when patients believe a rare occurrence (an ICD shock) will happen frequently, which may contribute to avoidance. For example, patients might think they should avoid physical activity if they previously received a shock while exercising. These fears and subsequent avoidance behaviours may increase with the number of shocks. Over time, fear and avoidance may adversely alter lifestyle and diminish QoL [90]. Participating in an ICD-specific rehabilitation programme may encourage patients and lower their fear of exercising [91]. Research has also highlighted how the attitudes of patients are among the best predictors of QoL [92]. Shock can reduce the patients' faith in their safety and their future, or could serve as a reminder of their commitment to live. Therefore, actively reminding patients to think about the positive aspects of their life, their relationships, their everyday activities and their future can provide the patient with hopefulness and rewarding plans for the [93].

Device Indication and Time Since ICD Implantation

One feature that is unique across studies of patients with an ICD is the heterogeneity of medical histories and the reasons for device implantation. Indications for implantation of an ICD have expanded since the device was first introduced to prevent sudden cardiac death in patients who had experienced a previous cardiac arrest (secondary prevention), with current guidelines now also advocating its use in patients at risk for life threatening ventricular arrhythmias (primary prevention). However, there is no evidence to suggest that patients receiving an ICD for primary prophylaxis have subsequent poorer QoL or greater distress than patients receiving an ICD for secondary prophylaxis [39, 41, 86, 94–96].

Circumstances surrounding the implant of an ICD can impact the manner in which individuals adjust to the device and affect levels of psychosocial distress following implantation [85, 97]. Dunbar et al. [98] presented a model of the patient's trajectory that breaks the patient's experience into three major categories: pre implantation, post implantation—with early recovery and adjustment phases—and end of life. Each of these categories includes events, treatments and potential complications that can impact the psychological well-being and QoL of patients with an ICD. In most of them, anxiety and symptoms of depression tend to lessen over time [99, 100], being most prevalent during the first 3–6 months after implantation [41], while other studies suggest that patients who have lived with their ICD longer than 1 year are more depressed compared with those who have received their ICD more recently [37]. However, in a large sample with >3000 patients who had their ICD implanted from 1 to 23 years, no correlation was found between time since implantation and psychosocial distress, suggesting that patients are stable across time [39].

Impact on Ventricular Arrhythmias and Mortality

Symptoms of depression and anxiety, as well as more stable personality traits such as type-D personality, are especially important to identify since they not only influence daily functioning but are also associated with an increased risk of ventricular arrhythmias [101, 102] and mortality [103], independently of traditional biomedical risk factors. Patients with a higher level of depression [104] as well as anxiety [105–107] have been found to be more likely to have arrhythmias treated with ICD shocks than those with a lower level of distress. We know little about the mechanisms that may explain the association between emotional distress and worse prognosis in patients with an ICD. One potential mechanism involves the autonomic nervous system, which may be deregulated in patients with an ICD [108]. Abnormalities in autonomic cardiovascular regulation, such as impaired baroreflex response and decreased heart rate variability [HRV] (i.e. increased sympathetic and/or decreased parasympathetic activity), have been shown to be independent risk factors for sudden cardiac death in post myocardial infarction patients [109, 110]. In the general cardiac population, there is evidence to suggest that HRV is decreased in patients with clinical levels of depression [111] and anxiety [112] as compared to patients without emotional distress. Moreover, HRV might be an important mediator in the relationship between emotional distress and mortality in cardiac patients [110, 113]. However, to date, only one study has investigated the relationship between emotional distress and HRV in ICD patients [114]. A shift towards sympathetic dominance and reduced vagal activity has been observed in ICD patients with emotional distress. This may trigger the development of ventricular tachycardia, resulting in a poorer prognosis [115].

It has been indicated that emotional distress is related to all-cause as well as cardiac-related mortalities in patients with an ICD. Particularly, general negative mood, somatic symptoms of depression [116], ICD-related concerns [101], a type-D personality [101] and an impaired QoL [117] are associated with mortality in patients with ICDs. Several behavioural and clinical factors may serve as mediators in the relationship between negative mood and mortality. Results among cardiac patients suggest that patients who were depressed displayed poor medication adherence and physical inactivity. Patients with mood disorders may have more comorbidities than patients without mood disorders. The relationship between negative emotions and mortality may be explained by the increased risk of arrhythmias and ICD shocks in patients with chronic levels of negative emotions [102] and depression [118]. Shocks have also been found to be related to mortality [116, 119]. The increased arrhythmia risk in these distressed patients may again be related to disturbed autonomic balance.

Managing Psychosocial Distress in Patients with ICD

Following implantation, patients are usually discharged from the hospital within 48 hours (in some ICD clinics as early as after 24 hours), leaving them little opportunity to raise questions and concerns. Remote monitoring makes follow-up easier for both patients and healthcare professionals, and may improve timeliness of management. However, a consequence of remote follow-up has been a decrease in the amount of time healthcare professionals may spend in face-to-face follow-up consultations with patients [120]. To ensure the patient is coping, interventions such as simple follow-up telephone calls and basic ICD-specific patient education should be implemented as a routine. Explaining how the device functions and what to do in the event of a shock, having a so-called "shock-plan" significantly reduces ICD-related anxiety and concerns [35, 121, 122]. Patients cannot control the shocks but they can learn to control their reactions, furthermore knowledge and preparedness can be empowering for patients. Open communication is the key, that is why "the shock-plan" should be developed collaboratively between patients and healthcare professionals. The plan should also be described and discussed with all family members [93].

ICDs are associated with a multitude of psychosocial issues, including anxiety and depression, especially in the first months or year after implantation. Unfortunately, there is a tendency for patients with an ICD to conceal their concerns because of embarrassment, lack of insight or the restricted nature of their symptoms [30]. It is therefore important that healthcare professionals actively ask their patients about their psychological state and functioning as soon as the device is implanted and consistently during routine follow-up care. Those who have received shock therapy might need special intervention that focuses on concerns about future shocks, since they are at higher risk for developing anxiety and/or depressive symptoms [79]. Because ICD-related concerns can change with experience and with time, it is important to assess concerns regularly. The patients should be assessed regularly even if they have not experienced a shock, since device-related distress can occur also in the absence of shocks. By discussing concerns and common reactions to the ICD, potential anxiety or depression can be prevented or alleviated. Adequate information provision and psycho-education can help as such. Surveys among patients with ICD have namely indicated that many patients have insufficient knowledge as to why they were implanted with an ICD, its possible side effects and benefits, and lack knowledge about ethical and practical issues at the end-of-life [123–125]. Demographically, it has have been found that especially women, older patients, those living alone and those with lower education levels tend to have insufficient knowledge, while those with shock experience are more knowledgeable, suggesting that healthcare professionals spend more time educating patients in these conditions [123]. When discussing the issues surrounding ICD implantation with patients and their families, healthcare professionals can facilitate optimal understanding and adaptation, and detect possible psychosocial concerns. However, for education to be effective, it should be tailored to patients' preferences and needs, which thus requires healthcare professionals to have insights into patients' health and social characteristics, understanding, attitudes and skills.

A scientific statement from the American Heart Association [35] emphasizes the importance of educational and psychological interventions to improve outcomes for patients with ICDs as well as their families. If difficulties adapting to the ICD are manifested, the patient might be referred to a mental health professional for evaluation and treatment of the psychosocial distress. The initial treatment goal is to relieve anxiety and depressive symptoms. These are likely to persist, however, if the patient's irrational beliefs, avoidance and conditioning are not addressed. Treatment and prophylaxis of distress often involves a combination of psycho-education and support groups using for example storytelling [35, 98, 126]. Optimal medical therapy and the provision of psychological support are key to the effective management of patients' biopsychosocial functioning. These interventions can improve mental status, QoL, and increase feelings of security by allowing ICD patients to discuss their fears and expectations related to their ICDs. Supportive group therapy is particularly useful in younger patients that may not have any friends in the same age group with whom they can discuss their problems [127].

To reduce anxiety and depressive symptoms, patients need to address irrational beliefs, avoidance and conditioning. Cognitive behavioural therapy [CBT] is often used to identify and correct maladaptive or irrational beliefs about ICDs and shocks, and to eliminate avoidance behaviours that serve as negative reinforcement. The treatment of symptoms of anxiety and depression with CBT has shown to improve patients' mental status as well as reduce the number of arrhythmias, which in turn decrease the propensity for shocks [128–132]. CBT typically begins with psycho-education about the ICD to help patients realize that their thoughts about the device might be irrational. It usually addresses stress management, problem solving techniques, avoidance behaviour, and how to resume work and social activities. Strategies include keeping a daily log of ICD related thoughts and cognitive re-structuring. Exposure therapy can help patients re-engage in activities they had been avoiding because of irrational fears. Clinical trials have also shown yoga and mindfulness to be effective in addressing both psychological and physical components that are present in illnesses such as cardiovascular diseases [133, 134]. These include cardiovagal function, sympathetic activation, oxidative stress, coagulation profiles, and symptoms of anxiety and depression. Yoga, relaxation training, including in deep-breathing techniques, could be particularly beneficial for ICD patients since they may help reduce the arousal response to an ICD shock [135].

References

1. Magyar-Russell G, Thombs BD, Cai JX, Baveja T, Kuhl EA, Singh PP, et al. The prevalence of anxiety and depression in adults with implantable cardioverter defibrillators: a systematic review. J Psychosom Res. 2011;71(4):223–31.
2. Thombs BD, Bass EB, Ford DE, Stewart KJ, Tsildis KK, Patel U, et al. Prevalence of depression in survivors of acute myocardial infarction. J Gen Intern Med. 2006;21:30–8.
3. Moser DK, Dracup K, Evangelista LS, Zambroski CH, Lennie TA, Chung ML, et al. Comparison of prevalence of symptoms of depression, anxiety, and hostility in elderly patients with heart failure, myocardial infarction, and a coronary artery bypass graft. Heart Lung. 2010;39:378–85.
4. Sears SF, Conti JB. Quality of life and psychological functioning of ICD patients. Heart. 2002;87:488–93.
5. Pedersen SS, Theuns DA, Erdman RA, Jordaens L. Clustering of device-related concerns and type D personality predicts increased distress in ICD patients independent of shocks. Pacing Clin Electrophysiol. 2008;31:20–7.
6. Stein D. Generalised anxiety disorder. Rethinking diagnosis and rating. CNS Spectr. 2005;10(12):930–4.
7. American Psychiatric Association. Diagnostic and statistical manual of mental disorders. Washington, DC: American Psychiatric Association (APA); 2013.
8. Pedersen SS, van Domburg RT, Theuns DA, Jordaens L, Erdman RAM. Concerns about the implantable cardioverter defibrillator: a determinant of anxiety and depressive symptoms independent of experienced shocks. Am Heart J. 2005;149(4):664–9.
9. Hegel MT, Griegel LE, Black C, et al. Anxiety and depression in patients receiving implanted cardioverter-defibrillators: a longitudinal investigation. Int J Psychiatry Med. 1997;27:57–69.
10. Ford J, Finch JF, Woodrow LK, Cutitta KE, Shea JA, Fischer A, et al. The Florida Shock Anxiety Scale (FSAS) for patients with implantable cardioverter defibrillators: testing factor structure, reliability, and validity of a previously established measure. Pacing Clin Electrophysiol. 2012;35:1146–53.
11. Frizelle DJ, Lewin B, Kaye G, Moniz-Cook ED. Development of a measure of the concerns held by people with implanted cardioverter defibrillators: the ICDC. Br J Health Psychol. 2006;11:293–301.
12. Kroenke K, Spitzer RL, Williams JB. The patient health questionnaire-2: validity of a two-item depression screener. Med Care. 2003;41(11):1284–92.
13. Zigmond AS, Snaith RP. The hospital anxiety and depression scale. Acta Psychiatr Scand. 1983;67(6):361–70.
14. Beck AT, Ward CH, Mendelson M, Mock J, Erbaugh J. An inventory for measuring depression. Arch Gen Psychiatry. 1961;4:561–71.

15. Beck AT, Epstein N, Brown G, Steer RA. An inventory for measuring clinical anxiety: psychometric properties. J Consult Clin Psychol. 1988;56:893–7.
16. Derogatis LR. Brief Symptom Inventory (BSI)-18. Administration, scoring and procedures manual. Minneapolis: NCS Pearson; 2001.
17. von Kanel R, Baumert J, Kolb C, Cho EY, Ladwig KH. Chronic posttraumatic stress and its predictors in patients living with an implantable cardioverter defibrillator. J Affect Disord. 2011;131:344–52.
18. Weiss DS, Marmar CR. The impact of event scale—revised. In: Wilson JP, Keane TM, editors. Assessing psychological trauma and PTSD. New York: Guilford Press; 1997. p. 399–411.
19. Ladwig KH, Baumert J, Marten-Mittag B, Kolb C, Zrenner B, Schmitt C. Posttraumatic stress symptoms and predicted mortality in patients with implantable cardioverter-defibrillators: results from the prospective living with an implanted cardioverter-defibrillator study. Arch Gen Psychiatry. 2008;65:1324–30.
20. Rahmawati A, Chishaki A, Sawatari H, Tsuchihashi-Makaya M, Ohtsuka Y, Nakai M, et al. Gender disparities in quality of life and psychological disturbance in patients with implantable cardioverter-defibrillators. Circ J. 2013;77:1158–65.
21. Pedersen SS, Van Den Broek KC, Van Den Berg M, Theuns DA. Shock as a determinant of poor patient-centered outcomes in implantable cardioverter defibrillator patients: is there more to it than meets the eye? Pacing Clin Electrophysiol. 2010;33(12):1430–6.
22. Denollet J. DS14: standard assessment of negative affectivity, social inhibition, and type D personality. Psychosom Med. 2005;67(1):89–97.
23. James JE, Albarran JW, Tagney J. The experiences of ICD patients and their partners with regards to adjusting to an imposed driving ban: a qualitative study. Coron Health Care. 2001;5(2):80–8.
24. Johansson I, Strömberg A. Experiences of driving and driving restrictions in recipients with an implantable cardioverter defibrillator: the patient perspective. J Cardiovasc Nurs. 2010;25(6):E1–E10.
25. Schuster PM, Phillips S, Dillon DL, Tomich PL. The psychosocial and physiological experiences of patients with an implantable cardioverter defibrillator. Rehabil Nurs. 1998;23: 30–7.
26. Pelletier D, Gallagher R, Mitten-Lewis S, McKinley S, Squire J. Australian implantable cardiac defibrillator recipients: quality-of-life issues. Int J Nurs Pract. 2002;8:68–74.
27. Albarran JW, Tagney J, James JE. Partners of ICD patients: an exploratory study of their experiences. Eur J Cardiovasc Nurs. 2004;3:201–10.
28. Eckert M, Jones T. How does an implantable cardioverter defibrillator (ICD) affect the lives of patients and their families. Int J Nurs Pract. 2002;8:152–7.
29. Craney J, Powers M. Factors related to driving in persons with an implantable cardioverter defibrillator. Prog Cardiovasc Nurs. 1995;10:12–7.
30. Tagney J, James JE, Albarran JW. Exploring the patient's experiences of learning to live with an implantable cardioverter defibrillator (ICD) from one UK Centre: a qualitative study. Eur J Cardiovasc Nurs. 2003;2:195–203.
31. Baessler C, Murphy S, Gebhardt L, Tso T, Ellenbogen K, Leman R. Time to resumption of driving after implantation of an automatic defibrillator (from the Dual chamber and VVI Implantable Defibrillator [DAVID] trial). Am J Cardiol. 2005;95:665–6.
32. Sears SF, Conti JB. Understanding implantable cardioverter defibrillator shocks and storms: medical and psychosocial considerations for research and clinical care. Clin Cardiol. 2003;26:107–11.
33. Jenkins LS, Powell JL, Schron EB, McBurnie MA, Bosworth-Farrell S, Moore R, et al. Partner quality of life in the antiarrhythmics versus implantable defibrillators trial. J Cardiovasc Nurs. 2007;22:472–9.
34. van den Broek KC, Habibović M, Pedersen SS. Emotional distress in partners of patients with an implantable cardioverter defibrillator: a systematic review and recommendations for future research. Pacing Clin Electrophysiol. 2010;33(12):1442–50.

35. Dunbar SB, Dougherty CM, Sears SF, Carroll DL, Goldstein NE, Mark DB, et al. Educational and psychological interventions to improve outcomes for recipients of implantable cardioverter defibrillators and their families: a scientific statement from the American Heart Association. Circulation. 2012;126(17):2146–72.
36. Thylén I. Younger implantable cardioverter defibrillator (ICD) patients' quality-of-life, psychosocial concerns, and experience of the device. The EuroHeartCare Congress 2014-04-04. Stavanger; 2014.
37. Friedmann E, Thomas SA, Inguito P, Kao CW, Metcalf M, Kelley FJ, et al. Quality of life and psychological status of patients with implantable cardioverter defibrillators. J Interv Card Electrophysiol. 2006;17:65–72.
38. Vazquez LD, Kuhl EA, Shea JB, Kirkness A, Lemon J, Whalley D, et al. Age-specific differences in women with implantable cardioverter defibrillators: an international multi center study. Pacing Clin Electrophysiol. 2008;31:1528–34.
39. Thylen I, Dekker RL, Jaarsma T, Stromberg A, Moser DK. Characteristics associated with anxiety, depressive symptoms, and quality-of-life in a large cohort of implantable cardioverter defibrillator recipients. J Psychosom Res. 2014;77(2):122–7.
40. Wójcicka M, Lewandowski M, Smolis-Bak E, Szwed H. Psychological and clinical problems in young adults with implantable cardioverter-defibrillators. Kardiol Pol. 2008; 66(10):1050–8.
41. Bilge AK, Ozben B, Demircan S, Cinar M, Yilmaz E, Adalet K. Depression and anxiety status of patients with implantable cardioverter defibrillator and precipitating factors. Pacing Clin Electrophysiol. 2006;29:619–26.
42. Johansen JB, Pedersen SS, Spindler H, Andersen K, Nielsen JC, Mortensen PT. Symptomatic heart failure is the most important clinical correlate of impaired quality of life, anxiety, and depression in implantable cardioverter-defibrillator patients: a single-centre, cross-sectional study in 610 patients. Europace. 2008;10:545–51.
43. Jacq F, Foulldrin G, Savoure A, Anselme F, Baguelin-Pinaud A, Cribier A, et al. A comparison of anxiety, depression and quality of life between device shock and nonshock groups in implantable cardioverter defibrillator recipients. Gen Hosp Psychiatry. 2009;31:266–73.
44. Thylén I, Strömberg A, Lindberg R, Moser DK. Octo-nonagenerians' outlook on life and death when living with an implantable cardioverter defibrillator: a cross-sectional study. Manuscript. 2017.
45. McDonough A. The experiences and concerns of young adults (18-40 years) living with an implanted cardioverter defibrillator (ICD). Eur J Cardiovasc Nurs. 2009;8(4):274–80.
46. Larimer K, Durmus J, Florez E. Experiences of young adults with pacemakers and/or implantable cardioverter defibrillators. J Cardiovasc Nurs. 2016;31(6):517–22.
47. Fortin M, Lapointe L, Hudon C, Vanasse A, Ntetu AL, Maltais D. Multimorbidity and quality of life in primary care: a systematic review. Health Qual Life Outcomes. 2004;2:51.
48. Hoogwegt MT, Kupper N, Jordaens L, Pedersen SS, Theuns DA. Comorbidity burden is associated with poor psychological well-being and physical health status in patients with an implantable cardioverter-defibrillator. Europace. 2013;15:1468–74.
49. Lee DS, Tu JV, Austin PC, Dorian P, Yee R, Chong A, et al. Effect of cardiac and noncardiac conditions on survival after defibrillator implantation. J Am Coll Cardiol. 2007;49:2408–15.
50. Theuns DA, Schaer BA, Soliman OI, Altmann D, Sticherling C, Geleijnse ML, et al. The prognosis of implantable defibrillator patients treated with cardiac resynchronization therapy: comorbidity burden as predictor of mortality. Europace. 2011;13:62–9.
51. van den Akker M, Buntinix F, Metsemakers JFM, Roos S, Knotterus JA. Multimorbidity in general practice: prevalence, incidence, and determinants of co-occurring chronic and recureent diseases. J Clin Epidemiol. 1998;51:367–75.
52. Brettschneider C, Leicht H, Bickel H, Dahlhaus A, Fuchs A, Gensichen J, et al. Relative impact of multimorbid chronic conditions on health-related quality of life—results from the multicare cohort study. PLoS One. 2013;8:e66742.
53. Chan PS, Birkmeyer JD, Krumholz HM, Spertus JA, Nallamothu BK. Racial and gender trends in the use of implantable cardioverter defibrillators among Medicare beneficiaries between 1997 and 2003. Congest Heart Fail. 2009;15:51–7.

54. Peterson PN, Daugherty SL, Wang Y, Vidaillet HJ, Heidenreich PA, Curtis JP, et al. Gender differences in procedure-related adverse events in patients receiving implantable cardioverter-defibrillator therapy. Circulation. 2009;119:1078–84.
55. Lin G, Meverden RA, Hodge DO, Uslan DZ, Hayes DL, Brady PA. Age and gender trends in implantable cardioverter defibrillator utilization: a population based study. J Interv Card Electrophysiol. 2008;22:65–70.
56. Bhavnani SP, Pavuluri V, Coleman CI, Guertin D, Yarlagadda RK, Clyne CA, et al. The gender-paradox among patients with implantable cardioverter-defibrillators: a propensity-matched study. Pacing Clin Electrophysiol. 2013;36:878–84.
57. van der Heijden AC, Thijssen J, Borleffs CJ, van Rees JB, Hoke U, van der Velde ET, et al. Gender-specific differences in clinical outcome of primary prevention implantable cardioverter defibrillator recipients. Heart. 2013;99:1244–9.
58. Miller J, Thylen I, Moser DK. Gender disparities in symptoms of anxiety, depression, and quality of life in defibrillator recipients. Pacing Clin Electrophysiol. 2015:1–11.
59. Brouwers C, van den Broek KC, Denollet J, Pedersen SS. Gender disparities in psychological distress and quality of life among patients with an implantable cardioverter defibrillator. Pacing Clin Electrophysiol. 2011;34:798–803.
60. Morken IM, Norekval TM, Bru E, Larsen AI, Karlsen B. Perceptions of healthcare professionals' support, shock anxiety, and device acceptance among implantable cardioverter defibrillator recipients. J Adv Nurs. 2014;70:2061–71.
61. Habibovic M, van Den Broek KC, Theuns DA, Jordaens L, Alings M, van der Voort PH, et al. Gender disparities in anxiety and quality of life in patients with an implantable-cardioverter defibrillator. Europace. 2011;13:1723–30.
62. Spindler H, Johansen JB, Andersen K, Mortensen P, Pedersen SS. Gender differences in anxiety and concerns about the cardioverter defibrillator. Pacing Clin Electrophysiol. 2009;32: 614–21.
63. Starrenburg A, Pedersen SS, van Den Broek KC, Kraaier K, Scholten M, van den Palen J. Gender differences in psychological distress and quality of life in patients with an ICD 1-year postimplant. Pacing Clin Electrophysiol. 2014;37:843–52.
64. Marshall P, Ketchell A, Maclean J. Comparison of male and female psychological outcomes related to implantable cardioverter defibrillators (COMFORTID). Eur J Cardiovasc Nurs. 2012;11:313–21.
65. Merchant FM, Jones P, Wehrenberg S, Lloyd MS, Saxon LA, Group TAS. Incidence of defibrillator shocks after elective generator exchange following uneventful first battery life. J Am Heart Assoc. 2014;3:e001289.
66. van der Heijden AC, Borleffs CJ, Buiten MS, Thijssen J, van Rees JB, Cannegieter SC, et al. The clinical course of patients with implantable cardioverter-defibrillators: extended experience on clinical outcome, device replacements, and device-related complications. Heart Rhythm. 2015;12(6):1169–76.
67. Klein RC, Raitt MH, Wilkoff BL, Beckman KJ, Coromilas J, Wyse DG, et al. Analysis of implantable cardioverter defibrillator therapy in the Antiarrhythmics Versus Implantable Defibrillators (AVID) Trial. J Cardiovasc Electrophysiol. 2003;14(9):940–8.
68. Erkapic D, Sperzel J, Stiller S, Meltendorf U, Mermi J, Wegscheider K, et al. Long-term benefit of implantable cardioverter/defibrillator therapy after elective device replacement: results of the INcidence free SUrvival after ICD REplacement (INSURE) trial – a prospective multicentre study. Eur Heart J. 2013;34(2):130–7.
69. Alsheikh-Ali AA, Homer M, Maddukuri PV, Kalsmith B, Estes NAI, Link MS. Time-dependence of appropriate implantable defibrillator therapy in patients with ischemic cardiomyopathy. J Cardiovasc Electrophysiol. 2008;19:784–9.
70. Bardy GH, Lee KL, Mark DB, Poole JE, Packer DL, Boineau R, et al. Amiodarone or an implantable cardioverter-defibrillator for congestive heart failure. N Engl J Med. 2005;352(3):225–37.
71. Moss AJ, Zareba W, Hall WJ, Klein H, Wilber DJ, Cannom DS, et al. Prophylactic implantation of a defibrillator in patients with myocardial infarction and reduced ejection fraction. N Engl J Med. 2002;346:877–83.

72. Wathen MS, DeGroot PJ, Sweeney MO, Stark AJ, Otterness MF, Adkisson WO, et al. Prospective randomized multicenter trial of empirical antitachycardia pacing versus shocks for spontaneous rapid ventricular tachycardia in patients with implantable cardioverter-defibrillators: pacing fast ventricular tachycardia reduces shock therapies (PainFREE Rx II) trial results. Circulation. 2004;110:2591–6.
73. Wilkoff BL, Williamson BD, Stern RS, Moore SL, Lu F, Lee SW, et al. Strategic programming of detection and therapy parameters in implantable cardioverter-defibrillators reduces shocks in primary prevention patients: results from the PREPARE (Primary Prevention Parameters Evaluation) study. J Am Coll Cardiol. 2008;52(7):541–50.
74. Kamphuis HC, Verhoeven NW, Leeuw R, Derksen R, Hauer RN, Winnubst JA. ICD: a qualitative study of patient experience the first year after implantation. J Clin Nurs. 2004;13:1008–16.
75. Carroll DL, Hamilton GA. Quality of life in implanted cardioverter defibrillator recipients: the impact of a device shock. Heart Lung. 2005;34:169–78.
76. Ahmad M, Bloomstein L, Roelke M, Bernstein AD, Parsonnet V. Patients' attitudes toward implanted defibrillator shocks. Pacing Clin Electrophysiol. 2000;23(6):934–8.
77. Thylén I, Moser DK, Chung ML, Miller J, Fluur C, Strömberg A. Are ICD recipients able to foresee if they want to withdraw therapy or deactivate defibrillator shocks? IJC Heart Vessels. 2013;1:22–31. doi:10.1016/j.ijchv.2013.11.001.
78. Lemon J, Edelman S, Kirkness A. Avoidance behaviors in patients with implantable cardioverter defibrillators. Heart Lung. 2004;33:176–82.
79. Thylen I, Moser DK, Stromberg A, Dekker RA, Chung ML. Concerns about implantable cardioverter defibrillator shocks mediate the relationship between actual shocks and psychological distress. Europace. 2016;18(6):828–35. doi:10.1093/europace/euv220. Epub August 31, 2015.
80. Morken IM, Isaksen K, Karlsen B, Norekvål TM, Bru E, Larsen A. Shock anxiety among implantable cardioverter defibrillator recipients with recent tachyarrhythmia. Pacing Clin Electrophysiol. 2012;35:1369–76.
81. Palacios-Ceña D, Losa-Iglesias ME, Alvarez-López C, Cachón-Pérez M, Reyes RA, Salvadores-Fuentes P, et al. Patients, intimate partners and family experiences of implantable cardioverter defibrillators: qualitative systematic review. J Adv Nurs. 2011;67(12):2537–50.
82. Schulz SM, Massa C, Grzbiela A, Dengler W, Wiedemann G, Pauli P. Implantable cardioverter defibrillator shocks are prospective predictors of anxiety. Heart Lung. 2013;42:105–11.
83. Crossmann A, Pauli P, Dengler W, Kuhlkamp V, Wiedemann G. Stability and cause of anxiety in patients with an implantable cardioverter defibrillator: a longitudinal two-year follow-up. Heart Lung. 2007;36:87–95.
84. Freedenberg V, Thomas SA, Friedmann E. Anxiety and depression in implanted cardioverter-defibrillator recipients and heart failure: a review. Heart Fail Clin. 2011;7:59–68.
85. Kapa S, Rotondi-Trevisan D, Mariano Z, Aves T, Irvine J, Dorian P. Pyschopathology in patients with ICDs over time: results of a prospective study. Pacing Clin Electrophysiol. 2010;33:198–208.
86. Groeneveld PW, Matta MA, Suh JJ, Yang F, Shea JA. Quality of life among implantable cardioverter-defibrillator recipients in the primary prevention therapeutic era. Pacing Clin Electrophysiol. 2007;30(4):463–71.
87. Bostwick JM, Sola CL. An updated review of implantable cardioverter defibrillators, induced anxiety, and quality of life. Psychiatr Clin North Am. 2007;30:677–88.
88. Eifert GH, Zvolensky MJ, Lejuez CW. Heart-focused anxiety and chest pain: a conceptual and clinical review. Clin Psychol Sci Pract. 2000;7:403–17.
89. Schron EB, Exner DV, Yao Q, Jenkins LS, Steinberg JS, Cook JR, et al. Quality of life in the antiarrhythmics versus implantable defibrillators trial: impact of therapy and influence of adverse symptoms and defibrillator shocks. Circulation. 2002;105(5):589–94.
90. van Ittersum M, de Greef M, van Gelder I, Coster J, Brügemann J, van der Schans C. Fear of exercise and health-related quality of life in patients with an implantable cardioverter defibrillator. Int J Rehabil Res. 2003;26(2):117–22.

91. Berg SK, Pedersen BD, Svendsen JH, Zwisler AD, Kristensen L, Pedersen PU. COPE-ICD: patient experience of participation in an ICD specific rehabilitation programme. Eur J Cardiovasc Nurs. 2012;11(2):207–15.
92. Sears SF, Serber ES, Lewis TS, Walker RL, Conners N, Lee JT, Curtis AB, Conti JB. Do positive health expectations and optimism relate to quality of life outcomes in ICD patients? J Cardiopulm Rehab. 2004;24:324–331.
93. Sears SF, Shea JB, Conti JB. How to respond to an implantable cardioverter defibrillator shock. Circulation. 2005;111:e380–2.
94. Pedersen SS, Sears SF, Burg MM, van den Broek KC. Does ICD indication affect quality of life and levels of distress? Pacing Clin Electrophysiol. 2009;32:153–6.
95. Pedersen SS, Theuns DA, Muskens-Heemskerk A, Erdman RAM, Jordaens L. Type D personality but not implantable cardioverter-defibrillator indication is associated with impaired health-related quality of life 3 months post-implantation. Europace. 2007;9(8):675–80.
96. Sweeney MO, Wathen MS, Volosin K, Abdalla I, DeGroot PJ, Otterness MF, et al. Appropriate and inappropriate ventricular therapies, quality of life, and mortality among primary and secondary prevention implantable cardioverter defibrillator patients: results from the Pacing Fast VT REduces shock thErapies (PainFREE Rx II) Trial. Circulation. 2005;111: 2898–905.
97. Sears SF, Hauf JD, Kirian K, Hazelton G, Conti JB. Posttraumatic stress and the implantable cardioverter defibrillator patient: what the electrophysiologist needs to know. Circ Arrhythm Electrophysiol. 2011;2011:242–50.
98. Dunbar SB, Langberg JJ, Reilly CM, Viswanathan B, McCarty F, Culler SD, et al. Effect of a psychoeducational intervention on depression, anxiety, and health resource use in implantable cardioverter defibrillator patients. Pacing Clin Electrophysiol. 2009;32:1259–71.
99. van den Broek KC, Nyklicek I, Van der Voort PH, Alings M, Denollet J. Shocks, personality, and anxiety in patients with an implantable defibrillator. Pacing Clin Electrophysiol. 2008;31:850–7.
100. Thomas SA, Friedmann E, Gottlieb SS, Liu F, Morton PG, Chapa DW, et al. Changes in psychosocial distress in outpatients with heart failure with implantable cardioverter defibrillators. Heart Lung. 2009;38:109–20.
101. Pedersen SS, Van den Broek KC, Erdman RAM, Jordaens L, Theuns DAMJ. Pre-implantation implantable cardioverter defibrillator concerns and type D personality increase the risk of mortality in patients with an implantable cardioverter defibrillator. Europace. 2010;12(10): 1446–52.
102. van den Broek KC, Nyklícek I, Van der Voort PH, Alings M, Meijer A, Denollet J. Risk of ventricular arrhythmia after implantable defibrillator treatment in anxious type D patients. J Am Coll Cardiol. 2009;54(6):531–7.
103. Denollet J, Tekle FB, Pedersen SS, Van der Voort PH, Alings M, Van den Broek KC. Prognostic importance of distressed (type D) personality and shocks in patients with an implantable cardioverter defibrillator. Int J Cardiol. 2013;167(6):2705–9.
104. Whang W, Mittleman MA, Rich DQ, Wang PJ, Ruskin JN, Tofler GH, et al. Heart failure and the risk of shocks in patients with implantable cardioverter defibrillators: results from the Triggers Of Ventricular Arrhythmias (TOVA) study. Circulation. 2004;109:1386–91.
105. Dunbar SB, Kimble LP, Jenkins LS, et al. Association of mood disturbance and arrhythmia events in patients after cardioverter defibrillator implantation. Depress Anxiety. 1999;9: 163–8.
106. Burg MM, Lampert R, Joska T, et al. Psychological traits and emotion-triggering of ICD shock-terminated arrhythmias. Psychosom Med. 2004;66:898–902.
107. Fries R, Konig J, Schafers HJ, et al. Triggering effect of physical and mental stress on spontaneous ventricular tachyarrhythmias in patients with implantable cardioverter-defibrillators. Clin Cardiol. 2002;25:474–8.
108. Jankowska EA, Ponikowski P, Piepoli MF, Banasiak W, Anker SD, Poole-Wilson PA. Autonomic imbalance and immune activation in chronic heart failure—pathophysiological links. Cardiovasc Res. 2006;70(3):434–45.

109. Carpeggiani C, Emdin M, Bonaguidi F, Landi P, Michelassi C, Trivella MG, et al. Personality traits and heart rate variability predict long-term cardiac mortality after myocardial infarction. Eur Heart J. 2005;26(16):1612–7.
110. Carney RM, Blumenthal JA, Freedland KE, Stein PK, Howells WB, Berkman LF, et al. Low heart rate variability and the effect of depression on post-myocardial infarction mortality. Arch Intern Med. 2005;165(13):1486–91.
111. Krittayaphong R, Cascio WE, Light KC, Sheffield D, Golden RN, Finkel JB, et al. Heart rate variability in patients with coronary artery disease: differences in patients with higher and lower depression scores. Psychosom Med. 1997;59(3):231–5.
112. Martens EJ, Nyklíček I, Szabó BM, Kupper N. Depression and anxiety as predictors of heart rate variability after myocardial infarction. Psychol Med. 2008;38(03):375–83.
113. Stein PK, Domitrovich PP, Huikuri HV, Kleiger RE. Traditional and nonlinear heart rate variability are each independently associated with mortality after myocardial infarction. J Cardiovasc Electrophysiol. 2005;16:13–20.
114. Francis JL, Weinstein AA, Krantz DS, Haigney MC, Stein PK, Stone PH, et al. Association between symptoms of depression and anxiety with heart rate variability in patients with implantable cardioverter defibrillators. Psychosom Med. 2009;71(8):821–7.
115. Hoogwegt MT, Pedersen SS, Theuns DA, Kupper N. Relation between emotional distress and heart rate variability in patients with an implantable cardioverter-defibrillator. Psychophysiology. 2014;51(2):187–96.
116. van den Broek KC, Tekle FB, Habibović M, Alings M, van der Voort PH, Denollet J. Emotional distress, positive affect, and mortality in patients with an implantable cardioverter defibrillator. Int J Cardiol. 2013;165(2):327–32.
117. Kao CW, Friedmann E, Thomas SA. Quality of life predicts one-year survival in patients with implantable cardioverter defibrillators. Qual Life Res. 2010;19:307–15.
118. Whang W, Albert CM, Sears SF, et al. Depression as a predictor for appropriate shocks among patients with implantable cardioverter-defibrillators: results from the Triggers of Ventricular Arrhythmias (TOVA) study. J Am Coll Cardiol. 2005;45:1090–5.
119. Tung R, Zimetbaum P, Josephson ME. A critical appraisal of implantable cardioverter-defibrillator therapy for the prevention of sudden cardiac death. J Am Coll Cardiol. 2008;52:1111–21.
120. Pedersen SS, Knudsen C, Dilling K, Sandgaard N, Brock Johansen JB. Living with an implantable cardioverter defibrillator: patients' preferences and needs for information provision and care options. Europace 2016 Jun 5. pii: euw109. [Epub ahead of print] https://doi.org/10.1093/europace/euw109
121. Sears SF, Sowell LD, Kuhl EA, Kovacs AH, Serber ER, Handberg E, et al. The ICD shock and stress management program: a randomized trial of psychosocial treatment to optimize quality of life in ICD patients. Pacing Clin Electrophysiol. 2007;30:858–64.
122. Lane DA, Aguinaga L, Blomström-Lundqvist C, Boriani G, Dan GA, Hills MT, et al. Cardiac tachyarrhythmias and patient values and preferences for their management: the European Heart Rhythm Association (EHRA) consensus document endorsed by the Heart Rhythm Society (HRS), Asia Pacific Heart Rhythm Society (APHRS), and Sociedad Latinoamericana de Estimulación Cardíaca y Electrofisiología (SOLEACE). Europace. 2015;17(12):1747–69. doi:10.1093/europace/euv233.
123. Stromberg A, Fluur C, Miller J, Chung ML, Moser DK, Thylen I. ICD recipients' understanding of ethical issues, ICD function, and practical consequences of withdrawing the ICD in the end-of-life. Pacing Clin Electrophysiol. 2014;37(7):834–42.
124. Groarke J, Beirne A, Buckley U, O'Dwyer E, Sugrue D, Keelan T, et al. Deficiencies in patients' comprehension of implantable cardioverter defibrillator therapy. Pacing Clin Electrophysiol. 2012;35:1097–102.
125. Yuhas J, Mattocks K, Gravelin L, Remetz M, Foley J, Fazio R, et al. Patients' attitudes and perceptions of implantable cardioverter-defibrillators: potential barriers to appropriate primary prophylaxis. Pacing Clin Electrophysiol. 2012;35:1179–87.

126. Dickerson SS, Posluszny M, Kennedy MC. Help seeking in a support group for recipients of implantable cardioverter defibrillators and their support persons. Heart Lung. 2000;29(2): 87–96.
127. Sears SFJ, Burns JL, Handberg E, Sotile WM, Conti JB. Young at heart: understanding the unique psychosocial adjustment of young implantable cardioverter defibrillator recipients. Pacing Clin Electrophysiol. 2001;24(7):1113–7.
128. Chevalier P, Cottraux J, Mollard E, Sai N, Brun S, Burri H, et al. Prevention of implantable defibrillator shocks by cognitive behavioral therapy: a pilot trial. Am Heart J. 2006;151(1):191. e1–6.
129. Irvine J, Firestone J, Ong L, Cribbie R, Dorian P, Harris L, et al. A randomized controlled trial of cognitive behavior therapy tailored to psychological adaptation to an implantable cardioverter defibrillator. Psychosom Med. 2011;73(3):226–33.
130. Kohn CS, Petrucci RJ, Baessler C, Soto DM, Movsowitz C. The effect of psychological intervention on patients' long-term adjustment to the ICD: a prospective study. Pacing Clin Electrophysiol. 2000;23:450–6.
131. Maia AC, Braga AA, Soares-Filho G, Pereira V, Nardi AE, Silva AC. Efficacy of cognitive behavioral therapy in reducing psychiatric symptoms in patients with implantable cardioverter defibrillator: an integrative review. Braz J Med Biol Res. 2014;47(4):265–72.
132. Qintar M, George JJ, Panko M, Bea S, Broer KA, St John J, et al. A prospective study of anxiety in ICD patients with a pilot randomized controlled trial of cognitive behavioral therapy for patients with moderate to severe anxiety. J Interv Card Electrophysiol. 2015;43(1): 65–75.
133. Cramer H, Lauche R, Haller H, Dobos G, Michalsen A. A systematic review of yoga for heart disease. Eur J Prev Cardiol. 2015;22(3):284–95.
134. Freedenberg VA, Thomas SA, Friedmann E. A pilot study of a mindfulness based stress reduction program in adolescents with implantable cardioverter defibrillators or pacemakers. Pediatr Cardiol. 2015;36(4):786–95.
135. Toise SC, Sears SF, Schoenfeld MH, Blitzer ML, Marieb MA, Drury JH, et al. Psychosocial and cardiac outcomes of yoga for ICD patients: a randomized clinical control trial. Pacing Clin Electrophysiol. 2014;37(1):48–62.

Chapter 4
Comparison of Health-Related Quality of Life Between Patients with Implantable Cardioverter Defibrillators and Pacemaker Recipients

Alena Kajanová, Martin Eisenberger, and Zuzana Řimnáčová

Abstract Both Implantable Cardioverter Defibrillators (ICD) and pacemakers are life-saving cardiac devices, however they may have a negative impact on Quality of Life (QoL). The implantation of an ICD may increase the risk of depression, anxiety or post-traumatic stress disorder. A few studies examining the devices used to regulate the heart rate report that sudden, but also lifelong mental disorders occur much more frequently in patients with ICDs than those with PM. Compared to healthy population, they experience more anxious states. As for depression, a slight prevalence can be seen in ICD patients as compared to PM patients and healthy population. After the implantation of the pacemaker, the patients' quality of life changes. Before implementation, patients fear a sudden heart failure or loss of conscience the most. After implantation, the stress related to fear of reduced self-sufficiency gradually disappears. If the patient is prepared for the operation in time and educated, as well as rehabilitated after the operation, anxiety and depression disappear as well. With increasing time elapsing from the operation, the problems decrease.

Keywords Pacemaker • Implantable cardioverter-defibrillator • Mental problems • Quality of life • Anxiety • Depression • Education • Self-help groups • Heart • Cardiac disease • Stress • Importance of nurse • HRQoL • Limitations • Loss of consciousness

---

A. Kajanová, Ph.D. (✉) • M. Eisenberger, M.D., Ph.D. • Z. Řimnáčová
Faculty of Health and Social Studies, University of South Bohemia in České Budějovice, České Budějovice, Czech Republic
e-mail: kajanova@zsf.jcu.cz

© Springer International Publishing AG 2017

R. Proietti et al. (eds.), *Psychological, Emotional, Social and Cognitive Aspects of Implantable Cardiac Devices*, DOI 10.1007/978-3-319-55721-2_4

Introduction

Implantable cardiovascular devices are battery-powered machines that are placed under the skin in order to treat or diagnose abnormal heart rhythms. Permanent implantable pacemakers are used to treat slow heart rhythms (bradycardias), whereas implantable cardioverter-defibrillators can treat some fast life-threatening arrhythmias, such as ventricular tachycardia or ventricular fibrillation [1]. Biventricular pacemakers are used to treat heart failure by resynchronizing the functions of both left and right ventricles [13]. These devices have been shown to improve cardiac symptoms and to prolong life in some patients. However, these devices can also impact negatively on patients' lives. The main reasons are the need for long-term follow-ups, concerns regarding malfunction, lifestyle restrictions and electrical shocks in patients with ICDs [2].

Permanent Pacemaker

A permanent pacemaker (PPM) is an implantable device that has been developed to treat cardiac disorders that cause the heart to beat slower. The main indications are sick sinus syndrome, which is caused by a malfunction of the sinus node (the heart's primary pacemaker) and atrio-ventricular block, in which the conduction between the atria and ventricles of the heart is impaired [3]. Guidelines that outline indications for cardiac pacing are available from both the American Heart Association [4] and the European Society of Cardiology [5]. At present, two types of pacing are in use: (a) single chamber pacemaker (VVI) with one pacing lead implanted in the right atrium and ventricle and (b) dual-chamber pacemaker (DDD) with two pacing leads implanted (one in the right ventricle and one in the right atrium). Remarkable advances have been made in pacemaker technology including reduced size, increased battery longevity and the addition of magnetic resonance imaging safe pacemakers [6].

Permanent pacemakers are implanted under the skin, most often in the right or left shoulder under the clavicle. This involves transvenous placement of one or more pacing electrodes within the chambers of the heart. The procedure is facilitated by fluoroscopy, which enables the physician to view the passage of the electrode lead. There are two types of fixation mechanisms at the tip of the pacing lead: (a) active fixation with a screw and (b) passive fixation with tines [7]. Some complications include bleeding, infection, dislodgement of the lead or pneumothorax [8]. The pacemaker battery usually lasts about 6–12 years, depending on type, programming and frequency of use. Pacemakers monitor the heart's native electrical rhythm and, when the pacemaker does not detect a heartbeat, it will send a short low voltage pulse. Patients with PPM should have follow-ups in the pacemaker clinic every 6–12 months but some pacemakers can be reviewed via transtelephonic monitoring [9]. Although these technologies provide some comfort to patients, they offer only limited data and don't permit changes to be made to the pacemaker from a remote centre. Most patients with permanent pacemakers do not have any structural heart disease and, after the bradycardia has been treated, they lead a relatively normal life [10].

Biventricular Pacemaker

Biventricular pacemaker, or cardiac resynchronization therapy (CRT), is used for patients with heart failure due to left ventricular (LV) dysfunction [11]. Heart failure often has a poor prognosis, with about half of patients dying within 5 years from diagnosis [12]. An extra lead is inserted through the coronary sinus to pace the epicardial wall of the left ventricle. Biventricular pacing alters the negative natural course of ventricular failure through favorable ventricular remodeling with a reduction in ventricular volumes and improvement in ventricular function [13, 14]. CRT can involve either pacing (CRT-P) or defibrillation (CRT-D). Multiple indications exist for implanting a biventricular pacemaker and the indications are continuously being revaluated in order to include a broader range of patients [15]. CRT is recommended for patients with left ventricular dysfunction, e.g. after a heart attack, or for patients with dilated cardiomyopathy, with a QRS complex duration longer than 120 ms and signs of heart failure (shortness of breath, legs swelling etc.) [16]. Approximately one third of patients with heart failure fulfill the criteria. Biventricular pacing has been shown to improve cardiac symptoms and QoL, to reduce the number of hospitalizations and to reduce the risk of mortality [17]. Compared with traditional pacemakers, which have leads in the right atrium and right ventricle only, a biventricular pacemaker involves an additional lead and thus an increased potential for complications, which mostlyconsist in lead dislodgement and inability to implant the left ventricular lead [18]. Patients must be routinely assessed so that the function of the pacemaker can be optimized. However, one third of patients do not respond to the therapy [19].

Implantable Cardioverter-Defibrillator

An implantable cardioverter-defibrillator is a device that is capable of treating some fast life-threatening cardiac arrhythmias by giving high-energy electrical shocks [20]. The ICD is a first-line prophylactic therapy for patients at risk of sudden cardiac death due to ventricular fibrillation and ventricular tachycardia. These life-threatening arrhythmias mostly occur in patients after a heart attack or with inherited genetic diseases [21]. In addition to delivering electrical shocks, current devices can be programmed to deliver therapy via fast ventricular pacing [22]. The device constantly monitors the rate and rhythm of the heart and delivers the therapy when the heart rate exceeds a preset number. Unfortunately, the device can deliver painful shocks also when there are no abnormal heart beats (inappropriate shocks) and this may have a negative impact on patients' overall condition [23]. On the other hand, the failure to deliver a shock may be due to failure to sense, lead fracture or inadvertent ICD deactivation. Although there are some controversies over ICD deactivation, it can be done in case of inappropriate shocks, during resuscitation and in the end-of-life care in some cases [24]. The implantation process of an ICD is similar to that of a pacemaker, although both the ICD lead and the generator are slightly larger, technological advances have reduced the size of the pulse generator tremendously. A new generation of devices are able to dispense with the transvenous lead system and still obtain satisfactory defibrillation [25]. Device battery longevity has also increased; early devices lasted 2 years or less, while current devices are expected to last 6 years or longer [26]. It has been shown that ICDs improve mortality and morbidity [27], but both the appropriate and inappropriate shocks are painful and may have a negative impact on patients' QoL [28].

It has been shown that the ICDs are underused in some countries including the United States [29]. As with a pacemaker, living with an ICD does impose some restrictions on patient's lifestyle. However, some limitations are specific for patients with an ICD: they are not allowed to use some electro-magnetic equipment, such as magnetic mattress pads or magnetic resonance imaging, and it is advisable that mobile phones be carried in a pocket far from the ICD [30].

Quality of Life, Anxiety and Depression in Patients with ICD

It is indispensable to deal with the mental state of ICD patients with regard to QoL and psychological well-being [49]. Any impairment of the mental state, for example due to anxiety and depression, may lead to impairment of the physical state, and vice versa. It has also been proved that mental complications increase the risk of premature mortality of ICD patients [31].

Quality of Life

As for the mental state of ICD patients, a number of negative displays have been described [32], most frequently depressive and anxious states [33] or post-traumatic stress disorder [31] and stress as such [34]. The outputs of the studies dealing with this topic record ambiguous results; the range of incidence of mental problems varies—for example for depressive disorders, individual authors report 24–33%, and for anxious disorders, 24–27.5% [35]. According to Dunbar et al. [34] up to 21% patients suffer from post-traumatic stress disorder. On the other hand, we rarely find psychosexual problems, panic disorders and other problems, although some of them may occur in form of isolated symptoms like pessimism, sleeping disorder or sadness [36]. Patients are also afraid of becoming a burden to their families [49].

The relatively great heterogeneity of the study results may be explained by the use of different methodologies (they usually include measurement with the help of BDI—Beck Depression Inventory, BAI—Beck Anxiety Inventory, TMAS, DIPS, HADS, Zung Self-Rating Depression Scale—Zung SDS), questionnaires are used in most cases, as well as by the size and structure of the research sets. However the degree of problems is serious in any case. Additionally, anxiety and depression are frequently present in the same patient [37].

Comparing the ICD patients to patients with other cardio-vascular diseases, the difference in the incidence of mental disorders is not too distinctive [38].

Factors that induce mental disorders are well known. They include fear from a painful electric discharge [39], so called shock anxiety [40], and fear that the device will fail to give the discharge in time when needed, as well as fear from the size of the device [41]. These disorders become worse as the number of discharges increases [42], five and more discharges per year being crucial, and in case of resuscitation experience [39]. A big problem consists in the fact that a vicious circle emerges when the patient gets more and more discharges associated with increasing fear. Different co-morbidities have a negative effect on the mental state as well [34]. The demographic variables include lower age [39], female gender [32] and unemployment [43]. It must be taken into consideration that some socio-demographic variables constitute risk factors of mental problems even in healthy population—for example unemployed people and women are generally more frequently anxious [44]. In case of employed patients, their field of employment/profession must be taken into consideration. An inadequate job may cause stress, anxiety and depression, while an adequately chosen job may increase self-confidence, self-realization and improve mental well-being. It is very probable that an adequate intervention in the form of reintegration in the working process may reduce depression and anxiety.

Within the mental variables, we attribute high level of risk particularly to the anxious personality type, so called type D, both in the actual patient and in the patient's partner [45]. The concept of D personality comes from J. Denollet, a Belgian psychologist. D means distressed and D type persons are characterized by a tendency to experience negative emotions and simultaneously to suppress the expression of such emotions and of the related behavior in social interactions. It is thus a combination of two personality characteristics, the tendency to experience negative emotions and the tendency to be socially inhibited. The D personality type tends to inhibit the displays of his/her own personality. Such people constantly worry about something, feel unhappy, judge circumstances negatively and experience chronic mental tension [46]. Some authors even speculate that persons with D personality type have less access to social support, due to their inhibitions in social contacts, which probably increases their tendency to develop cardio-vascular diseases [47]. In 2005, Johan Denollet presented the last (for now) version of the questionnaire aimed at ascertaining the characteristics of D type personality [48]. The scale (DSl14) has 14 items, seven to ascertain negative effectiveness and seven to ascertain social inhibition.

Patients who use negative coping strategies are at higher risk [49]. The available studies [50] state that ICD patients are more frequently inclined to use problem focused coping strategies when managing stress related to physical (body) stressors. Emotionally based strategies are used by ICD patients in case of mental and social stress. Lidová et al. [51] their study confirmed the general predominance of positive coping strategies in ICD patients. However, the choice of the coping strategy did not influence the incidence of the patient's mental problems (anxieties or depressions).

On the contrary, a protective factor can be seen in the time elapsed from implantation (the longer the time, the lower the problems), particularly if the time has exceeded 1 year [52], in implantation without general anaesthesia [53] and satisfaction with the therapy [54]. We also know that patients who have accepted the ICD have less of a possibility to suffer from mental problems [55]. A significant protective factor consists in social support from family and friends [37]. Women, despite suffering more frequently from mental problems, show faster adaptation to the device after the operation [43].

Lidová et al. [43] found a strong correlation between scores of depression and anxiety recorded the day after ICD implantation and those of a re-test performed after 9 months. Although they constitute two different clinical units and different questionnaires were used for their assessment, both factors can be found in ICD patients concurrently. The key question for this study and for further studies dealing with the patients' mental state after implantation remains whether depression and anxiety are a state or a personality feature. In view of the fact that the respondents were not tested by a personality questionnaire and that it was not investigated whether they were treated with depression/anxiety in the past, it cannot be excluded that a part of them may have suffered from such mental problems already before the ICD implantation, which could distort the results of many studies in this area.

Quality of Life of ICD Patients

The quality of life constitutes one of the indicators of subjective experience and assessment of a life situation. For this reason, it is commonly used in interventions in health and social spheres. In these spheres, the quality of life also constitutes an important indicator of assessment of the care provided. A group of experts from the World Health Organization (WHO [56]) defined the quality of life as individual perception of an individual's life situation in the context of the cultural and value system in which the individual lives and in relation to the individual's goals, expectations, standards and interests [57].

The assessment of the quality of life and the effort to objectify it with the help of questionnaires has multiple reasons. One of them consists in the increasing pressure to provide the best possible health care to all patients, in spite of limited funds. The data acquired with the help of questionnaires may provide useful information on the quality of the care provided and help choose the most efficient therapy [58]. The assessment of the quality of life should be a routine part of clinical studies, but also of common clinical practice. The questionnaires assessing it should constitute a standard part of all studies that evaluate the cost-effectiveness of new therapeutic procedures. The advantage of standardized questionnaires consists in the opportunity to compare the patients' quality of life in the course of therapy, e.g. at its beginning, after a specific time, after healing, etc. The quality of life is also the basic criteria of analysis of the usefulness of therapy costs [59].

As for the quality of life (hereinafter referred to only as "QoL"), we also find discrepancies among individual studies. While some studies report changed QoL only in a low number of patients [60], others speak of its deterioration. In such cases, we can speak of temporarily reduced QoL shortly before and some 2 months after implantation. In the course of time, the quality of life improves again, and after about a year, it is even comparable to standard population [61]. In psychological studies assessing the of QoL researchers use an identical questionnaire, SF-36 (Short-Form Health-Survey Questionnaire) in order to avoid distorted results due to different methodologies. It is a tool that is frequently used in different comparative studies since it allows to compare the QoL of different patient groups [62]. According to the above mentioned author, QoL of ICD patients and QoL of patients with the same diagnoses, treated pharmacologically, do not differ with statistical significance.

The reduced QoL of such patients is primarily related to the mental problems described above. In this respect, worsened QoL can be seen in the dimensions of mental health rather than those of physical health. Godemann et al. [63] state that depression and anxiety rank among the most important variables that contribute to reducing the quality of life.

Further, the reduced QoL is related to reduced physical activities (particularly sports), employment and driving [64]. Freedenberg et al. [65] state that more than a fourth of economically active patients lose or change their job after implantation. Unlike the mental factors, the physical ICD factors, for example in form of the number of discharges, do not play any considerable role [63].

Potential Improvement of QoL of ICD Patients and Elimination of Their Mental Problems

The prevention of mental problems and reduced QoL can be achieved in several ways. Firstly, through comprehensive and personality-focused educational programs and professional counselling. A central role is played by the nurse who can eliminate the patient's fears and uncertainties through daily contact with him [66]. Qualitative studies show that patients who have actively searched for information on their disease and on ICDs suffered from lower degree of uncertainty and had less mental problems as well [67]. Patients are interested and at the same time made uneasy by questions like: how will the shock feel like, how painful it will be, what specific restrictions will the ICD bring, will there be any cognitive changes? [55].

Of course, education should start before the implantation. Additionally to the health care staff, different handbooks and booklets, issued by the defibrillator manufacturers for patients, can be useful provided they describe in an understandable way not only the surgical intervention, but also the post-operation care and restrictions, the technical parameters of the device and other information that could be useful to the patients. A self-contained part is devoted to mental problems and possible ways for coping with them.

A program suggested to ICD patients called Mindfulness Based Stress Reduction (MBSR)—is a structured psycho-educational program that includes meditation, yoga, and group support [65].

In general, the educational program should be carried out in three phases—before the intervention, after the intervention before discharge from the hospital, and on a day case basis within regular checks of the device, meetings and workshops. In each phase we selected the information so that the scope, content and communication is personalized and respects the process of coping with, and adapting to the disease and the implantation of the ICD device ("coping"). During the course of the personal educational interview with the patient, we hand over written materials including phone and e-mail contacts [68].

The physician should select endangered patient groups for example according to personality types and provide them with specific psychological therapeutic care. Such groups may be face-to-face groups or Internet groups. An adequate psychological approach consists primarily in cognitive-behavioral therapeutic procedures aimed to work on automatic ideas [32]. Techniques of positive psychology, aimed at assuming control of oneself, are suitable as well [69].

Patients who have mental problems already should get adequate pharmacotherapy as well [32]. Self-help groups in which patients can share their experience concerning fears and anxieties, as well as discuss health problems have provided useful support [70]. The authors point out that self-help groups are especially important in case of young patients who do not have any peers of the same age with whom to share their problems.

Quality of Life, Anxiety and Depression in Patients with PM

Quality of Life of Pacemaker Patients

A great number of Czech and foreign studies deal with the topic of how the QoL of pacemaker patients changes. Pacemaker-using therapy was discovered somewhere around 1950. The first implantation was carried out in 1958 [71]; since then, great progress has been made in pacemaker research, implantation and life with a pacemaker. In the past, the pacemaker constituted mere human life rescue [90]; in older references, we can read that it extended the mean lifespan or reduced morbidity and a mortality [72]; however, at present, the pacemaker implantation allows people to return to their original life, to their jobs, work, sports, hobbies [91]; further, many studies research the operation taking more and more into account the quality of life [72].

Before actual implantation of the pacemaker, the patient should be educated as extensively as possible, either by a nurse or by the physician. The patient receives all information in oral form and in the form of booklets. The Biotronik Company points out that each patient should have (and has) the opportunity to contact his or her physician at any time. This is also revealed by the research of Kučerová [73] who found that most patients primarily contact their families or friends, but more than 30% of the interviewed persons report to contact their physicians in case of need and in case of questions and to have great confidence in them.

Presently the technology of the pacemakers at such a high level that it is able to adapt the heart rhythm exactly to the activities performed by the individual at a given moment. Biotronik points out in its educational material that their device is even able to respond to unexpected situations, to fright, excitement, etc., accelerating the heart rate and increasing the blood pressure [90].

What has Changed from the QoL Perspective

In spite of reduced mortality, and other indisputable benefits of pacemaker implantation, many studies do not completely agree that the patients' quality of life is significantly increased; therefore the question as to whether quality of life increases after the operation cannot be answered in a convincing way [64]. Nevertheless, a lot of new studies keep coming out and many researchers keep dealing with this topic.

The study carried out in the Czech Republic on 150 patients did not find any significant difference between the quality of life before and after the operation. This may be due to the fact that the research was repeated only 6–10 weeks after implantation. The first quality-of-life questionnaires were collected 7–10 days before the pacemaker implantation. The evaluation of the questionnaires and the comparison of the questionnaires before and after operation did not show any statistically significant difference in the quality of life. However, the study showed that the operation had an impact on two individual quality-of-life items—on the level, structure and quality of social support and on localization of the patients' control [72].

The study made by Malm et al. [74] gave results on health-related quality of life issues. The respondents reported, with respect to HRQoL, that the symptoms that had required the pacemaker implantation (longer walking, housework, ...) were considerably reduced. The respondents reported that the symptoms either decreased or completely disappeared. Thanks to that, they were able to manage everyday life situations again, for example not getting out of breath when climbing stairs.

The study made by Kučerová [73] that primarily examined pacemaker patients over 60 years of age showed that although they have some limitations (they still cannot go for longer walks, etc.), they are very satisfied with their life.

Chen et al. [88] examined the quality of life of patients before the implantation and the quality of life 2, 4 and 6 months after implantation. The patients before the implantation had approximately 62.5 points on a QoL scale ranging up to 97 points. In the course of the subsequent months, the quality of life improved, reaching a peak by the end of the fourth month. The quality of life improved primarily in the areas of sleep, appetite, physical activities, working capability. The research shows that the time elapsed from the operation may be a protective factor. Malm et al. [71] researched the HRQoL conditioned by the pacemaker implantation of 697 patients aged between 65 and 84 years. All patients experienced an increase of health-related quality of life within several years after the operation, which confirms the assumption that the longer the time elapsed from the operation, the higher the patient's quality of life.

The study examining child patients was focused on prevention of loss of consciousness before the operation and short-term pulmonary arrest. The questionnaires of the study were also completed by the children's parents. It turned out that the operation and the adequately configured pacemaker constitute a good prevention of loss of consciousness and of pulmonary arrest. The patients' and their parents' strain in everyday life was reduced and the subjective quality of life was increased [75].

Biotronik writes in its information booklet for patients that after the intervention, patients can return to their daily routine immediately. Nevertheless, they point out the need to observe regular check-ups, to take the necessary medicines, to carry the pacemaker card when on travels and to contact the physician each time the patient notices any irregularities with respect to the pacemaker. If the patient has any questions, the attending physician must be contacted [91]. The same results were also found by the study carried out by Súkeníková [76]. The respondents from her study manage a higher amount of common activities after PM implantation and they perceive an improvement primarily in physical fitness.

Patients can evaluate the quality of life also from their subjective perspective which is often a very valid indicator. Malm et al. [77] used a lot of methods to investigate HRQoL; one of the methods consisted in letting the patients assess their health by themselves. They also assessed the quality of life from the perspective of demographic data, etc. The results are more than interesting. They found that patients living with a pacemaker for 3–7 years have better health-related quality of life, which confirms the original assumption of the time elapsed from operation as a protective factor. Another finding stated that men living in a household with a woman or having their own household have better HRQoL. Women, on the contrary, evaluated their HRQoL as poorer compared to men. The same applied to older patients as compared to younger ones.

These finding have also been reported by Avlund et al. [78]. According to them, it is very important that individuals maintain functional abilities and social participation, for they can compensate each other in relation to quality of life. They explain this by stating that women have less opportunities to manage daily activities and that their dependency on the assistance of other people is six times higher than in men. They also point out the need of rehabilitation and of more social activities these types of patients (women, lonely persons, aged persons in pension, etc.) [77].

Malm (2005) writes in his study that support groups for women, lonely and very old persons with reduced health-related quality of life are more than desirable.

These kinds of patients should have access to information on how to face difficult situations so they can quickly return to normal life. He adds that patients achieve social and emotional well-being provided they experience understanding, empathic therapy and insight in their specific situation.

Subjective feelings and subjective quality of life were examined by Súkeníková [76]. She found that the most serious feelings reported by the patients are related to finding that their heart does not work as it should, as well as to the fear that their heart could fail. Thanks to the implantation of pacemakers, the stress caused by such fears is reduced in most patients.

A short-term study took place in Žilina (Slovak Republic) just after pacemaker implantation. The patients reported lowest quality of life from a psychological aspect, while high quality of life was reported in the area of family relations. Even better quality of life was found in married patients. Another finding stated that older patients perceive their quality of life far worse than younger patients. Older patients reported that the disease had a negative effect on them or that the development of the disease and subsequent operation and convalescence was complicated by other diseases [79].

In a few cases, the quality of life worsened. The quality of life was described as bad more frequently by patients who had experienced a discharge of their device [64]. The study made by Lauberg [80] reports that the patients' quality of life had changed (worsened) the most from a psychological aspect. The study was focused on PM patients who were checked 3 months after implantation and then 2 years after the operation. The patients checked 3 months after implantation had experienced fear due to the long interval between the two checks, which had a negative impact on their mental state. Over that long period, anxiety or depression may be experienced. These initial problems, fears and anxieties may lead to more serious problems. The study points out and emphasizes that patients should have the opportunity to discuss problems and psychological topics.

The restrictions that the patients must abide by may also contribute to worsening quality of life. There are places where a pictogram indicates that persons with pacemakers are not allowed to enter. Furthermore, some devices can interfere with the pacemaker and cannot be used by PM patients or can be used only upon consulting the physician or the PM manufacturer (induction cooktops, firearms, drills, etc.) [90].

As for sports activities, a PM individual should avoid contact sports where a blow to the pacemaker could occur.

A study that examined the devices that help restore normal heart rhythm reports that sudden, but also lifelong mental disorders occur much more frequently in patients with ICD (implantable cardioverter-defibrillators) than in those with PM (pacemaker) (27 vs. 11%). As compared to healthy population, they experience more anxious states. As for depression, a slight prevalence can be seen in ICD patients as compared to PM patients and healthy population (10 vs. 4%).

Nevertheless, a multi-variance analysis carried out, taking into account the disease, demographic differences, exposure to beta blockers, restrictions of physical activity and hospitalization concluded that the device type (ICD or PM) did not constitute the cause of mental diseases [81].

Pacemaker-Related Mental Problems

The fact that the human heart does not work as it should is a very stressing factor in itself. When people learn that they suffer from a disease that may cause a sudden heart failure or stoppage accompanied by loss of consciousness, they can't think about anything else [76].

Balvínová [82] found that if a nurse concentrates on appropriately educating the patient after a heart disease is detected, the patient is able to absorb the information better and faster. The patient is able to cope better with the situation if the nurse is obliging, patient and explains and answers all of the patient's questions. Stress is also reduced if the patient is informed on what will happen before, during and after the forthcoming intervention. That includes everything concerning the pacemaker, i.e. how it works, what restrictions there are, as well as the prospect of returning to common activities after the wound has healed and after the patient has passed a short convalescence. Balvínová [82]

The implantation of a permanent pacemaker implies strong mental pressure for the patient; the patient must adapt to another rhythm of life and, in a specific period, has restricted activities. This may cause some psychiatric disorders. Aydemir et al. (2006) researched 84 patients with a permanent pacemaker, examining their psychiatric morbidity and depression-related symptoms. The Hamilton Depression Rating Scale (mHDRS) was used to determine the depressive symptoms. Sixteen (19.1%) patients had a psychiatric diagnose; there were adaptation disorders, depressive episodes, as well as clinical depression. The depression was significantly more serious in women than in men. The most frequent symptoms included problems at work, in routine home activities (53.6%), mental anxiety (48.8%), loss of energy (42.9%) and sleeplessness (39.3%).

Patients who had not been educated in advance showed more significant loss of energy than patients who had been educated. The study was compared to common population and it was found that depressed mood, psychic anxiety, and somatic concerns and symptoms were more frequent in patients with permanent pacemakers than in the general population. The symptoms, resembling an anxious-depressive disorder, were related primarily to fears related to the permanent pacemaker, however this was due to the fact that the population included patients who had not been informed in advance and did not have sufficient knowledge of the device.

The improved mental condition after implantation of the pacemaker was studied by Kolterer et al. [75]. Their study was devoted primarily to loss of conscience, the thing most feared by patients. After the implantation of the pacemaker, its good adjustment and avoidance of possible risk situations, such danger completely disappeared and the patients could return to their normal life.

Cenková [83] examined in 99 patients whether their psycho-social well-being returned, improved or worsened after implantation of the pacemaker. She found that in more than 70% of the cases, the mental condition of the patients improved and some of the patients even got rid of the stress caused by sleeplessness and related sleep problems.

A study that examined the devices that help restore normal heart rhythm reports that sudden, but also lifelong mental disorders occur much more frequently in patients with ICD (implantable cardioverter-defibrillators) than in those with PM (pacemaker) (27 vs. 11%). As compared to healthy population, they experience more anxious states. As for depression, a slight prevalence can be seen in ICD patients as compared to PM patients and healthy population (10 vs. 4%).

Nevertheless, a multi-variance analysis carried out, taking into account the disease, demographic differences, exposure to beta blockers, restrictions of physical activity and hospitalization concluded that the device type (ICD or PM) did not constitute the cause of mental diseases [81].

A more recent study investigated similarly 69 ICD patients and 71 PM patients. In total, there were 140 participants. Truton and Emily [84] examined the group for incidence of depression and anxiety and compared the two groups and their potential differences. According to her results, the two groups did not differ much from each other; nevertheless, some differences were described. People with ICD had substantially more PTSD symptoms, they were generally more afraid of the threats of their existing disease and of other diseases and their consequences and were more emotionally engaged. In conclusion, it was suggested again that anxious patients should not hesitate to ask for psychological care and support.

In Mexico, a study was carried out on patients who attended cognitive-behavioral therapy after pacemaker implantation due to cardiac arrhythmia. Therapy was performed once a week over a 6-week period due to patients' persisting anxiety and depression, 11 patients were observed and the results showed a very significant improvement. Of the 45.5% of the patients that had suffered from depression, only 9.1% of them kept suffering from it after therapy. A similar situation could be found in anxious conditions experienced by 81.8% of the patients. After therapy, the figure dropped to 45%. Thanks to the improved mental state of the patients, their physical health improved as well [85].

It is much better for patients to have the opportunity to speak of their mental state and to consult with an expert rather than to deny it and avoid dealing with it. The same opinion is expressed by Bose et al. [86] who tried to study how avoiding and denying a health condition affects depressive and anxious patients who suffered from chronic heart failure. Their study demonstrates unambiguously that avoidance as a style of coping with the disease has a negative impact on the depressive and anxious states of the patients. The examined patients denied their troubles and problems in order to be able to continue engaging in activities they were used to, or they started drinking alcohol or taking drugs to forestall thinking of the ever-present problem.

A year before, Bose [87] published a study in which she started dealing with chronic heart failure and its deep impacts on the patient's life. She pointed out that individuals dealing with the disease have a poor quality of life, suffering from depressions and anxieties, which often leads to re-hospitalizations. Despite these things, which are known, psycho-social factors only rarely lead to therapy and increased care of the patient. Therefore her study focused on coping with such states, as well as intervention by a nurse to educate the patient. A special training—Coping Effectiveness Training (CET) was created for the purpose of teaching patients how to manage stress. During the study, she also found that younger male patients often resorted to alcohol to help them manage the stress afflicting them. As for CET, the results were excellent. The intervention increased the patients' feeling of control of the disease, which is important for mental well-being. Patients who had suffered from slight or no symptoms of depression and anxiety experienced a reduction of the negative perception of their restrictions. A similar research was attempted in China. The research set consisted of 114 patients (68 males and 46 females) who had undergone a pacemaker transplantation. The patients were divided into two groups—a control group and a group where an intervention was carried out. The nurses cared for both groups using different approaches. For the control group, there was only routine work of general nurses. For the intervention group, there was another procedure, that took place from January 2014 to January 2015. The results of the two groups were subsequently compared and evaluated by using a self-assessment method for depression and anxiety and an additional questionnaire. The results showed that the intervention carried out in the second group was very effective. That group was able to cope much better with the situation, compared with the control group. In conclusion the intervention made a significant difference.

There is one more area that should be dealt with and that is not readily discussed in general by patients. It consists in fear of reduced sexual function. The fear of a sexual disorder and of a cardio-vascular attack caused by sexual activity may lead to depression and loss of self-esteem. The physicians should strongly support rehabilitation programs. Such programs contribute to increase the patient's physical capability and self-esteem.

Conclusions

Both the ICD and the pacemaker can significantly prolong the life of implanted patients. On the other hand, they may also cause mental problems and reduce QoL in some patient groups. Clinical physicians should thus inform their patients of these potential consequences when considering the ICD implantation. However, such complications are not unsolvable. Many studies point out that psychological and educational interventions may improve QoL of both ICD and PM patients [88]. The knowledge of the particularities of the target patient group, for example with regard to personality and mental health, could result in more efficient interventions [89].

A markedly specific target group are younger patients, particularly adolescents. Although they are few in both the ICD and PM populations, they are considerably at risk of mental problems and reduced quality of life [65].

References

1. Zareba W. Implantable cardioverter defibrillator therapy in postinfarction patents. Curr Opin Cardiol. 2004;19(6):619–24.
2. Duru F, et al. How different from pacemaker patients are recipients of implantable cardioverter-defibrillators with respect to psychosocial adaptation, affective disorders, and quality of life? Heart. 2001;85:375–9.
3. Alt E, Volker R, Wirtzfeld A, Ulm K. Survival and follow-up after pacemaker implantation: a comparison of patients with sick sinus syndrome, complete heart block, and atrial fibrillation. Pacing Clin Electrophysiol. 1985;8(6):849–55.
4. Epstein AE. ACC/AHA/HRS 2008 guidelines. J Am Coll Cardiol. 2008;51:21.
5. Vardas PE. Guidelines for cardiac pacing. Eur Heart J. 2007;28(18):2256–95.
6. Santini L. Evaluating MRI—compatible pacemakers. Pacing Clin Electrophysiol. 2013;36(3): 270–8.
7. Furman S, Pannizzo F, Campo I. Comparison of active and passive adhering leads for endocardial pacing. Pacing Clin Electrophysiol. 1979;2(4):417–27.
8. Ellenbogen KA, et al. Complications arising after implantation of DDD pacemakers: the MOST experience. Am J Cardiol. 2003;92(6):740–1.
9. Burri H. Remote monitoring and follow-up of. Europace. 2009;11(6):701–9.
10. Wood MA, Ellenbogen KA. Cardiac pacemakers from the patient's perspective. Circulation. 2002;105:2136–8.
11. Singh JP, Gras D. Biventricular pacing: current trends and future strategies. Eur Heart J. 2012;33(3):305–13.
12. Roger VL, et al. Trends in heart failure incidence and survival in a community-based population. JAMA. 2004;292(3):344–50.
13. Abraham WT, et al. Cardiac resynchronization in chronic heart failure. N Engl J Med. 2002;346:1845–53.
14. Abraham WT, et al. Cardiac resynchronization therapy for heart failure: biventricular pacing and beyond. Curr Opin Cardiol. 2002;17(4):346–52.
15. Tracy CM, et al. 2012 ACCF/AHA/HRS focused update of the 2008 guidelines for device-based therapy of cardiac rhythm abnormalities. J Am Coll Cardiol. 2012;60(14):1297–313.
16. Brignole M, et al. 2013 ESC Guidelines on cardiac pacing and cardiac resynchronization therapy. Eur Heart J. 2013;34(29):2281–329.
17. Moss AJ. Cardiac resynchronization therapy. N Engl J Med. 2009;363(25):2385–95.
18. van Rees JB, de Bie MK, Thijssen J, Borleffs CJ, Schalij MJ, van Erven L. Implantation-related complications of implantable cardioverter-defibrillators and cardiac resynchronization therapy devices: a systematic review of randomized clinical trials. J Am Coll Cardiol. 2011;58(10):995–1000.
19. Auricchio A, Prinzen FW. Non-responders to cardiac resynchronization therapy: the magnitude of the problem and the issues. Circ J. 2011;75(3):521–7.
20. DiMarco JP. Implantable cardioverter defibrillators. N Engl J Med. 2003;349:1836–47.
21. Trappe HJ, Brugada P, Talajic M, Della Bella P, Lezaun R, Mulleneers R, Wellens HJ. Prognosis of patients with ventricular tachycardia and ventricular fibrillation: role of the underlying etiology. J Am Coll Cardiol. 1988;12(1):166–74.
22. Weber M, Block M, Bansch D, Castrucci M, Gradaus R, Schriever C, Breithardt G, Bocker D. Antitachycardia pacing for rapid VT during ICD charging: a method to prevent ICD shocks. Pacing Clin Electrophysiol. 2001;24(3):345–51.
23. Deyell MW, et al. Prognostic impact of inappropriate defibrillator shocks in a population cohort. Heart. 2013;99(17):1250–5.
24. Pitcher D, et al. Cardiovascular implanted electronic devices in people towards the end of life, during cardiopulmonary resuscitation and after death: guidane from the Resuscitation Council (UK), British Cardiovascular Society and National Council for Palliative Care. Heart. 2016;102(Suppl 7):A1–A17.

25. Lewis GF, Gold MR. Safety and efficacy of the subcutaneous implantable defibrillator. J Am Coll Cardiol. 2016;67(4):445–54. doi:10.1016/j.jacc.2015.11.026.
26. Zanon F, et al. Device longevity in a contemporary cohort of ICD/CRT-D patients undergoing device replacement. J Cardiovasc Electrophysiol. 2016;27(7):840–5.
27. Bardy GH. Sudden Cardiac Death. N Engl J Med. 2005;352(3):225–37.
28. Mastenbroek MH, Pedersen SS, van der Tweel I, Doevendans PA, Meine M. Results of ENHANCED implantable cardioverter defibrillator programming to reduce therapies and improve quality of life (from the ENHANCED-ICD study). Am J Cardiol. 2016;117(4): 596–604.
29. Birnie DH, et al. Use of implantable cardioverter defibrillators. Can Med Assoc J. 2007; 177(1):41–6.
30. Lampert R. Managing with pacemakers and implantable cardioverter defibrillators. Circulation. 2013;128:1576–85.
31. Habibović M, van den Broek KC, Alings M, Van der Voort PH, Denollet J. Posttraumatic stress 18 months following cardioverter defibrillator implantation: shocks, anxiety, and personality. Health Psychol. 2012;31(2):186–93.
32. Irvine J, Firestone J, Ong L, Cribbie R, Dorian P, Harris L, et al. A randomized controlled trial of cognitive behavior therapy tailored to psychological adaptation to an implantable cardioverter defibrillator. Psychosom Med. 2011;73(3):226–33.
33. Maryniak A, Szumowski Ł, Orczykowski M, Przybylski A, Walczak F. Anxiety and depression among the patients with frequent implantable cardioverter–defibrillator discharges. Int J Cardiol. 2009;132(2):e80–1.
34. Dunbar S, et al. Educational and psychological interventions to improve outcomes for recipients of implantable cardioverter defibrillators and their families. Circulation. 2012;126: 2146–72.
35. Kajanova A, Bulava A, Eisenberger M. Factors influencing psychological status and quality of life in patients with implantable cardioverter-defibrillators. Neuro-endocrinology letters. 2014;35(1):54–8.
36. Heller S, Ormont MA, Lidagoster L, Sciacca RR, Steinberg S. Psychosocial outcome after ICD implamtation: a current perspective. Pacing Clin Electrophysiol. 1998;21:1207–17.
37. Pedersen SS, van den Broek KC, Sears SF Jr. Psychological intervention following implantation of an implantable defibrillator: a review and future recammendations. Pacing Clin Electrophysiol. 2007;30:1546–54.
38. Kitzlerová E, Anders M, Kautzner J, Dohnalová A. Evaultation of psychopatology in patiens with paroxymal supraventricular tachycardia. Exp Clin Cardiol. 2007;12(1):42–5.
39. Francis JL, Weinstein AA, Krantz DS, Haigney MC, Stein PK, Stone PH, et al. Association between symptoms of depression and anxiety with heart rate variability in patients with implantable cardioverter defibrillators. Psychosom Med. 2009;71(8):821–7. doi:10.1097/PSY.0b013e3181b39aa1.
40. Kuhl EA, Dixit NK, Walker RL, Conti JB, Sears SF. Measurement of patient fears about implantable cardioverter defibrillator shock: an initial evaluation of the florida shock anxiety scale. Pacing Clin Electrophysiol. 2006;29(6):614–8.
41. Bourke JP, Turkington D, Thomas G, McComb JM, Tynan M. Florid psychopathology in patients receiving shocks from implanted cardioverter-defibrillators. Heart. 1997;78(6):581–3. doi:10.1136/hrt.78.6.581.
42. Freedenberg V, Thomas SA, Friedmann E. Anxiety and depression in implanted cardioverter-defibrillator recipients and heart failure: a review. Heart Fail Clin. 2011;7(1):59–68.
43. Lidová L, Kajanová A, Eisenberger M. Vývoj depresivity a úzkosti u pacientů s implantabilními kardiovertery-defibrilátory. Česka Slov Psychiatr. 2016;112(3)
44. Willerton J. The psychology of relationships. New York: Palgrave Macmillan; 2010. p. 196.
45. Starrenburg AH, Kraaier K, Pedersen SS, van Hout M, Scholten M, van der Palen J. Association of psychiatric history and type d personality with symptoms of anxiety, depression, and health status prior to ICD implantation. Int J Behav Med. 2013;20(3):425–33.

46. Štejfa M, editor. Kardiologie. Praha: Grada; 2007.
47. Denollet J, Pedersen S. Type D personality, cardiac events, and impaired quality of life: a review. Eur J Cardiovasc Prev Rehabil. 2003;10(4):241–8.
48. Denollet J. DS14: standard assessment of negative affectivity, social inhibition, and Type D personality. Psychosom Med. 2005;67(1):89–97.
49. Sears SF Jr, Conti JB. Quality of life and psychological functioning of ICD patients. Heart. 2002;87:488–93.
50. Kuiper R, Nyamathi MA. Stressors and coping strategies of patients with automatic implantable cardioverter defibrillators. J Cardiovasc Nurs. 1991;5(3):65–76.
51. Lidová L, Kajanová A, Eisenberger M. Coping strategies for patients with ICD. IJAS; 2015.
52. Sears SF, Camm AJ, Todaro JF, Lewis TS, Sotile W, Conti JB. Examining the psychosocial impact of implantable cardioverter defibrillators: a literature review. Clin Cardiol. 1999;22(7):481–9.
53. Petrowski K, Wintermann GB, Petzold C, Strasser RH, Guenther M. Pre-hospital discharge testing of defibrillator without anesthesia. Psychosom Med. 2013;75(7):640–9.
54. Sears SF, Conti JB. Understanding implantable cardioverter defibrillator shocks and storms: medical and psychosocial considerations for research and clinical care. Clin Cardiol. 2003;26(3):107–11.
55. Tagney J, James JE, Albarran JW. Exploring the patient's experiences of learning to live with an implantable cardioverter defibrilator (ICD) from one UK centre: a qualitative study. Eur J Cardiovasc Nurs. 2003;2:195–203.
56. World Health Organization. The World Health Report 1998. Life in the 21st century: A vision for all, 1998. http://www.who.int/whr/1998/en/whr98_en.pdf.
57. Van Kamp I, et al. Urban environmental quality and human well-being towards a conceptual framework and demarcation of concepts; a literature study. Landsc Urban Plan. 2003;65(4):5–18.
58. Nelson EA. Health related quality of life measurement. EWMA J. 2002;2:5–7.
59. Slováček L, Slováčková B, Jebavý L, Blažek M, Kačerovský J. Kvalita života nemocných—jeden z důležitých parametrů komplexního hodnocení léčby. Vojen Zdrav Listy. 2004;73(1):6–9.
60. Stankoweit B, et al. Quality of life after implantation of an automatic cardioverter-defibrillator (ICD) – Results of an empirical study of 132 ICD patients. Zeitschrift fur Kardiologie. 1997;6:460–468.
61. Verkerk AJ, Vermeer AM, Smets EM, Dekker LR, Wilde AA, Van Langen IM, et al. Quality of life in young adult patients with a cardiogenetic condition receiving an ICD for primary prevention of sudden cardiac death. Pacing Clin Electrophysiol. 2015;38(7):870–7.
62. Schron EB, Exner DV, Yao Q, Jenkins LS, Steinberg JS, Cook JR, et al. Quality of life in the antiarrhythmics versus implantable defibrillators trial. Impact of therapy and influence of adverse symptoms and defibrillator shocks. Circulation. 2002;105:589–94.
63. Godemann F, Butter C, Lampe F, Linden M, Werner S, Behrens S. Determinants of the quality of life (QoL) in patients with an implantable cardioverter/defibrillator (ICD). Qual Life Res. 2004;13(2):411–6.
64. Tomzik J, et al. Quality of life in patients with an implantable cardioverter defibrillator: a systematic review. Front Cardiovasc Med. 2015;2:34.
65. Freedenberg VA, Thomas SA, Friedmann E. A pilot study of a mindfulness based stress reduction program in adolescents with implantable cardioverter defibrillators or pacemakers. Pediatr Cardiol. 2015;36(4):786–95.
66. Carroll LS, McGillion M, Arthur MH. Living with an implantable cardiac defibrillator: a model of chronic uncertainty. Res Theory Nurs Pract. 2014;28(1):71–86.
67. Eckert M, Jones T. How does an implantable cardioverter defibrilátor (ICD) affect the lives of patients and their families? Int J Nurs Pract. 2002;8:152–7.
68. Nečasová L, Sedláček K. Edukace pacientů s implantabilními kardiovertery-defibrilátory. 2016. http://www.cksonline.cz/21vyrocnisjezdcks/sjezd.php?p=read_abstrakt_program&idabstrakta=628. Accessed 3 May 2016.

69. Williams AM, Young J, Nikoletti S, McRae S. Getting on with life: accepting the permanency of an implantable cardioverter defibrilátor. Int J Nurs Pract. 2007;13:166–72.
70. Thomas SA, Friedmann E, Kelley FJ. Living with an implantable cardiverter-defibrillator. A review of the current literature related to psychosocial factors. AACN Clin Issues. 2001;12:156–63.
71. Malm D, et al. Health-related quality of life in pacemaker patients: a single and multidimensional self-rated health comparison study. Can J Cardiovasc Nurs. 2003;2(4):291–302.
72. Kebza V. Psychosociální determinanty zdraví. Praha: Academia, 2005. ISBN 80-200-1307-5.
73. Kučerová M. Kvalita života u pacientů s trvalým kardiostimulátorem. Bakalářská práce, Univerzita Karlova; 2008.
74. Malm D, Karlsson JE, Fridlund B. Effects of a self-care program on the health-related quality of life of pacemaker patients: a nursing intervention study. Can J Cardiovasc Nurs. 2007;17(1):15–26.
75. Kolterer B, et al. Improved quality of life after treatment of prolonged asystole during breath holding spells with a cardiac pacemaker. Ann Pediatr Cardiol: 2015;8(2):113–117.
76. Súkeníková V. Kvalita života po aplikaci kardiostimulátoru. Bakalářská práce, Západočeská univerzita v Plzni; 2014.
77. Malm D, et al. Regaining Normalcy in Relatives of Patients with a Pacemaker. Open Journal of Nursing. 2014;3(4). doi:10.4236/ojn.2014.43018.
78. Avlund K, et al. Active life in old age. Combining measures of functional ability and social participation. Dan Med Bull. 1999;46(4):345–9.
79. Kurucová R, et al. Quality of life of patients with a permanent pacemaker. Ošetřovatelství a porodní Asistence. 2014;5(1):15–20.
80. Lauberg A. Pacemaker patients' perspective and experiences in a pacemaker outpatient clinic in relation to test intervals of the pacemaker. Eur J Cardiovasc Nurs. 2014;13(1):72.
81. Webster G, et al. Psychiatric functioning and quality of life in young patients with cardiac rhythm devices. Pediatrics. 2014;133(4):e964–72.
82. Balvínová H. The influenece of the permanent carcdiac stimulator on the life of the client. Bachelor's thesis, University of South Bohemia in České Budějovice; 2010.
83. Cenková H. Patients' satisfaction after implantation of a pacemaker. Bachelor's thesis, Masaryk University; 2014.
84. Turton, Emily L. Psychological distress beyond anxiety and depression in a population with cardiac devices: inclusive of those with pacemakers. Doctoral thesis, University of Surrey, 2015. http://epubs.surrey.ac.uk/808576/.
85. Figueroa C, Alcocer L, Ramos B. Psychological intervention to modify anxiety, depression and quality of life in patients with an implantable pacemaker. Psychology. 2016;7:374–81. doi:10.4236/psych.2016.73040.
86. Bose CN, et al. Patterns and the mediating role of avoidant coping style and illness perception on anxiety and depression in patients with chronic heart failure. Scand J Caring Sci. 2016;30(4):704–13. doi:10.1111/scs.12297.
87. Bose CN. Coping and emotional well-being in patients with chronic heart failure. Dissertation, Karolinska Institutet; 2015.
88. Chen MY, Lin PH, Kao CW. The effects of psycho-educational intervention on quality of life in patients with implantable cardioverter defibrillators: a meta-analysis. In: 43rd biennial convention, Las Vegas, Nevada, USA, 7–11 November 2015; 2015
89. Manzoni GM, Castelnuovo G, Compare A, Pagnini F, Essebag V, Proietti R. Psychological effects of implantable cardioverter defibrillator shocks. A review of study methods. Front Psychol. 2015;6:39.
90. Biotronik SE, et al. Brožury pro pacienty. 2009a. http://www.biotronik.com/wps/wcm/connect/en_cz_web/biotronik/sub_top/patients/treatments_en/#jump. Accessed 5 May 2016.
91. Biotronik SE, et al. Co byste měli vědět o svém kardiostimulátoru. 2009b. http://www.biotronik.com/files/AFA53F3DC5E87A9CC1257A160036A975/$FILE/Patientbrochure_IPG_CS.pdf. Accessed 5 May 2016.

Chapter 5
Psychological Indices in Patients After Multiple Shocks with Implantable Cardioverter Defibrillator (ICD) and Psychotherapy

Ludmila Peregrinova and Jochen Jordan

Abstract We deliver an overview of the psychological reactions and distress in ICD-patients (implantable cardioverter defibrillator), especially after experiencing multiple consecutive shocks. Psychodiagnostic assessment will be discussed. After reviewing the scientific literature concerning psychological interventions we describe the most important areas of coping and adjustment, indicating helpful psychological tools for the treatment of psychiatric disorders following ICD-shocks. Finally, we present a case study of a specific psychological treatment as part of an inpatient multimodal therapy setting (psychocardiological rehabilitation) for a patient, who had experienced about 35 ICD-shocks, and his partner.

Keywords Implantable cardioverter defibrillator (ICD) • Multiple consecutive ICD-shocks • Posttraumatic stress disorder (PTSD) • Psychotherapy • Eye movement desensitization and reprocessing (EMDR)

Psychological Reactions and Emotional Distress in Patients Following ICD-Shocks

The implantation of an ICD (implantable cardioverter defibrillator) is often performed suddenly leaving the patient hardly any time for information and mental preparation. This requires a high ability to adapt in patients as well as their environment [1]. Coping with the disease after an ICD-implantation occurs without complications and patients develop positive feelings towards the ICD-therapy and consider

L. Peregrinova (✉) • J. Jordan
Department of Psychocardiology, Kerckhoff Clinic,
Benekestr. 2-8, 61231 Bad Nauheim, Germany
e-mail: l.peregrinova@kerckhoff-klinik.de; jochen_jordan@t-online.de

© Springer International Publishing AG 2017

R. Proietti et al. (eds.), *Psychological, Emotional, Social and Cognitive Aspects of Implantable Cardiac Devices*, DOI 10.1007/978-3-319-55721-2_5

it protective against death [2]. There are several factors that can significantly affect etiopathology and coping, such as progression of the cardiac disease, ICD-events (e.g. complications, shocks, pain, replacement of the ICD), personality traits (ability to adapt, coping strategies) and the reaction of the environment (partner, doctors, paramedics). The most indicated mental stress in patients after an ICD-implantation is the concern about ICD-shocks, physical paresthesia, limited mobility and quality of life as well as dependence on the ICD [2–4]. There are also behavior modifications to be considered, that have being observed in some patients. It has been reported that 41% of patients avoid sexual activities after an ICD-implantation and 50% of patients (≤40 years old) avoid physical activities [5]. The reasons can be diverse, e.g. fear of exhaustion, fear of ICD-shocks. Some patients are anxious that the ICD will trigger during sexual activity. Coping with this new situation requires internal and external resources, adaptive coping strategies and a supportive social network. After all, 96% of the patients stick to their decision and 98% would recommend this type of therapy to others who are in the same situation [6].

However, when patients experience multiple consecutive shocks or several episodes of shocks it becomes exceptionally problematic (in 25% of all ICD-patients; [2]). The number of shocks released yearly influences the degree of mental stress [3, 7]. During the ICD-shocks, thus in acute situations, patients feel helpless, a loss of control, they feel as though they are at the ICD's mercy and are often in violent pain ("… like a kick from a horse in the chest…" [8]). Almost all patients report having fear of dying in these moments ("…this time the defibrillator won't make it, the fight is lost …" [8]).

The stress inducing factors in these critical situations are:

- unexpectedness of the event (the event happens unexpectedly)
- unavoidability of the event (the affected person cannot avoid the situation)
- being at the mercy of it (the affected person is at the mercy of the circumstances)
- high intensity (the event is experienced as physically and mentally intensive)
- being pulled out of life activity (the affected person is being pulled out of his existing life)
- restricted or limited perception (the perception of affected people is highly limited)
- lifelong dependence (the life of affected people depends on the ICD).

For days and even weeks after, patients can experience intense and recurrent fears, panic attacks, nervousness, helplessness and hopelessness, depression and feelings of being insufficient (symptoms of acute stress disorder). Patients also report flashbacks in the context of premature beats, increase of heart frequency or blood pressure, intrusions/constrictions [9]. Many isolate themselves socially and emotionally and develop a pronounced avoidance behavior. Classical conditioning, learned helplessness and causal attribution are helpful models for explaining this behavior [10, 11]. In general, one avoids speaking about the experience as well as places and people, who are associated with the shock experience [12]. Further, nightmares, insomnia, recurring memories of the experiences can occur, but also future troubles, drifting thoughts, restricted emotional perception and depression [9]. Many patients and their partners report limited future prospects and personal plans, the evaluation of their life and future changes. In order for the disease to be coped with adequately, the reactions of partners and family are relevant as well ("... my wife doesn't know what to do and runs finally in an open store. We are in France and she doesn't speak any French ..." [8]). Many partners and children, who were present during the shocks, develop psychopathological problems of adjustment that needed to be addressed. Reactions of paramedics and the physicians are not less relevant for the development of mental stress after ICD-shocks ("...Give yourself a boot and continue living as you did before! ..." [8]). Helpless, angry, desperate or depressive partners but also trivialized, generalized and unclear comments by doctors can trigger strong symptoms of stress and trauma. These aspects should be considered during evaluation and be included in the treatment setting [9].

Prevalence of Psychiatric Disorders and Psychodiagnostic Assessments

The diagnosis of mental diseases in ICD-patients is often complicated. In individual cases it is not always clear whether the mental impairment developed because of the underlying cardiovascular disease or because of the ICD-implantation [2]. The prevalence of mental disorders among ICD-patients fluctuates depending on the diagnostic criteria and measures used. Approximately 11–28% of all ICD-patients are afflicted with apparent depression and approx. 11–38% has anxiety disorders [11, 13]. Data on patients' subjectively experienced depressive moods and anxiety is way more. A total of 13% of ICD-patients are also developing symptoms of PTSD (post-traumatic stress disorder) [1]. The prevalence of anxiety, depression and PTSD in patients after an ICD-implantation however decreases within 1 year [14]. However approx. 10% of those patients are still showing striking psychopathological symptoms 1 year after implantation [14]. A study that was performed with about 300 patients about 6 months after the ICD-implantation reports a prevalence of 13% showing PTSD [15]. Risk factors in favor of PTSD 3 months after the ICD-implantation are Type-D-personality, high level of anxiety before the implantation and ICD-shocks within this period of time. Six months after implantation it is the high level of anxiety about the implantation, preimplantation anxiety and ICD-concerns, that can trigger PTSD [15].

It becomes especially problematic when patients experience multiple consecutive shocks. After these experiences approximately 20% suffer from depression, approx. 66% suffer from anxiety and approx. 13% suffer from symptoms of PTSD [11, 14, 16]. Patients who've experienced ICD-shocks are showing overall higher PTSD-values compared to patients without ICD-shocks [14] and a higher PTSD-prevalence than all other cardiac patients [17]. However, the prevalence of trauma symptoms fluctuates after the shocks and ranges somewhere between 20 and 40% [18].

The diagnostic assessment of psychiatric disorders after ICD-shocks is quite complicated and is being encoded differently, so far there are no specific standardized measuring methods for this particular subgroup of patients. Most commonly self-assessment tools are used to diagnose depression ("Beck depression inventory" (BDI), [19]), anxiety ("Hospital Anxiety and Depression Scale" (HADS), [20]; "The State-Trait Anxiety Inventory" (STAI), [21]) and trauma-symptoms ("Impact of Event Skala" (IES), [22]). The results are interpreted on the item-level [23]. The symptom-profiles of patients taken from the found case reports are similar to those of panic-patients and treatment corresponds to the diagnostics of anxiety and panic disorders as well as agoraphobia [16, 24]. This assumption is being supported by studies that have found that the anxiety of these patients does not correlate primarily with the discharge of the ICD, but with catastrophic thoughts and hypochondriac introspection [16]. It is part of a detailed diagnostic to define whether it is a panic disorder, agoraphobia or disorders as consequence of trauma as well as the question of an existing pre-trauma (e.g. as a result of a previous cardiac arrest) and the anamneses of the partners, who were present in the acute situation and also experienced high levels of mental stress, must. One of the most important factors is the clarification of the patient's attribution patterns i.e. what the patient thinks causes the ICD-shocks (adequate and inadequate shocks; potassium deficiency, too much stress). These convictions sustain the hyper-vigilance, hyper-arousal and flashbacks and intensify the avoidance behavior. For the therapeutic work with the patient it is furthermore necessary to have identified the individual defense mechanisms of the affected person (denial, repression, rationalization, regression).

In an acute critical situation, directly during or after an experienced ICD-shock, it is helpful for the patient to experience his overexcitement (shivering, screaming, and crying) and the physiological sensation allowed or endured by the person present. This reduces the patient's overexcitement, relieves and stabilizes him and releases his helplessness taking him back to normality. So, the medical staff should be trained to react appropriately and adequately in these situations as to prevent potential trauma. Table 5.1 shows the most important behavior patterns when dealing with affected patients (q.v. [25]). During the future procedure and the medical interview, the doctor should convey a sense of security, not by using flowery phrases such as "It'll be ok" or "Well, I guess you're just lucky", but through empathetic and active listening (verbal and non-verbal), psycho-education (cognitive-behavioral), by empowering the patient to use self-calming techniques and personal coping strategies as well as the organization of further help relief. The experience of ICD-shocks can shatter the previous self-concept and world-view of affected people and their relatives; therefore, the doctor in charge should be accepting and understanding of their way of experiencing things, their feelings and individual needs. He should be prepared and sensibilized to constantly evaluate the mental state of ICD-patients after the shock experience and when necessary, to begin with relevant screenings for anxiety, depression and trauma symptoms (for key questions, q.v. [12]). Table 5.2 shows the key aspects of differentiated anamneses of mental stress after ICD-shocks (modified according to [18]).

Table 5.1 Crisis intervention

• Create transparency and orientation
– Introduction of oneself (who am I)
– Education about the measures (inform about the next actions, what am I doing now; what is the meaning of this measure)
• Calm and professional actions
– A leaning forwards posture (go to the same height level as the patient, don't approach from behind; if possible, try to establish a "light" physical contact (shoulder)
– Speech (adapt your speech speed to the affected patient)
• Reduce the sense of loss of control and helplessness
– Integrate the patient actively in the procedure—i.e. breathing techniques, to press down the band-aid
– Help while changing the clothes (i.e. after he/she wets the bed)
• Promote ability to act of present persons
– Assign tasks, involve in the procedures
– Involve in the communication and the distribution of information

Table 5.2 Specific aspects of an anamneses guideline after an ICD-shock

• Disease development
• Reasons for an ICD-implantation
• Experience and the previous experience with the device
• How do partners deal with the disease and the ICD
• Other illnesses, especially heart disease that runs in the family
• Numbers of ICD-shocks and other circumstances
• The situation setting during the multiple shocks
– Objective situational factors (people that are present; who has done and organized what; when did the ambulance arrive; which measures were performed)
– Subjective coping possibilities (to be at the situation's mercy)
• The effects of the ICD-therapy on the partners/family
• The structure and the acceptance level of the social network
• Biography: in the first place also the topic of the mental self-government and tendencies of dependence respectively
• Kind and extent of the developed avoidance behavior since then
• Defense mechanisms
• Dealing with earlier critical situations and helplessness
• Resilience
– Individual coping mechanisms and existing resources
• Trauma map (taken from the trauma therapy)

Psychological Interventions Following First ICD-Implantation

Lüderitz and Wolpert [26] already defined some helpful practical guidelines that consent to perform a comprehensible medical and patient-oriented education before an ICD-implantation. In addition to the preparatory and educational interviews/

talks before an ICD-implantation there are multiple possibilities for psychosocial care of affected patients after implantation, that include, singular or combined, the following aspects: psycho-educational interventions, relaxation techniques, cognitive behavioral therapy, offers for group therapy, individual counseling and crisis intervention as well as self-help groups (for an overview see [1, 27]). Most studies are using randomized, controlled designs; however, there are deviations in type of intervention and effect sizes [28]. The article from Ginzburg et al. [1] delivers an overview of five studies that are offering effective psychoeducational/psychotherapeutic group therapy to ICD-patients and also presents a new ambulant training program for patients and their partners after the first implantation of an ICD [9]. All interventions have one specific focus: medical education; exchange with other patients; psychoeducation for dealing with anxiety, avoidance behavior and depression; dealing with stress and stressful life events; learn and practice relaxation techniques; re-establishment of the integrity of the body; role models; dealing with ICD-shocks (emergency plan); exchange among relatives (q.v. Table 5.3). The advantage of a group intervention is the time and cost effectiveness of the process itself, therefore, it can be performed within rehabilitation as well as in an ambulant setting [1]. Another positive factor of group sessions is that patients have the possibility to experience an intensive exchange with each other. This allows them to perceive their own reactions and experiences as something "normal" and they learn to deal with non unexceptional events; that alone allows gaining emotional

Table 5.3 Compilation of the most important aspects of a psychological intervention

Doctor's attitude towards the patient
• Sensitive relationship with the patients
• Convey a feeling of security
• Give the patients the possibility to reflect
• Requirements for an interview:
– Calm setting
– The patient dictates the speed of the interview
– Paraphrase/listen actively
– Open body language facing the patient
– Reflect feelings
• Reestablish a sense of normality and a (new) life's plan with the patient and the relatives
Psychological Intervention
• Psychoeducation
• Stress management
• Relaxation techniques
Settings
• Individual and family counseling
• Group interventions
• Cardiac rehabilitation
• Self-help groups
• Outpatient physical training programs

de-escalation [1]. Patients who go through such programs achieve a very good acceptance of the ICD and in the end show a better quality of life and personal life planning. It seems that treating the anxiety disorder within those group sessions can reduce the likelihood of an ICD-shock, however only temporary [29]. Strictly psychoeducational programs with the receipt of information for record, telephone helpline or self-help groups don't seem to have any significant effect on the reduction of mental impairments; in contrast, gender-specific issues, elements of cognitive behavior therapy and cardiac rehabilitation lead to an improved acceptance of the device itself, they reduce anxiety, depression and the experience of stress and improve lastingly the quality of life of patients and their families ([30–38], overview in [28]). Furthermore, the clinical experience shows that those patients who took part in these interventions (after the first implantation) can cope much better with the mental consequences of ICD-shocks, i.e. these patients can cope well with the disease after ICD-shocks as patients who were not prepared.

Psychotherapeutic Treatments of Psychiatric Disorders in Patients After Multiple ICD-Shocks

The aim of a psychotherapeutic intervention can be different and goes by the primary symptomatology. So far there are no randomized case control studies covering the treatment of this subgroup of patients, much less the treatment of their partners and affected persons. The scientific literature provides some articles (often singular case studies) about psychotherapeutic/psychiatric treatments of patients with anxiety disorders or trauma symptoms after multiple ICD-shocks. The most heterogeneous reports describe briefly the psychotherapeutic techniques, however, they do not explain it in detail ([39]: "behavior program", [40]: "stress management", [41]: "psycheducation, individual and family counseling interview"; [42]: "supportive therapy"). All reports describe positive treatment progress for the affected patients. It is particularly evident that the therapeutic interventions in almost all cases are being accompanied by psychopharmacological treatments. Only some cases integrate therapy on physical functions. One of the most revealing papers is the case study performed by Benninghoven et al. [24]. It provides very detailed information about the disorders, the diagnostic assessment and biography of the patient and delivers insights into the psychotherapeutic treatment concept for a psychiatric disease after an ICD-shock. The patient was admitted to a psychosomatic university hospital in close cooperation with cardiology so that his anxiety disorder could be treated successfully. So we know, that cognitive restructuring, psycho-education, imaginative techniques and hypnotherapy are all absolutely reasonable therapy options for the described psychopathological symptoms of ICD-patients [41, 43]. So far, a CBT—cognitive behavioral therapy—has shown to be the most successful treatment. There's a review by Maia et al. [44] of multiple studies that confirm the effectiveness of this method for treating psychiatric disorders of ICD-patients (however not necessarily after ICD-shocks). There are no particular patterns for

ICD-shocks and the patients experiences them as being something random and unpredictable, the situation is therefore especially stressful, traumatizing and associated with feelings of helplessness and fears of dying. Thus, the primary aim is the reduction of the mental stress resulting from the heart disease and the ICD-implantation (ICD-Shocks). Within the cognitive behavioral therapy (CBT) the patient is invited to keep a journal and record the negative and stressing thoughts and feelings, in order to analyze and work on these later with the therapist (cognitive restructuring). Furthermore, the patient learns new stabilizing techniques and coping-strategies in order to reduce distress and improve his quality of life. By processing the avoidance behavior, the patient is supposed to learn how to return to participate in daily routines and how to boost his activity level (as far as it is compatible with the heart disease). However, almost all patients suffer from some anxiety after ICD-shocks; in particular the fear of having new shocks remains real. The psychodynamic therapeutic treatment approach has its main focus on the trauma syntheses. This therapeutic concept, mostly based on trauma model (without conflict and structural pathology), includes the following steps: stabilization (build up and activation of internal and external resources), trauma debriefing and reintegration [45]. If it takes the experience of trauma into consideration, then it should also be discussing the therapy of traumatic experiences.

Clinical Evidence of Trauma-Focused Approach

Many life threatening cardiac events, such as an acute heart disease, cardiac infarction and surgical interventions often have a mental impairment as a result. It is already known, that EMDR (eye movement desensitization and reprocessing) is an effective, non-invasive treatment when dealing with depression, anxiety and PTSD-symptoms after such events, which is well accepted by patients [46–48]. The psychotherapeutic treatment of affective disorders after ICD-shocks can be supported by an extensive expertise in that area. The manual for this therapy by Jordan et al. [9] was developed systematically and was derived from a stationary and multimodal high dose of focal therapy. This therapy was constantly extended and modified based on previous projects, so that the current status of clinical experiences and pretreatments is being supported by treatments of approximately 80 patients. The first 50 patients received different components of this therapy (elements of CBT, elements of psychodynamic imaginative trauma therapy, imaginative stabilization technique, relaxation technique, elements of cardiac rehabilitation). Therefore, the final concept had to be reviewed. The experience so far shows, that this treatment averages from one to three weeks. Therefore, the final manual was implemented in a stationary setting of 25 patients and its effect was analyzed in a 1-year-follow-up. For this matter standardized test series with four points in time to measure were implemented. All patients underwent a stationary psychocardiological treatment (q.v. case study). At this point the measurements confirm a significant decline in symptoms of PTSD, anxiety and depression for all cases. We can also conclude that memories and especially fears of the future marginally exist, which is absolutely comprehensible, as the possibility of new ICD-shocks can't be excluded and the patients are being reminded of the finitude and their own death. Finally, the results indicate that after 1 year the patients are convinced and are able by all means to handle critical situations by themselves and can cope with the new life situation and the traumatizing ICD-experiences.

Case Study

Below we will describe a typical case from our years of experience in psychotherapeutic work with patients who suffered from trauma symptoms after ICD-shocks.

Anton is a 60 years old man, married and due to heart failure an early retired engineer. He describes the quality the relationship with his partner as very good. Anton and his wife, who is a 56 year old teacher, live in a house that they own. They don't have any financial problems or other social troubles. During the past 2–3 months he could not pursue any of his hobbies, such as photography, the outdoors or walking his dog, because of massive fear of being alone; his wife had to be constantly present. No critical life events were found in his biography.

Medical History and Psychopathological Symptoms

In November of 2012 the patient survived a heart attack. A CRT-ICD (ICD with a cardiac resynchronization function) was implanted, for secondary prevention (dilated cardiomyopathy, ejection fraction 40%). In January of 2013, one single adequate shock followed. At this particular time, Anton reported no psychopathological symptoms. His attitude was "My ICD saved my life." In February of 2013, the ICD delivered 15 shocks. The in-hospital admission screening revealed a recurrent ventricular tachyarrhythmia (VT), which resulted in a cardiac ablation and reprogramming of the ICD. Emotional stress, anxiety and insomnia followed this event. At this point, Anton did not feel the need to seek professional psychological support. In April of 2013, the patient experienced recurrent VTs and ICD-shocks again. From that point on, Anton has been suffering from intrusive recollections, especially flashbacks of the ICD-shocks, feelings of hopelessness and inferiority, fear of the future, fear of darkness and fear of dying, as well as panic attacks. The psychometric tools confirmed a high level of hyperarousal, physical and emotional exhaustion, and extreme avoidance behavior, lack of interest and social withdrawal, sleep and concentration disorders. All these symptoms indicated an impressive emotional suffering in the patient, accompanied by an increased psychophysiological arousal within the last 3 months.

Measurement

We used the method SCID [49] in order to perform the clinical diagnostics. Furthermore, the IES-R was applied. Both tools were applied to assess post-traumatic stress symptoms. To record anxiety and depression we used the HADS and BDI. To measure the severity of depressive symptoms we used the BDI. The patient fulfilled the criteria in order to be diagnosed with PTSD. SCID (positive, severity code 3) and IES confirmed this diagnose; furthermore, critical values of depression and anxiety were observed. Anton's wife fulfilled the criteria for the diagnose of PTSD SCID (positive, severity code 3), IES, no pathological values of depressions and anxiety were found.

Treatment

The psychotherapeutic treatment was carried out together with the inpatient cardiac rehabilitation. The physical program comprised of supervised exercises on the ergometer, deep-breathing exercises, and group and endurance workouts. Relaxation techniques such as meditation, autogenous training and progressive muscle relaxation were performed daily. The patient participated in supervised discussions about balanced diet and healthy life conditions. In the context of psychotherapeutic treatment Anton's treatment plan included ten individual sessions of psychotherapy (emotional support, stabilization exercises, psychoeducation, cognitive restructuring and activation on internal and external resources) and three EMDR sequences for confrontation [50, 51]. We used bilateral brain stimulation—tapping: while sitting, the patient puts the palm of his hands on his knees and the therapist alternatingly taps the back of the patient's hands. Anton's wife was his chaperon and present during the rehabilitation and she also received minimal psychotherapeutic treatment from a different therapist.

In the following chapter we describe Anton's EMDR treatment in detail:

Before starting the confrontation with painful memories (ICD-shocks), the procedure of EMDR and the standard protocol were explained. Then the stabilization techniques were established. While preparing the EMDR phase, we focused developing attachment security, therapeutic alliance and patient's acceptance of this technique. Due to Anton's high physical activity (increased heart rate, blood pressure, tremble, and perspiration) he was instructed in regards to the breathing technique, working on mindfulness and imagination of internal resources. Many ICD-patients can't do the "butterfly-hug", a common tool; probably because of the placement and location of the ICD itself (near the left shoulder). The breath-and-count technique (breathe in through the nose and count from 1 to 4 inwardly; exhale through the mouth and count from 4 to 1 inwardly) and finding one's "inner safe place" (such as a resort in the mountains for example) were the most effective methods for our patient to distance himself from emerging distress and for self-reassurance. We assumed that these techniques would be useful in enhancing tolerance during the EMDR-confrontation.

The target memory with the highest level of disturbance was the last sequence of 20 multiple ICD-shocks in April. The first session of EMDR took place 10 days after this event. The SUD scale (Subjective Units of Disturbance, range 1 (minimum strain)–10 (maximum strain)) was 10. Anton considered the first shock within that sequence as not critical. The subsequent shocks however were experienced as being extremely negative and life threatening. He thought that he'd be dying and felt helpless: "I'm going to die! I feel helpless!" Due to the fast increase in psychophysiological arousal we started with the first shock soon after (typically it should be started with/right after the worst part of the target memory, which, in our case, is the second shock). Despite the extensive exploration, description and stabilization, the patient stopped this sequence early with a "stop signal" as soon as he recollected the initial shock from this electrical storm. He cried and said: "I'm scared of repeated ICD-shocks!" Due to the patient's distress when continuing with this sequence (increased heart rate) we finished it with the breath-and-count technique and finding his inner safe place. During the next 5 days we focused the therapy on activity and improvement of physical functions and resilience as well as the regulation of sleep quality. After repeated relaxation and stabilization, we started the second confrontation of the previous target memory. The duration of the sequences was increased subsequently and eventually, Anton fully tolerated the EMDR session and the SUD scale fell from the initial 10 to 6 at the end of the session. Due to his dysfunctional thought pattern and the fact that his emotional arousal could influence the technique and the functioning of the ICD ("If I discompose, my heart rate will increase heavily and my ICD will trigger a shock!") it was a very important experience of achievement, encouragement, of being in control of his actions and of increase of security. The third treatment session lead to a decrease of the SUD scale from 6 to 0.

After the stabilization, we focused on the next memory target: 15 ICD-shocks in February (2 months before the therapy). This session resulted in an overall reduction of the SUD-scale from 10 to 0. The total time of both effective EMDR sessions took about 75 min each. For some patients the most recent event represents the worst experience. While exploring and processing the trauma it becomes evident that not the last event (ICD-shock) is basic but another previous experience (e.g. reanimation before the ICD implantation). Even though in our patient it was not indicated, we need to mention that clinical work sometimes evidences cases, in which it is necessary to process these "not remembered" patient experiences, such as cardiopulmonary reanimation.

An essential component of psychotherapeutic work was the psychoeducation, the knowledge transfers about the dysregulation mechanisms of autonomic nervous system in PTSD and review and debriefing of critical incidents (ICD-shocks). Clinically positive effects were observed. (negative/full remission), IES (−1.31), BDI = 7, HADS(A) = 6, HADS(D) = 1. The values all stabilized towards the discharge date. In the follow-up measurements 12 months later, the results were confirmed and Anton has reported a higher self-efficacy and the resumption of his hobbies.

The reevaluation of the EMDR treatment and the psychotherapeutic intervention revealed some remaining discomfort regarding the eventuality of future ICD-shocks ("It could happen anytime!") In such cases, in order to treat this feeling of insecurity, we use the technique of "future projection" as the last step of our treatment model. Not all patients achieve the value 0 in the SUD scale. Some residual (real) fear remains according to clinical experience. This is probably associated with the increased mindfulness and body perception, with the patient understanding of the life threatening disease and with the ambivalent experiences of ICD-shocks (…" save the life and recall attention to the finiteness" …). In spite of the SUD scale = 0 of our patient, the measured values indicate a functional fear and an adequate acceptance of the device therapy, which sometimes threatens the patient.

Treatment of Anton's Wife

There were no previous traumatic experiences detected while reporting the biography. First, there was a narrative description of the situation (15 shocks in February, SUD = 10), that Anton's wife experienced as very wearing and stressful: "My husband wakes up at night saying he's not feeling well. I turn on the lights; he's holding his chest and is pale. I am asking what's wrong and before I even get to finish my question, he starts to scream and is twitching heavily and his whole body lifts. I've never seen anything like that before and I don't understand what is going on. I yell ("Anton, Anton, what is wrong with you…"), he's not reacting. I am thinking it must be the defibrillator. I pick up the phone but the battery is dead. What am I supposed to do now? I am confused. The defibrillator keeps on triggering shocks, 5, 6, 7 times. I can't watch it and he still doesn't react. I run out in the street and scream for help. The neighbors are right there to help. I can't remember anything that happened afterwards. She felt helpless and alone in that situation. Sometime after that event she suffered from nightmares (…" I am in a room that is decorated with all white curtains; I am walking around that room and I am in panic. I am looking for my husband while screaming for help, but he's nowhere to be found. Then I wake up soaked in sweat…"). Till this day, she can't speak about that event without bursting into tears and shaking while hawing. Furthermore, she avoids speaking about it while her husband is present ("I don't want my husband to see me like that! He's having enough of his own worries"). Since that event she also experienced her husband being clinging, dependent, "a different man" and felt very restricted in her own personal freedom. After the first contact and an established relation of some sort, anamneses and stabilization (inner safe place: the swing in the backyard of her parents; biofeedback) we started with short sequences (10–15 s, as defined by Constant Installation of Present Orientation and Safety (CIPOS-technique)). She couldn't bear more. Additionally, we instructed her to have at least 2 h of personal time daily (going out to the city, go for a swim or read), to be active and do sports on a daily basis (Nordic Walking) and to go for a walk in the park right after the EMDR session. Her husband tolerated it without any problems. After four CIPOS-sessions, she could bear 30 s and endured a full EMDR-session (SUD = 3). At the end we performed a future projection ("I see myself at the cemetery at my husband's funeral"). Surprisingly, it resulted in her being more courageous to speak about death with her husband. Anton was also more open and relieved; together, they made arrangements in the case of him and her dying.

Discussion

After the treatment, Anton and his wife reported to be satisfied with the psychotherapy and the reduction of physiological arousal. They were more active and participated in daily life and showed interest and the ability to regain strength. Anton had more trust in his physical condition and could be alone. This relieved his wife and she regained her freedom. At the end of Anton's cardiac rehabilitation, he appeared to be more encouraged and he reported to have normal quality of sleep. Overall, the anxiety and depressive symptoms, such as post-traumatic stress, were reduced significantly.

Our case study shows that cardiac (ICD-) patients who suffer from traumatic symptoms tolerate EMDR treatment and are grateful to benefit from psychotherapy with a therapist who has competence in treating cardiac diseases. This is an indispensable qualification for a psychotherapist in psychocardiology. The fact that a cardiologist was available at all times certainly helped Anton in stabilizing and establishing a feeling of security and confidence. The emotional stabilization and the intensive preparation of the patient before the confrontation treatment (often it is more intensive than usual) was a crucial factor of the treatment. In this case, Anton was scared of how his body would react during the confrontation. Therefore, in those cases it is advisable to conduct a test-EMDR session (before the actual confrontation) to process a less stressful event from the patient's biography. The patient got used to the technique of EMDR and gained confidence with it. In the context of cardiac rehabilitation an important factor of the treatment is active physical therapy, which allows the patient to exercise under supervision in order to experience and finally to accept the increasing heart rate. Thus, repetitive training should be considered and carried out to improve body awareness and the workout capacity of the patient. This has to accompany all possible psychological interventions. According to our clinical experience during therapy, ICD-patients prefer the tapping-stimulation technique due to the fact that many of them suffer from side effects of the medication, which causes visual impairments. Anton received recurrent shocks before the treatment, causing him constant feelings of insecurity. In the course of the treatment he regained confidence. In general, it is crucial for patients to continue the psychotherapeutic treatment after being discharged from the hospital in order to stabilize acquired knowledge and to transfer it into everyday life (outpatient). Apparently the treatment also helped reduce the wife's symptoms and gave both of them the possibility of being more open and honest with each other (showing respect towards the impairments of one other). The results conclude that anxiety (fear of death, fear of shocks or malfunctions of the device) never disappears entirely. These marginal difficulties endure and the symptoms can increase with a temporary progression of the disease (new ICD-shocks, ICD complications) or stressful life events (death of a family member, hospitalization). It should be noted that the determining factor for a fast and intensive effect of the EMDR-therapy is the process of providing safety, sensitive therapeutic attitude and attachment in order to provide the patient with an opportunity to review his experiences and associated feelings.

References

1. Ginzburg D,·Tavenaux M, Sperzel J, Boukacem A, Hamm C,·Jordan J (2011) Ein ambulantes Schulungsprogramm für Betroffene und Partner nach Erstimplantation eines implantierten Kardioverter/Defibrillators (ICD). Herzschr Elektrophys 22:157
2. Leithäuser B, Jordan J. Mental comorbidities in patients with ICD. Aktuel Kardiol. 2015;4(06):387–91.
3. Lüderitz B, Jung W, Deister A, Marneros A, Manz M. Patient acceptance of the implantable cardioverter defibrillator in ventricular tachyarrhythmias. Pacing Clin Electrophysiol. 1993;16(9):1815–21.
4. Schöhl W, Trappe HJ, Lichtlen PR. Akzeptanz und Lebensqualität nach Implantation eines automatischen Kardioverter/Defibrillators. Z Kardiol. 1994;83:927–32.
5. Dubin AM, Batsford WP, Lewis RJ, Rosenfeld LE. Quality-of-life in patients receiving implantable cardioverter defibrillators at or before age 40. Pacing Clin Electrophysiol. 1996;19(11):1555–9.
6. Lüderitz B, Jung W, Deister A, Manz M. Patient acceptance of implantable cardioverter defibrillator devices: changing attitudes. Am Heart J. 1994;127(4):1179–84.
7. Morris PL, Badger J, Chmielewski C, Berger E, Goldberg RJ. Psychiatric morbidity following implantation of the automatic implantable cardioverter defibrillator. Psychosomatics. 1991;32:58–64.
8. Anonymous. A different person in 2 minutes. Herzschr Elektrophys. 2011;22(3):132–9. doi:10.1007/s00399-011-0137-y.
9. Jordan J, Tischer G, Peregrinova L, Kirsch H. Manual for the psychotherapeutic treatment of acute and post-traumatic stress disorders following multiple shocks from implantable cardioverter defibrillator (ICD). Psychosoc Med. 2013;10:1–17. ISSN: 1860-5214.
10. Lemon J, Edelmann S, Kirkness A. Avoidance behaviors in patients with implantable cardioverter defibrillators. Heart Lung. 2004;33(3):176–82.
11. Sears SF, Todaro JF, Lewis TS, Sotile W, Conti JB. Examining the psychosocial impact of implantable cardioverter defibrillators: a literature review. Clin Cardiol. 1999;22(7):481–9.
12. Sears SF, Hauf JD, Kirian K, Hazelton G, Conti JB. Posttraumatic stress and the implantable cardioverter-defibrillator patient. What the electrophysiologist needs to know. Circ Arrhythm Electrophysiol. 2011;4:242–50.
13. Ladwig KH, Lederbogen F, Albus C, Angermann C, Borggrefe M, Fischer D, Fritzsche K, Haass M, Jordan J, Jünger J, Kindermann I, Köllner V, Kuhn B, Scherer M, Seyfarth M, Völler H, Waller C, Herrmann-Lingen C. Position paper on the importance of psychosocial factors in cardiology: update 2013. Ger Med Sci. 2013;12. doi:10.3205/000194.
14. Kapa S, Rotondi-Trevisan D, Mariano Z, Aves T, Irvine J, Dorian P, Hayes DL. Psychopathology in patients with ICDs over time: results of a prospective study. Pacing Clin Electrophysiol. 2010;33:198–208.
15. Versteeg H, Theuns DA, Erdman RA, Jordaens L, Pedersen SS. Posttraumatic stress in implantable cardioverter defibrillator patients: the role of pre-implantation distress and shocks. Int J Cardiol. 2011;146(3):438–9.

16. Pauli P, Wiedemann G, Dengler W, Blaumann-Benninghoff G, Kühlkamp V. Anxiety in patients with an automatic implantable cardioverter defibrillator: what differentiates them from panic patients? Psychosom Med. 1999;61(1):69–76.
17. Ladwig KH, Baumert J, Marten-Mittag B, Kolb C, Zrenner B, Schmitt C. Posttraumatic stress symptoms and predicted mortality in patients with implantable cardioverter-defibrillators: results from the prospective living with an implanted cardioverter-defibrillator study. Arch Gen Psychiatry. 2008;65(11):1324–30.
18. Jordan J, Titscher G, Kirsch H. Behandlungsmanual zur Psychotherapie von akuten und posttraumatischen Belastungsstörungen nach ICD-Mehrfachschocks. Herzschr Elektrophys. 2011;22:189–201.
19. Hautzinger M, Bailer M, Worall H, Keller F. Beck-Depressions-Inventar (BDI). Testhandbuch. 2. Aufl ed. Bern: Hans Huber; 1995.
20. Herrmann C, Buss U, Snaith RP. Hospital anxiety and depression scale – Deutsche version (HADS-D). Bern: Hans Huber; 1995.
21. Spielberger CD, Rickman RL. Assessment of state and trait anxiety in cardiovascular disorders. In: Byrne DG, Rosenman RH, editors. Anxiety and the heart. New York: Hemisphere; 1990. p. 73–92.
22. Maercker A, Schützwohl M. Erfassung von psychischen Belastungsfolgen: Die Impact of Event Skala-revidierte Version (IES-R). Diagnostica. 1998;44:130–41.
23. Crösmann A. Früherkennung und Prävention von Angststörungen bei Patienten mit implantierbarem Kardioverter-Defibrillator (ICD). Inaugural-Dissertation Philosophische Fakultät III Julius-Maximilians-Universität Würzburg; 2005.
24. Benninghoven D, Kunzendorf S, Heberlein I, Jantschek G. Angststörungen bei Patienten mit implantiertem Kardioverter-Defibrillator (ICD). Fallstudie einer psychotherapeutischen Behandlung. Psychotherapeut. 2006;51:206–13.
25. Hausmann C. Notfallpsychologie und Traumabewältigung. Ein Handbuch. 3rd ed. Wien: facultas.wuv; 2003.
26. Lüderitz B, Wolpert C. The patient's informed consent for pacemakers and ICD implantation: how to write and how to explain it. Z Kardiol. 2003;92(5):377–83.
27. Salmoirago-Blother E, Ockene IS. Methodological limitations of psychosocial interventions in patients with an implantable cardioverter-defibrillator (ICD). A systematic review. BMC Cardiovasc Disord. 2009;9:56.
28. Pedersen SS, van den Broek KC, Sears SF. Psychological intervention following implantation of an implantable defibrillator: a review and future recommendations. Pacing Clin Electrophysiol. 2007;30:1546–54.
29. Chevalier P, Cottraux J, Mollard E, NanYao S, Brun S, Burri H, Restier L, Adeleine P. Prevention of implantable defibrillator shocks by cognitive behavioral therapy: a pilot trial. Am Heart J. 2006;151(1):191e1–6.
30. Badger JM, Morris PL. Observations of a support group for automatic implantable cardioverter-defibrillator recipients and their spouses. Heart Lung. 1989;18(3):238–43.
31. Dougherty CM, Lewis FM, Thompson EA, Baer JD, Kim W. Short-term efficacy of a telephone intervention by expert nurses after an implantable cardioverter defibrillator. Pacing Clin Electrophysiol. 2004;27(12):1594–602.
32. Edelman S, Lemon J, Kirkness A. Educational intervention for patient with automatic implantable cardioverter defibrillators. Aust J Adv Nurs. 2007;24(3):26–32.
33. Fitchet A, Doherty PJ, Bundy C, Bell W, Fitzpatrick AP, Garratt CJ. Comprehensive cardiac rehabilitation programme for implantable cardioverter defibrillator patients: a randomised controlled trial. Heart. 2003;89(2):155–60.
34. Frizelle DJ, Lewin RJ, Kaye G, Hargreaves C, Hasney K, Beaumont N, et al. Cognitive-behavioural rehabilitation programme for patients with an implanted cardioverter defibrillator: a pilot study. Br J Health Psychol. 2004;9(3):381–92.
35. Kohn CS, Petrucci RJ, Baessler C, Soto DM, Movsowitz C. The effect of psychological intervention on patients' long-term adjustment to the ICD: a prospective study. Pacing Clin Electrophysiol. 2000;23(4):450–6.

36. Molchany CA, Peterson KA. The psychosocial effects of support group intervention on AICD recipients and their significant others. Prog Cardiovasc Nurs. 1994;9(2):23–9.
37. Sneed NV, Finch NJ, Michel Y. The effect of psychosocial nursing intervention on the mood state of patients with implantable cardioverter defibrillators and their caregivers. Prog Cardiovasc Nurs. 1997;12(2):4–14.
38. Vasquez L, Conti JB, Sears SF. Female-specific education, management, and lifestyle enhancement for implantable cardioverter defibrillator patients: the FEMALE-ICD study. Pacing Clin Electrophysiol. 2010;33:1131–40.
39. Kuiper R, Nyamathi AM. Stressors and coping strategies of patients with automatic implantable cardioverter defibrillators. J Cardiovasc Nurs. 1991;5(3):65–76.
40. Urizar GG, Sears SF, Handberg E, Conti JB. Psychosocial intervention for a geriatric patient to address fears related to implantable cardioverter defibrillator discharges. Psychosomatics. 2004;45(2):140–4.
41. Pycha C, Gulledge AD, Hutzler J, Kadri N, Maloney J. Psychological responses to the implantable defibrillator: preliminary observations. Psychosomatics. 1986;27:841–5.
42. Mello MF, Batista F. Post-traumatic stress disorder in a patient with an implant cardioverter-defibrillator. Int J Psychiatry Clin Pract. 2001;5(4):291–2.
43. Stockdale LL. The effect of audiotaped guided imagery relaxation exercises on anxiety levels in male automatic implantable cardioverter defibrillator recipients. 1990. Dissertation abstracts international 51/09-B 4270 (1990).
44. Maia ACCO, Braga AA, Soares-Filho G, Pereira V, Nardi AE, Silva AC. Efficacy of cognitive behavioral therapy in reducing psychiatric symptoms in patients with implantable cardioverter defibrillator: an integrative review. Braz J Med Biol Res. 2014;47(4):265–72.
45. Wöller W, Reddemann L. Trauma und Persönlichkeitsstörungen: Psychodynamisch-integrative Therapie. Stuttgart: Schattauer; 2006.
46. Arabia E, Manca ML, Solomon RM. EMDR for survivors of life-threatening cardiac events: results of a pilot study. J EMDR Pract Res. 2011;5(1):1–13.
47. Moghadam MB, Moghadam AB, Salehian T. Efficacy of Eye Movement Desensitization and Reprocessing (EMDR) on depression in patients with Myocardial Infarction (MI) in a 12-month follow up. Iran J Crit Care Nurs. 2015;7(4):221–6.
48. Urtz A. EMDR in the treatment of trauma after acute heart disease; 2011. PIOe_04_11_Urtz.pdf. p. 314–21.
49. Wittchen HU, Zaudig M, Fydrich T. Structured clinical interview for DSM-IV. Göttingen: Hogrefe; 1997.
50. Shapiro F. The Role of Eye Movement Desensitization and Reprocessing (EMDR) Therapy in Medicine: Addressing the Psychological and Physical Symptoms Stemming from Adverse Life Experiences. The Permanente Journal. 2014;18:71–77.
51. Hofmann A. EMDR. Praxishandbuch zur Behandlung traumatisierter Menschen. 2014 Stuttgart, Georg Thieme.

Chapter 6
Sexual Function in Adults with Implantable Cardioverter-Defibrillators/Pacemaker Recipients

Moshe Rav Acha and Tal Hasin

Abstract Sexual function is an important component of quality of life. The present chapter examines issues concerning sex and implantable electronic devices, including sexual dysfunction and safety concerns. Performing sex involves a 3–5 metabolic equivalent effort, a gradual increase in catecholamines with a modest and short increase in heart rate and blood pressure. Overall sexual activity is safe, especially if response to moderate physical activity tested normal. Pathology based research suggests a mild increased in the incidence of myocardial infarction, specifically in men performing extra-marital sex. However, significant arrhythmia that may lead to activation of an implanted defibrillator is extremely rare. Sexual dysfunction is prevalent in patients with a cardiovascular disease including those with implantable devices. Patients with pacemakers may have sexual dysfunctions which seem attributable to older age, and not to the device. Heart failure patients implanted with a resynchronization device may benefit from improved sexual function and consequently better quality of life. Despite these low risks, "sexual avoidance" is prevalent among patients with implanted defibrillators and has several causes such as fear, anxiety and altered body image. Sex and sexuality should be actively addressed during medical consultation to relieve unjustified fears and provide patients with adequate information and treatment.

Keywords Sex • Physiology • Cardiovascular disease • Coronary artery disease • Heart failure • Pacemaker • Intra-cardiac defibrillator • Cardiac resynchronization device • Sudden cardiac death • Myocardial infarction • Avoidance • Consultation

M. Rav Acha, M.D., Ph.D. • T. Hasin, M.D. (✉)
Department of Cardiology, Shaare Zedek Medical Center,
12 Hans Beyth Street, POB 3235, Jerusalem 9103102, Israel
e-mail: ravacha.moshe@gmail.com; hasint@szmc.org.il

© Springer International Publishing AG 2017

R. Proietti et al. (eds.), *Psychological, Emotional, Social and Cognitive Aspects of Implantable Cardiac Devices*, DOI 10.1007/978-3-319-55721-2_6

Introduction

Sexuality Among Healthy Subjects

Sexual function is an important aspect of general health and quality of life, both in healthy and diseased persons. Normal sexuality involves the desire, ability and satisfaction in performing sex and requires complex social, psychological and physiological capacities. Inability or dysfunction in performing sex is often interrelated with anxiety and depression [1, 2] and is associated with increased morbidity [3] and mortality. Nevertheless, this important aspect of life is often neglected in patient care [3] due to barriers both on behalf of the patient and the physician/caregiver.

The physiological demands involved during sex have mostly been studied among healthy young adults performing heterosexual vaginal intercourse with their usual sexual partner. The various stages of sexual activity include foreplay and arousal, intromission to climax with orgasm and subsequently recovery. Physical manifestations include the ability to sustain erection in men. In women physiological ability is less demonstrable and may be manifested with vaginal lubrication [4]. Sexual activity provokes adrenergic activation with an increase of epinephrine and norepinephrine during intercourse which peaks with orgasm and rapidly declines thereafter. Prolactin also increases with orgasm lasting some 30 min after [5–7]. In 1966, Masters and Johnson [8] reported 11 years of observational studies involving 382 female volunteers, 18–78 years, and 312 male volunteers, 21–89 years. They observed that the intensity of the physiologic responses to sexual activity was proportional to the degree of sexual tension. Respiratory rates progressively increased to a high of 40 per minute, heart rate to 110–180 beats/min, and a 80 mmHg (systolic) and 50 mmHg (diastolic) increase in blood pressure, all peaking at the time of the subject's orgasm. However, these studies were performed in the laboratory and not in the participants' familiar environment. Later studies performed in more familiar environments with the aid of continuous monitoring or telemetry devices deduced that during usual sexual activity heart rate reaches 60–70% of the age predicted maximal [9] and physical stress is modest, comparable with stage II of the standard multistage Bruce treadmill protocol for men and stage I for women [10] in the range of 3–5 metabolic equivalents [11]. The physiological demands of sexual activity may differ with the type of activity performed and the position used. Non-coital activity is less strenuous. For coital intercourse, woman on top is less demanding physically than man on top according to one [12] but not another [13] report.

Sexuality Among Patients with Cardiovascular Disease

Patients with a cardiovascular disease frequently encounter sexual dysfunction [14]. This is attributable to the older age of this population, risk factors, vascular dysfunction leading to impotence, psychological and social implications of the disease and possible side effects of cardiovascular medications. Fear of harm after myocardial infarction [11] or an arrhythmic event and angina related to sexual activity ("angina d'amour") [15] may lead to abstinence from sexual activity. A specific case is made for heart failure since many of the capacities necessary to maintain sexuality function work abnormally in these patients [16, 17]. Several medications used to treat cardiovascular disease have been implicated to cause sexual dysfunction but clear causality has not been established. Beta adrenergic blockers probably have only a minor effect [18], mediated mostly by the patient's knowledge of their potential side effect [19, 20]. Antihypertensive medication such as Acebutolol, Amlodipine Maleate, Doxazosin Maleate and Enalapril Maleate were not associated with increased sexual dysfunction compared to placebo [21]. As treatment of cardiovascular disease becomes more advanced, patients are currently treated with multiple electronic devices, which have potential implications on sexuality.

Cardiac Implantable Electronic Devices

Cardiac implantable electronic devices (CIED) are used for various heart diseases. Pacemakers are known to prevent bradycardia-related symptoms and death. Implantable cardiac defibrillators (ICD) are used to prevent arrhythmic death in patients with ischemic, dilated and various other cardiomyopathies [22–25]; channelopathies such as Long QT syndrome, Brugada and others [26]. ICD implantation for primary and secondary prevention of sudden cardiac death is a common practice in today's medicine. Cardiac re-synchronization devices (CRT) or cardiac re-synchronization devices with defibrillator (CRTD) are indicated for symptomatic patients with advanced ischemic and dilated cardiomyopathy, low ejection fraction and wide complex ECG [27, 28] with a proven survival benefit. CIED's were shown not only to improve cardiac patient's survival but their quality of life as well [29, 30]. Although the contribution of normal sexual activity to one's well-being is widely known, sexual activity was rarely assessed post CIED and was usually omitted from the post-ICD patient educational process [31, 32]. The aim of the present chapter is to discuss sexual function among patients with CIED's summarizing existing data regarding the probability of ventricular arrhythmia and ICD shocks and device related sexual dysfunction (including the prevalent "sexual avoidance" phenomenon) [2, 33].

SCD and ICD Shocks Associated with Sexual Activity

Studies examining the physiologic response of the cardiovascular system during normal sexual activity (usually with stable partners) show only modest exertion and a heart rate increase similar to that observed during everyday activities supporting the overall safety of this activity [12, 34, 35]. However, meta-analysis autopsy studies and case-crossover studies suggest an increased risk of sudden cardiac death (SCD). Multiple autopsy studies [36–39] suggest that the majority of SCD during sexual activity happens in men, usually during extramarital sexual activity. The dominant cardiovascular pathology found in these sex-related SCD was myocardial infarction (MI). Other studies have documented sex-related SCD in men with coronary artery disease (CAD) without evidence of MI, suggesting that sex plays a role in CAD related ischemia and left ventricular hypertrophy [40, 41]. The apparent conflict between physiological and pathological studies might reflect the difference between healthy individuals and CAD patients. Patients with cardiovascular pathologies were found to have more than a twofold relative risk for MI during or shortly after sexual activity [36, 40–42]. Notably, not everyone agrees with this distinction as some studies found a similar relative risk for MI associated with sexual activity among healthy individuals and patients with CAD [43]. The difference in cardiovascular stress between intra-marital and extramarital intercourse was proposed to explain the results of the autopsy studies in which the majority of coital deaths occurred during or shortly after extramarital intercourse [36, 38]. Despite a potential reporting bias (death during extramarital sex is more prone to be reported compared to "usual" marital sex) these reports suggest that extramarital intercourse might be more physically demanding with potential increased psychological stress leading to increased risk.

Autopsy studies showed sex-MI association to be more prevalent in men. Men may be more physically active during sexual activity and exhausted by sexual intercourse compared to women [36]. Women have more non-cardiac SCD compared to men and this tendency may translate into sex-related mortality [40]. Indeed, in a Korean study of SCD related to sexual activity including 14 fatalities, only five women were reported compared to nine men. The dominant etiology of SCD in these men was CAD while 3/5 women in this study died due to subarachnoid hemorrhages [39].

Case-crossover studies investigating the association between sexual activity and MI or SCD, showed a statistically significant association of such activity with MI [43–45]. Although these studies did not show direct association between sexual activity and SCD, it is reasonable to assume that some of the sex-related MI's resulted in SCD. In contrast to autopsy studies, the case-crossover studies did not differentiate between intra and extramarital sexual activities. Nevertheless, the case-crossover studies do note that although there was a significant relative risk for MI during sexual activity, its absolute risk increment was extremely low due to the relatively infrequent nature of such triggers and their transient effect. This sex-related absolute risk increase was estimated as 2–3 per 10,000 person-years for MI and 1 per 10,000 person-years for SCD [43, 44].

The concept that patients with an ICD might receive defibrillation during sexual activity is a cause of anxiety and distress for both the patient and spouse. Although the fear of sex-induced ICD shocks is spread among ICD recipients it seems to lack supportive evidence-based data. There is very little published data, with but a few cases to suggest any meaningful effect of sexual activity on ICD-documented tachyarrhythmic events [46, 47]. Based on the vast majority of the published literature, arrhythmic SCD was not correlated with sexual activity (in contrast with SCD as a consequence of myocardial infarction) [36, 43–45]. An ECG monitoring study performed during sexual activity among 88 men with CAD revealed ectopic activity exacerbation in a minority of patients, and in this minority the arrhythmia consisted of simple ectopy, similar to that observed during non-sexual daily activities [48].

Examining patients at high risk for arrhythmia during exercise may reflect on the overall risk during sex. Patients with long QT syndrome (LQT) and Catecholaminergic Polymorphic Ventricular Tachycardia (CPVT) are known to be particularly prone to cardiac events during sympathetic activation such as with anxiety, mental stress and physical exertion [49–51]. Therefore, it would be reasonable to assume that sympathetic surge during sexual activity might lead to increased cardiac events among these patients. Loar et al. [52] reviewed the Mayo Clinic cohort of LQT and CPVT patients for arrhythmic events. Their work included 402 LQT patients and 43 CPVT patients who were routinely asked about cardiac events during daily activities including sexual activity. To note that 97/402 (24%) of the LQT cohort and 10/43 (26%) CPVT had an ICD implanted. During a mean follow-up period of 5 years, 45/402 (11%) of LQT patients experienced SCD or ICD shock, but none occurred during sex. There were 5/43 (12%) CPVT patients who experienced SCD or ICD shock and two of these happened during sexual activity. The authors extrapolated the probability of sex-related SCD or ICD shock from the published national estimates of intercourse frequency, resulting with an overall event rate of only 0.005% for CPVT patients. The above study suggests a very low risk of sex-related cardiac arrhythmic events among CPVT patients and even more so among LQT patients. Moreover, a literature review till that year did not reveal any other cases of sex related cardiac events among LQT patients. In conclusion, significant arrhythmia leading to ICD discharge related to sexual activity is extremely rare, even in patients at risk.

Device Related Sexual Dysfunction

CIED Related Sexual Avoidance

Avoidance of sexual activity is well documented in patients with ICDs, nearly half of these patients avoid sex [31, 32, 53, 54]. There are multiple issues contributing to this phenomenon, including:

- Inadequate communication about sex between cardiovascular patients and their health providers. Some of it is related to the widespread belief that sex and intimacy are not to be discussed with others. Indeed, a study focusing on sex-related discussions among cardiac patients revealed that only a small minority of patients discussed sex issues with their physicians [32, 55].
- Decrease in desire for sexual activity, which frequently occurs in CIED recipients [31, 32, 53]. Reduced interest in sex post ICD implant has occurred in 29%

of ICD recipients and 39% of their partners [32]. Some of it may be related with anxiety, depression, or a change in body image as previously described in CIED recipients [32, 56].

- Fear of sex-induced ICD shocks occurs in above 40% of ICD recipients and their partners [32, 54, 57]. Usually, these fears consist in fears related to the consequence of ICD shock during sex (creating a scene) and fears related to triggering device shocks during specific acts as sex, exercise, etc. [54]. As discussed previously in this chapter, there is little evidence to support this fear, since the probability of sex-induced MI or arrhythmia is extremely low in healthy people and although greater among cardiac patients, the overall risk is still very low even in these patients [43–45]. Nevertheless, this fear is common in ICD recipients as revealed by numerous studies, far beyond its real occurrence and was shown to negatively affect quality of life [31, 32, 58]. This shock-related anxiety was quantitatively assessed in adults with congenital heart disease who were implanted with ICDs [54], revealing a high level of shock related anxiety according to the Florida shock anxiety scale [59]. Moreover, in that same study, a higher level of shock-related anxiety was associated with significantly poorer sexual function scores in both men and women [54], emphasizing the role of shock-related anxiety and fear in the sexual avoidance phenomenon of ICD recipients.

Cardiac Pacemaker and Resynchronization Devices: Impact on Sexual Activity

A limited number of studies examined the impact of cardiac permanent pacemakers (PPM) on sexual activity, however these results may be influenced by the prevalence of sexual dysfunction in the older population [3] which consists mostly of PPM recipients. The majority of the studies that examined the impact of PPM on quality of life have concentrated on the geriatric population, and sexual activity was not addressed [60–62]. According to those few studies that examined the impact of PPM on quality of life in a relatively younger (20–60 year old) and more sexually active population, there was no change in sexual activity in most patients (68%), with 8% describing improvement and 8% describing some deterioration in their sexual activity post implantation [63]. On the whole, this study suggests that PPM implants have no adverse impact on sexual activity in the majority of patients. Although 11% of patients in the above study described anxiety or fear of pacing failure after PPM implant, this did not impact their sexual lives [63]. Similar results were found in another study that included older patients (median age 71 years old) most patients had subsided their sexual activity during the period of bradycardia-related symptoms, however the majority resumed the same level of sexual activity they had prior to implantation of the PPM [64]. Lastly, a non-significant improvement in sexual function was found in 42 patients implanted with a PPM [65]. Taken together, evidence from these small observational studies suggests that patients implanted with a PPM maintain the sexual life quality they had prior to device implantation.

The impact of Cardiac resynchronization devices (CRT/CRTD) on sexual function in heart failure (HF) patients is more complicated. As mentioned above, many HF patients suffer from erectile dysfunction due to various reasons including, underlying atherosclerosis, neurologic pathology, endothelial dysfunction, hormonal deficiencies, drug side effects, psychological factors and increased peripheral vasoconstriction [66]. Moreover, depression, anxiety, and usage of various HF drugs might decrease libido among HF patients [66]. In a study describing health complains of HF patients scheduled for resynchronization therapy, fatigue and sexual problems were ranked as their most severe health complains [67]. Sildenafil citrate, a selective inhibitor of cGMP, can improve exercise capacity and erectile dysfunction in patients with HF [68, 69]. Patients with advanced NYHA III/IV HF were considered at high-risk for coitus-induced cardiovascular events according to the second Princeton Consensus guidelines, which recommends that sexual activity in these patients should be postponed until they are treated and stabilized [70]. Cardiac resynchronization therapy was shown in many studies to improve cardiac ejection fraction, HF symptoms, NYHA functional capacity, quality of life and survival of NYHA III/IV HF patients [28, 71, 72]. However, its impact on sexual function in general and patients' libido and erectile function specifically were rarely addressed in the initial studies. A recent study [73] examined the effect of cardiac resynchronization devices on libido and erectile function in 31 HF patients. The patients' libido and erectile dysfunction prior and 6 months after resynchronization device implant were evaluated using both the internationally validated Sexual Health Inventory for Men (SHIM) questionnaire and the aging male symptoms rating scale. A significant increase in the SHIM score and a decrease in the aging male symptoms score were found at 6 months post resynchronization device implant, indicating a significant improvement in erectile function and libido [73]. A significant correlation was found between LVEF increase and erectile dysfunction improvement [73]. Similar findings were described in a case report of a HF patient with long-standing erectile dysfunction who experienced significant improvement of his sexual function following biventricular pacing device implantation [74]. The authors suggested that resynchronization therapy improves sexual function of advanced HF patients by increasing their exercise capacity, improving endothelial function and arterial blood flow and decreasing peripheral vasoconstriction.

Maintaining Sexuality and Intimacy with a CIED

There are numerous obstacles to resuming a normal and enjoyable sexual activity after CIED implant. An effective communication strategy between patients and health-care professionals in general and specifically a routine discussion with one's health provider regarding sexual activity is of prior importance. Early identification of ICD shock-related anxiety or lack of desire for resuming normal sexual activity should pave the way for targeted interventions such as educational initiatives, professional sexual counseling and psychological referral. Patient education should include some explanation of how the device functions, events that potentially may trigger a shock and their realistic probability to occur, and a simple plan of action in the rare event of an ICD shock. Indeed, performing a routine educational program and a cognitive behavioral therapy to all ICD recipients was found beneficial in a study including 29 women implanted with an ICD [30]. However, without underscoring the importance of sexual activity with your partner, one needs to remember that sex is only one part of an intimate relation with your significant other, which include other acts as holding hands, kissing, hugging, etc. Although many think exclusively of sex when discussing intimacy, there is much more to intimacy than just intercourse. Moreover, it is important to remember that intimacy is a continuing process and not just a single event. At the end of the day, a lack of sex will usually not damage a close relationship as long as other acts of intimacy are kept. Thus, even if one feels lack of desire for sex or fear from sex-induced ICD shocks, it is of crucial importance to maintain intimacy.

References

1. Kriston L, Gunzler C, Agyemang A, Bengel J, Berner MM, Group SS. Effect of sexual function on health-related quality of life mediated by depressive symptoms in cardiac rehabilitation. Findings of the SPARK project in 493 patients. J Sex Med. 2010;7(6):2044–55.
2. Friedman S. Cardiac disease, anxiety, and sexual functioning. Am J Cardiol. 2000;86(2A): 46F–50F.
3. Lindau ST, Schumm LP, Laumann EO, Levinson W, O'Muircheartaigh CA, Waite LJ. A study of sexuality and health among older adults in the United States. N Engl J Med. 2007; 357(8):762–74.
4. Masters WH. The sexual response cycle of the human female: vaginal lubrication. Ann N Y Acad Sci. 1959;83:301–17.
5. Kruger T, Exton MS, Pawlak C, von zur Muhlen A, Hartmann U, Schedlowski M. Neuroendocrine and cardiovascular response to sexual arousal and orgasm in men. Psychoneuroendocrinology. 1998;23(4):401–11.
6. Exton NG, Truong TC, Exton MS, Wingenfeld SA, Leygraf N, Saller B, et al. Neuroendocrine response to film-induced sexual arousal in men and women. Psychoneuroendocrinology. 2000;25(2):187–99.
7. Exton MS, Bindert A, Kruger T, Scheller F, Hartmann U, Schedlowski M. Cardiovascular and endocrine alterations after masturbation-induced orgasm in women. Psychosom Med. 1999;61(3):280–9.
8. Masters WH, Johnson VE, New York Academy of Medicine. In: Masters WH, Johnson VE, editors. Human sexual response. 1st ed. Boston: Little, Brown and Company; 1966. xiii, 366 pp.
9. Masini V, Romei E, Fiorella AT. Dynamic electrocardiogram in normal subjects during sexual activity. G Ital Cardiol. 1980;10(11):1442–8.
10. Palmeri ST, Kostis JB, Casazza L, Sleeper LA, Lu M, Nezgoda J, et al. Heart rate and blood pressure response in adult men and women during exercise and sexual activity. Am J Cardiol. 2007;100(12):1795–801.
11. Hellerstein HK, Friedman EH. Sexual activity and the postcoronary patient. Arch Intern Med. 1970;125(6):987–99.
12. Bohlen JG, Held JP, Sanderson MO, Patterson RP. Heart rate, rate-pressure product, and oxygen uptake during four sexual activities. Arch Intern Med. 1984;144(9):1745–8.

13. Nemec ED, Mansfield L, Kennedy JW. Heart rate and blood pressure responses during sexual activity in normal males. Am Heart J. 1976;92(3):274–7.
14. Bohm M, Baumhakel M, Probstfield JL, Schmieder R, Yusuf S, Zhao F, et al. Sexual function, satisfaction, and association of erectile dysfunction with cardiovascular disease and risk factors in cardiovascular high-risk patients: substudy of the ONgoing Telmisartan Alone and in Combination with Ramipril Global Endpoint Trial/Telmisartan Randomized AssessmeNT Study in ACE-INtolerant Subjects with Cardiovascular Disease (ONTARGET/TRANSCEND). Am Heart J. 2007;154(1):94–101.
15. Drory Y, Shapira I, Fisman EZ, Pines A. Myocardial ischemia during sexual activity in patients with coronary artery disease. Am J Cardiol. 1995;75(12):835–7.
16. Hoekstra T, Lesman-Leegte I, Luttik ML, Sanderman R, van Veldhuisen DJ, Jaarsma T. Sexual problems in elderly male and female patients with heart failure. Heart. 2012;98(22):1647–52.
17. Mandras SA, Uber PA, Mehra MR. Sexual activity and chronic heart failure. Mayo Clin Proc. 2007;82(10):1203–10.
18. Ko DT, Hebert PR, Coffey CS, Sedrakyan A, Curtis JP, Krumholz HM. Beta-blocker therapy and symptoms of depression, fatigue, and sexual dysfunction. JAMA. 2002;288(3):351–7.
19. Silvestri A, Galetta P, Cerquetani E, Marazzi G, Patrizi R, Fini M, et al. Report of erectile dysfunction after therapy with beta-blockers is related to patient knowledge of side effects and is reversed by placebo. Eur Heart J. 2003;24(21):1928–32.
20. Cocco G. Erectile dysfunction after therapy with metoprolol: the Hawthorne effect. Cardiology. 2009;112(3):174–7.
21. Grimm RH Jr, Grandits GA, Prineas RJ, McDonald RH, Lewis CE, Flack JM, et al. Long-term effects on sexual function of five antihypertensive drugs and nutritional hygienic treatment in hypertensive men and women. Treatment of Mild Hypertension Study (TOMHS). Hypertension. 1997;29(1 Pt 1):8–14.
22. Moss AJ, Hall WJ, Cannom DS, Daubert JP, Higgins SL, Klein H, et al. Improved survival with an implanted defibrillator in patients with coronary disease at high risk for ventricular arrhythmia. Multicenter automatic defibrillator implantation trial investigators. N Engl J Med. 1996;335(26):1933–40.
23. Moss AJ, Zareba W, Hall WJ, Klein H, Wilber DJ, Cannom DS, et al. Prophylactic implantation of a defibrillator in patients with myocardial infarction and reduced ejection fraction. N Engl J Med. 2002;346(12):877–83.
24. Kadish A, Dyer A, Daubert JP, Quigg R, Estes NA, Anderson KP, et al. Prophylactic defibrillator implantation in patients with nonischemic dilated cardiomyopathy. N Engl J Med. 2004;350(21):2151–8.
25. Bardy GH, Lee KL, Mark DB, Poole JE, Packer DL, Boineau R, et al. Amiodarone or an implantable cardioverter-defibrillator for congestive heart failure. N Engl J Med. 2005;352(3):225–37.
26. Priori SG, Blomstrom-Lundqvist C, Mazzanti A, Blom N, Borggrefe M, Camm J, et al. 2015 ESC Guidelines for the management of patients with ventricular arrhythmias and the prevention of sudden cardiac death: the task force for the management of patients with ventricular arrhythmias and the prevention of sudden cardiac death of the European Society of Cardiology (ESC). Endorsed by: Association for European Paediatric and Congenital Cardiology (AEPC). Eur Heart J. 2015;36(41):2793–867.
27. Bristow MR, Saxon LA, Boehmer J, Krueger S, Kass DA, De Marco T, et al. Cardiac-resynchronization therapy with or without an implantable defibrillator in advanced chronic heart failure. N Engl J Med. 2004;350(21):2140–50.
28. Cleland JG, Daubert JC, Erdmann E, Freemantle N, Gras D, Kappenberger L, et al. The effect of cardiac resynchronization on morbidity and mortality in heart failure. N Engl J Med. 2005;352(15):1539–49.
29. Sears SF, Matchett M, Conti JB. Effective management of ICD patient psychosocial issues and patient critical events. J Cardiovasc Electrophysiol. 2009;20(11):1297–304.
30. Irvine J, Dorian P, Baker B, O'Brien BJ, Roberts R, Gent M, et al. Quality of life in the Canadian Implantable Defibrillator Study (CIDS). Am Heart J. 2002;144(2):282–9.

31. Vazquez LD, Sears SF, Shea JB, Vazquez PM. Sexual health for patients with an implantable cardioverter defibrillator. Circulation. 2010;122(13):e465–7.
32. Steinke EE, Gill-Hopple K, Valdez D, Wooster M. Sexual concerns and educational needs after an implantable cardioverter defibrillator. Heart Lung. 2005;34(5):299–308.
33. Lemon J, Edelman S, Kirkness A. Avoidance behaviors in patients with implantable cardioverter defibrillators. Heart Lung. 2004;33(3):176–82.
34. Bartlett RG Jr. Physiologic responses during coitus. J Appl Physiol. 1956;9(3):469–72.
35. Xue-Rui T, Ying L, Da-Zhong Y, Xiao-Jun C. Changes of blood pressure and heart rate during sexual activity in healthy adults. Blood Press Monit. 2008;13(4):211–7.
36. Niederseer D, Moller J, Niebauer J. Increased rates of myocardial infarction and deaths in men after sexual activity. Int J Cardiol. 2012;156(2):234–5.
37. Chen X, Zhang Q, Tan X. Cardiovascular effects of sexual activity. Indian J Med Res. 2009;130(6):681–8.
38. Parzeller M, Bux R, Raschka C, Bratzke H. Sudden cardiovascular death associated with sexual activity: a forensic autopsy study (1972–2004). Forensic Sci Med Pathol. 2006;2(2):109–14.
39. Lee S, Chae J, Cho Y. Causes of sudden death related to sexual activity: results of a medicolegal postmortem study from 2001 to 2005. J Korean Med Sci. 2006;21(6):995–9.
40. Gips H, Zaitsev K, Hiss J. Sudden cardiac death of a woman during extramarital sex: a case report and review of the literature. J Forensic Legal Med. 2010;17(4):186–7.
41. Parzeller M, Raschka C, Bratzke H. Sudden cardiovascular death in correlation with sexual activity—results of a medicolegal postmortem study from 1972–1998. Eur Heart J. 2001;22(7):610–1.
42. Kimmel SE. Sex and myocardial infarction: an epidemiologic perspective. Am J Cardiol. 2000;86(2A):10F–3F.
43. Muller JE, Mittleman MA, Maclure M, Sherwood JB, Tofler GH. Triggering myocardial infarction by sexual activity. Low absolute risk and prevention by regular physical exertion. Determinants of myocardial infarction onset study investigators. JAMA. 1996;275(18):1405–9.
44. Dahabreh IJ, Paulus JK. Association of episodic physical and sexual activity with triggering of acute cardiac events: systematic review and meta-analysis. JAMA. 2011;305(12):1225–33.
45. Baylin A, Hernandez-Diaz S, Siles X, Kabagambe EK, Campos H. Triggers of nonfatal myocardial infarction in Costa Rica: heavy physical exertion, sexual activity, and infection. Ann Epidemiol. 2007;17(2):112–8.
46. Fries R, Konig J, Schafers HJ, Bohm M. Triggering effect of physical and mental stress on spontaneous ventricular tachyarrhythmias in patients with implantable cardioverter-defibrillators. Clin Cardiol. 2002;25(10):474–8.
47. Safi AM, Rachko M, Yeshou D, Stein RA. Sexual activity as a trigger for ventricular tachycardia in a patient with implantable cardioverter defibrillator. Arch Sex Behav. 2002;31(3):295–9.
48. Drory Y, Fisman EZ, Shapira Y, Pines A. Ventricular arrhythmias during sexual activity in patients with coronary artery disease. Chest. 1996;109(4):922–4.
49. Leenhardt A, Denjoy I, Guicheney P. Catecholaminergic polymorphic ventricular tachycardia. Circ Arrhythm Electrophysiol. 2012;5(5):1044–52.
50. Schwartz PJ, Crotti L. QTc behavior during exercise and genetic testing for the long-QT syndrome. Circulation. 2011;124(20):2181–4.
51. Shamsuzzaman AS, Ackerman MJ, Kara T, Lanfranchi P, Somers VK. Sympathetic nerve activity in the congenital long-QT syndrome. Circulation. 2003;107(14):1844–7.
52. Loar RW, Bos JM, Cannon BC, Ackerman MJ. Sudden cardiac arrest during sex in patients with either catecholaminergic polymorphic ventricular tachycardia or long-QT syndrome: a rare but shocking experience. J Cardiovasc Electrophysiol. 2015;26(3):300–4.
53. Taylor HA Jr. Sexual activity and the cardiovascular patient: guidelines. Am J Cardiol. 1999;84(5B):6N–10N.
54. Cook SC, Valente AM, Maul TM, Dew MA, Hickey J, Jennifer Burger P, et al. Shock-related anxiety and sexual function in adults with congenital heart disease and implantable cardioverter-defibrillators. Heart Rhythm. 2013;10(6):805–10.

55. Bedell SE, Duperval M, Goldberg R. Cardiologists' discussions about sexuality with patients with chronic coronary artery disease. Am Heart J. 2002;144(2):239–42.
56. Dougherty CM. Longitudinal recovery following sudden cardiac arrest and internal cardioverter defibrillator implantation: survivors and their families. Am J Crit Care. 1994;3(2):145–54.
57. Pycha C, Calabrese JR, Gulledge AD, Maloney JD. Patient and spouse acceptance and adaptation to implantable cardioverter defibrillators. Cleve Clin J Med. 1990;57(5):441–4.
58. van Ittersum M, de Greef M, van Gelder I, Coster J, Brugemann J, van der Schans C. Fear of exercise and health-related quality of life in patients with an implantable cardioverter defibrillator. Int J Rehabil Res. 2003;26(2):117–22.
59. Kuhl EA, Dixit NK, Walker RL, Conti JB, Sears SF. Measurement of patient fears about implantable cardioverter defibrillator shock: an initial evaluation of the Florida Shock Anxiety Scale. Pacing Clin Electrophysiol. 2006;29(6):614–8.
60. Becker MC, Zucker IR, Parsonnet V, Gilbert L. Rehabilitation of the patient with a permanent pacemaker. Geriatrics. 1967;22(2):106–11.
61. Hesse KA. Meeting the psychosocial needs of pacemaker patients. Int J Psychiatry Med. 1975;6(3):359–72.
62. Rossel CL, Alyn IB. Living with a permanent cardiac pacemaker. Heart Lung. 1977;6(2):273–9.
63. Mickley H, Petersen J, Nielsen BL. Subjective consequences of permanent pacemaker therapy in patients under the age of retirement. Pacing Clin Electrophysiol. 1989;12(3):401–5.
64. Greene WA, Moss AJ. Psychosocial factors in the adjustment of patients with permanently implanted cardiac pacemakers. Ann Intern Med. 1969;70(5):897–902.
65. Chen HM, Chao YF. Change in quality of life in patients with permanent cardiac pacemakers: a six-month follow-up study. J Nurs Res. 2002;10(2):143–50.
66. Schwarz ER, Rastogi S, Kapur V, Sulemanjee N, Rodriguez JJ. Erectile dysfunction in heart failure patients. J Am Coll Cardiol. 2006;48(6):1111–9.
67. Ingadottir B, Thylen I, Jaarsma T. Knowledge expectations, self-care, and health complaints of heart failure patients scheduled for cardiac resynchronization therapy implantation. Patient Prefer Adherence. 2015;9:913–21.
68. Bocchi EA, Guimaraes G, Mocelin A, Bacal F, Bellotti G, Ramires JF. Sildenafil effects on exercise, neurohormonal activation, and erectile dysfunction in congestive heart failure: a double-blind, placebo-controlled, randomized study followed by a prospective treatment for erectile dysfunction. Circulation. 2002;106(9):1097–103.
69. Webster LJ, Michelakis ED, Davis T, Archer SL. Use of sildenafil for safe improvement of erectile function and quality of life in men with New York Heart Association classes II and III congestive heart failure: a prospective, placebo-controlled, double-blind crossover trial. Arch Intern Med. 2004;164(5):514–20.
70. Kostis JB, Jackson G, Rosen R, Barrett-Connor E, Billups K, Burnett AL, et al. Sexual dysfunction and cardiac risk (the Second Princeton Consensus Conference). Am J Cardiol. 2005;96(12B):85M–93M.
71. Anand IS, Carson P, Galle E, Song R, Boehmer J, Ghali JK, et al. Cardiac resynchronization therapy reduces the risk of hospitalizations in patients with advanced heart failure: results from the Comparison of Medical Therapy, Pacing and Defibrillation in Heart Failure (COMPANION) trial. Circulation. 2009;119(7):969–77.
72. Linde C, Leclercq C, Rex S, Garrigue S, Lavergne T, Cazeau S, et al. Long-term benefits of biventricular pacing in congestive heart failure: results from the MUltisite STimulation in cardiomyopathy (MUSTIC) study. J Am Coll Cardiol. 2002;40(1):111–8.
73. Vural A, Agacdiken A, Celikyurt U, Culha M, Kahraman G, Kozdag G, et al. Effect of cardiac resynchronization therapy on libido and erectile dysfunction. Clin Cardiol. 2011;34(7):437–41.
74. Domanski D, Rosanio S, Schwarz ER. Improved erectile function after cardiac resynchronization therapy in a patient with heart failure-a case report. J Sex Med. 2009;6(10):2910–4.

Chapter 7
Critical Appraisal of Cardiac Implantable Electronic Devices: Complications and Management

Arjun D. Sharma

Abstract Pacemakers, defibrillators and cardiac resynchronization devices (CIEDs) should not only meet regulatory requirements, but ideally also the expectations of medical staff and patients. Unfortunately, most of these clinical recommendations are fairly vague, and not related to specific products or malfunctions, but rather to some concept of overall performance. This may be entirely appropriate as the myriad of potential individual malfunctions can hardly be expected to be anticipated by medical staffs. This chapter will discuss some potential malfunctions, and how variable patient harms and complications may be for different malfunctions. The individual risks of patient harm considered together with their needs dictate recommendations for management of the malfunction.

Keywords Pacemakers • Defibrillators • Malfunctions • Complications

Product Performance Reports

There are several measures of performance, such as meeting regulatory requirements. Manufactures who are members of AdvaMed also produce Product Performance Reports according to definitions for standardized reporting (Fig. 7.1). These are available on-line for physicians and patients to view permitting them to compare the long term performance of CIEDs. Pulse generators, malfunctions are usually grouped, as with, or without therapy compromise, and may be listed by type of malfunction. Leads have additional clinical outcomes reported in the first 30 days' post implant, such as dislodgement, and perforation. Generally there are many potential malfunctions which may result in similar superficial manifestations and

A.D. Sharma, M.D., F.A.C.C.
94 Crocus Pl, St Paul, MN 55102, USA
e-mail: sharmarjun@gmail.com

© Springer International Publishing AG 2017

R. Proietti et al. (eds.), *Psychological, Emotional, Social and Cognitive Aspects of Implantable Cardiac Devices*, DOI 10.1007/978-3-319-55721-2_7

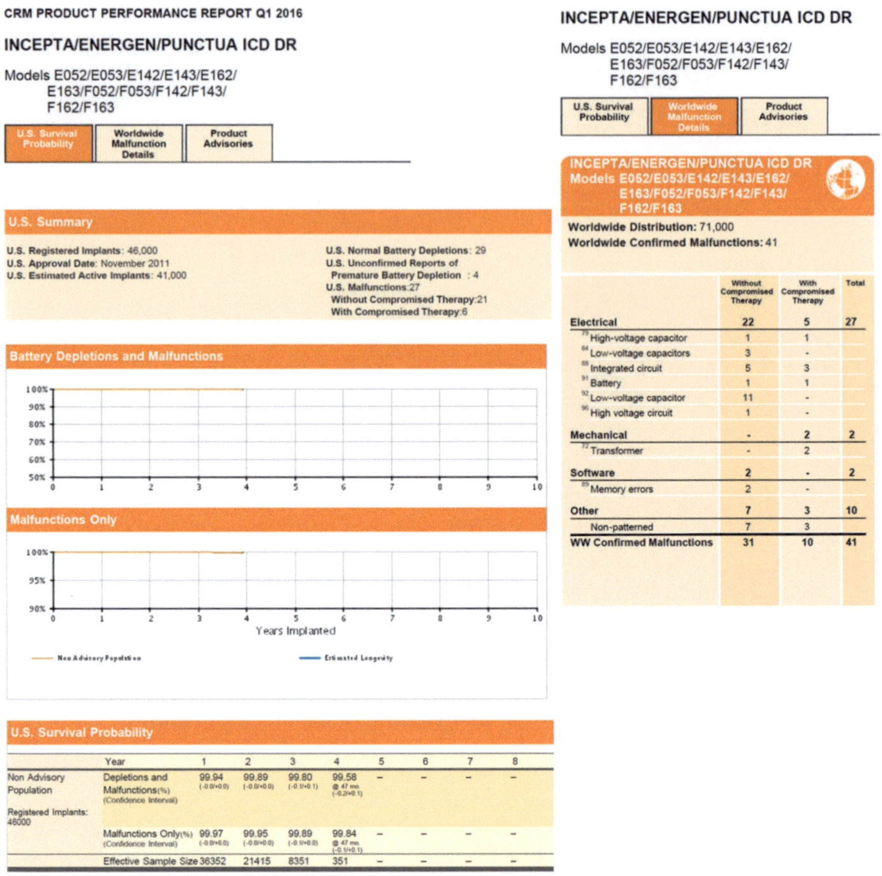

CRM PRODUCT PERFORMANCE REPORT Q1 2016

INCEPTA/ENERGEN/PUNCTUA ICD DR

Models E052/E053/E142/E143/E162/
E163/F052/F053/F142/F143/
F162/F163

U.S. Survival Probability | Worldwide Malfunction Details | Product Advisories

U.S. Summary

U.S. Registered Implants: 46,000
U.S. Approval Date: November 2011
U.S. Estimated Active Implants: 41,000

U.S. Normal Battery Depletions: 29
U.S. Unconfirmed Reports of Premature Battery Depletion : 4
U.S. Malfunctions:27
Without Compromised Therapy:21
With Compromised Therapy:6

Battery Depletions and Malfunctions

Malfunctions Only

U.S. Survival Probability

	Year	1	2	3	4	5	6	7	8
Non Advisory Population Registered Implants: 46000	Depletions and Malfunctions(%) (Confidence Interval)	99.94 (-0.0/+0.0)	99.89 (-0.0/+0.0)	99.80 (-0.1/+0.1)	99.58 @ 47 mo. (-0.2/+0.1)	–	–	–	–
	Malfunctions Only(%) (Confidence Interval)	99.97 (-0.0/+0.0)	99.95 (-0.0/+0.0)	99.89 (-0.1/+0.0)	99.84 @ 47 mo. (-0.1/+0.1)	–	–	–	–
	Effective Sample Size	36352	21415	8351	351	–	–	–	–

INCEPTA/ENERGEN/PUNCTUA ICD DR

Models E052/E053/E142/E143/E162/
E163/F052/F053/F142/F143/
F162/F163

U.S. Survival Probability | Worldwide Malfunction Details | Product Advisories

INCEPTA/ENERGEN/PUNCTUA ICD DR
Models E052/E053/E142/E143/E162/
E163/F052/F053/F142/F143/
F162/F163

Worldwide Distribution: 71,000
Worldwide Confirmed Malfunctions: 41

	Without Compromised Therapy	With Compromised Therapy	Total
Electrical	22	5	27
79 High-voltage capacitor	1	1	
84 Low-voltage capacitors	3	-	
88 Integrated circuit	5	3	
91 Battery	1	1	
92 Low-voltage capacitor	11	-	
96 High voltage circuit	1	-	
Mechanical	-	2	2
72 Transformer	-	2	
Software	2	-	2
89 Memory errors	2	-	
Other	7	3	10
Non-patterned	7	3	
WW Confirmed Malfunctions	31	10	41

Fig. 7.1 An example of a manufacturer product performance for a dual chamber defibrillator. Two pages have been combined to show overall life table performance and individual worldwide malfunctions. The life table analysis can only be done currently for the U.S. because patient data on death is available in the U.S. but not in other geographies

patient harms. Thus, an insulation failure, conductor fracture with intermittent loss of contact, intermittent cross talk may all be associated with inappropriate shocks in a defibrillator [1]. However, to clarify this, in the product performance reports, the products are listed by type of product, model, and actual malfunction. As a result of the variable patient manifestations, the best data on product performance does require detailed analysis of the products by engineering experts who can dismantle and electronically test the returned product. Unfortunately, and particularly for leads, it may pose incremental patient risk to extract the lead and return it, and accordingly, by AdvaMed convention leads are included in the Performance Report if there is adequate data from pulse generator interrogation, even if there is no returned product.

Lead Performance

Lead performance has been under greater regulatory scrutiny in the last decade because some lead recalls have become evident after some time, and consequentially have affected large numbers of patients long after initially going into service, and in most cases long after patient implant. Clinical events, as opposed to malfunction events are particularly important for leads in the first 90 days, with common issues like inability to place the lead (particularly Left Ventricular epicardial coronary venous leads), difficulty in obtaining adequate sensing and pacing values either acutely or after implant, perforation, and dislodgement. Over the longer term, insulation degradation (e.g. hydrolysis of polymers), weld or joint failures, and conductor fracture are issues that affect performance. For leads in particular, the performance is related to not only the device's characteristics, but also to the implant technique, and patient's characteristics (Fig. 7.2). Thus, some leads malfunction has been associated with medial subclavian cannulation resulting in crush between the clavicle and first rib. Patient factors which seem associated with lead malfunctions include young age, female gender, and increased ventricular contractility. However, other common issues are clinically based, and include progressive myocardial pathology post implant, such as myocardial infarction leading to loss of sensing and pacing functionality at the lead tissue interface. Some functional studies have shown loss of function overall at 10 years to be high for leads. In contrast, malfunction rates for leads may be expected to be overall about 1% per year, but critical malfunctions such as conductor fractures must occur at much lower rates to meet regulatory

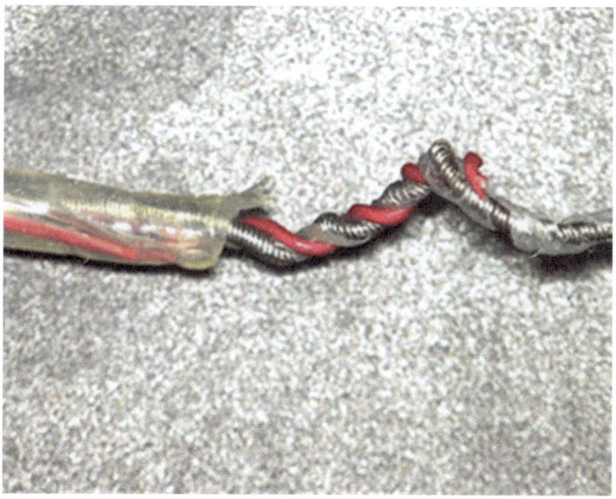

Fig. 7.2 Lead malfunction related to twiddler syndrome. In this syndrome the patient rotates the pulse generator repetitively, resulting in the leads being twisted, usually dislodging the leads from the heart, and in this case resulting in severe damage to the lead insulation with short circuit. This rare malfunction is usually entirely related to patient action

requirements, and when conductor fracture does occur, it usually is in association with clavicular first rib crush or an anchoring sleeve with a tight suture. Generally, since patient factors such as myocardial infarction or fibrosis at the lead tip tissue interface contribute to functional loss of lead pacing and sensing, these are not usually counted against the lead malfunction rate by manufacturers. It should be noted that with loss of lead function related to a clinical event, the patient still experiences all the same potential risks related to lead malfunction. Another characteristic of lead malfunction is that frequently, but not always, the malfunctions have a latency period of several years during which the lead appears to perform normally, and then as the lead ages, in part related to repetitive flexural stress, or degradation of the insulation, the lead malfunction rates increase exponentially later in the product's life. This non-linearity of lead malfunction rates makes a single malfunction rate quotation at 5 years highly misleading and incomplete, although it is consistent with accepted conventions.

Complications Related to Lead Malfunction

Pacemaker patient adverse events related to lead malfunction increase with factors such as: pacemaker dependence, ventricular lead failure (single and dual chamber devices), the abruptness of failure, and the lack of any detectable abnormality, such as non-physiologic signals or impedance change prior to malfunction. However, most patients do not have pacemaker dependence to the point of death with lead malfunction. Furthermore, with remote monitoring systems, there is often detectability of impending total lead failure with transient increases in impedance (open circuit) or reductions in impedance (with inner insulation failure) [1]. This intermittent manifestation of malfunction prior to complete and permanent loss of function is variable. For example, pacemaker lead failure which manifests as a high impedance, may trigger a polarity switch to the unipolar mode, which uses the inner conductor only, and if this conductor is still functioning, despite malfunction of the outer (anode) conductor, then the patient may have minimal symptoms. Symptoms may include palpitations (oversensing and undersensing), pre-syncope (brief loss of capture with pacemaker dependency), and syncope, prior to death if there is prolonged asystole (Fig. 7.3).

Defibrillator leads pose a higher risk of malfunction. This incremental risk is in part due to the greater structural and functional complexity of the lead, related to the high voltage portion of the lead which is used to deliver the shock to either cardiovert or defibrillate a patient. Failure to deliver sufficient energy to the cardiac tissue, either due to open circuit or short circuit, can result in death with no prior warning. It has been observed that the low amplitude test impedance measurements may fail to detect any abnormality, but when a high voltage shock is delivered for therapy, it may cause the insulation failure with current shunting, or

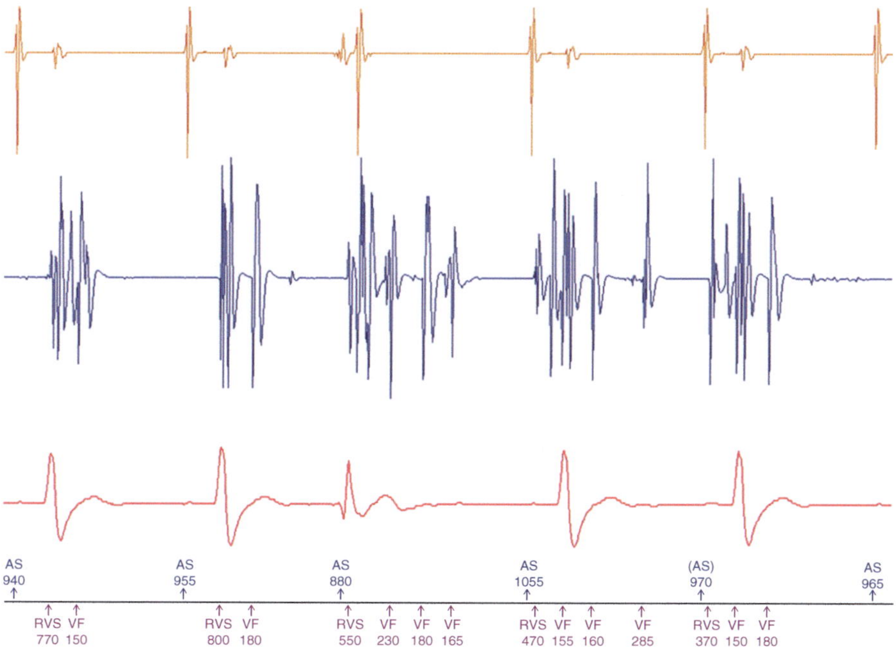

Fig. 7.3 Defibrillator lead malfunction. This lead, a part of a cardiac resynchronization system, demonstrates irregular high amplitude and high frequency content non-physiologic signals. These signals, related to lead malfunction, result in loss of cardiac resynchronization pacing and some inappropriate detections of tachycardia beats. Potential causes of this include intermittent break in the conductor continuity

disruption of the conductor with truncation of the high energy pulse (Fig. 7.4). The additional risk related to the pace/sense portion of a defibrillator lead is the oversensing of non-physiologic signals which may result in inappropriate shocks, induction of ventricular fibrillation with asynchronous shocks, and failure to detect ventricular tachyarrhythmias which also could result in death. Treatment of the malfunction can consist in either placement of an additional lead or extraction of the old lead and placement of a new lead. Extraction of leads is associated with small risks event in the hands of experienced physicians. On the other hand, leaving a failed lead in place may result in interference with sensing and or shocking, depending on the type of malfunction involved. Over time each additional lead across the tricuspid valve increases the risk of valve dysfunction, which can have serious consequences in patients with heart failure particularly in association with prior pulmonary hypertension. The physician needs to assess the risk of leaving a lead in place versus the risk of lead extraction in advising a patient on which approach to pursue. In the next chapter we consider the emotional impact that these difficult decisions with regards to leads extractions can have on patients.

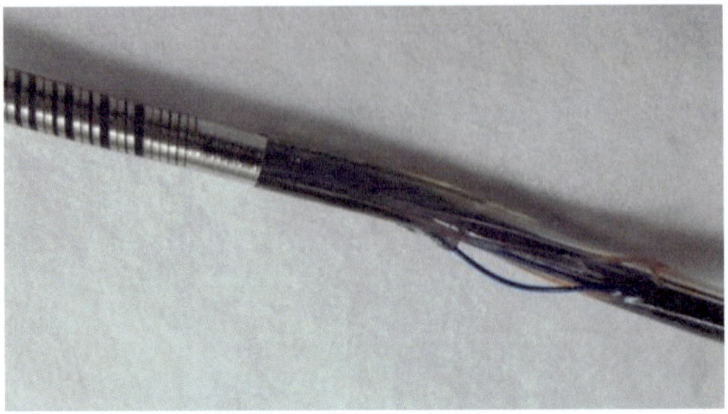

Fig. 7.4 A malfunction on a defibrillator lead. There is externalization of a high voltage conductor (*red arrow*). The insulation coating may be subject to subsequent flex failure, a high voltage short circuit between the distal and proximal conductor coil may occur. A high voltage coil is seen in close proximity to the conductor externalization. Mitigation for this externalization may take the form of taking the proximal conductor out of the circuit by programming shock vector to distal coil and can. However, the location of the external breech in conductor insulation in some cases can lead to shunting of current away from the myocardium, with the effect of leading to an increased energy requirement for successful defibrillation, even with removal of the proximal coil from the circuit

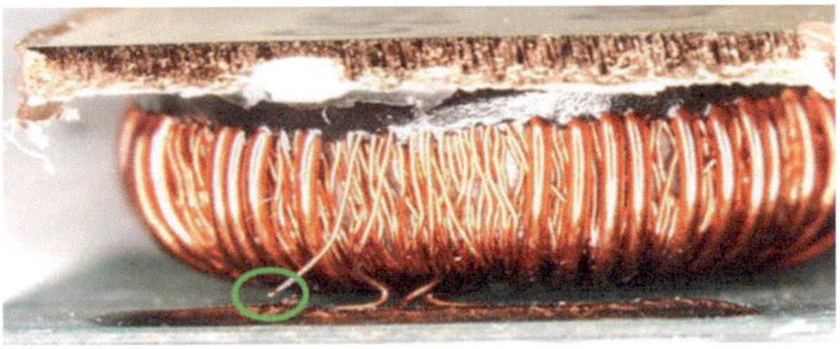

Fig. 7.5 An example of a pulse generator malfunction. The *green circle* shows the broken loose end of a transformer wire. Large primary windings and small secondary windings are seen. The loading of the secondary windings has to be done carefully. This transformer brings the delivered voltage up from the battery voltage of 2.8 V, to the voltage of about 800 V is delivered by the high voltage capacitor. Malfunction of the transformer results in inability to deliver high voltage defibrillation therapy and may be potentially life threatening. A short circuit in the transformer may release significant internal energy and damage other components

CIED Components

Pulse generators generically have batteries, capacitors, hybrid circuitry, analog and digital amplifiers, integrated circuitry, a transmission and receiving system, and memory [2]. The pulse generator and the leads are connected via feed through the header, which in turn connects to the leads. Malfunctions can occur with any of these components, many of which are rare and poorly understood by physicians and patients (Fig. 7.5). In general, the defibrillators with their high voltage circuitry

(ICD 800 V versus Pacemaker 7.5 V) tend to have higher malfunction rates of about 1% at 5 years compared to pacemakers, which tend to have rates less than 0.5% at 5 years. An FDA analysis suggested that half of all malfunctions are related to batteries and capacitors [3]. Some of these malfunctions may be detected by the safety architecture built into pulse generators, providing warning before all function is lost. Internal low impedance unanticipated circuits can trigger a high current consumption, which can automatically be detected by the pulse generator. Such current drain may occur, for example, through capacitors or the integrated circuits. In some capacitors the malfunction may have variable latency (occur late in product life) and a variable current drain, sometimes gradually draining the battery over the course of a year, which is generally detectable early, so that serious patient harm can be mitigated by device replacement. Other capacitors may have an infancy failure and may "heal" with use. Understanding of these failure modes is important for the device physician, as appropriate patient follow-up can often detect these issues long before therapy is actually compromised (i.e. no pacing or shock). In general, when a component failure is present and can or has impacted therapy delivery, management involves removal of the pulse generator when the risk of replacement of the generator is exceeded by the risk of leaving the generator in place. It was generally thought that generator replacements carried a very low risk, but the REPLACE trial [4] suggests that the risk is higher than commonly perceived by physicians, and needs to be considered in the management of some pulse generator malfunction issues.

Factors Affecting Patient Impact

The malfunction itself affects patient impact. Some malfunctions affect diagnostic information and may have minimal patient impact. As described earlier, at the opposite end of the spectrum, loss of high voltage defibrillator shock can result in sudden death in the worst case scenario. Early detectability of the malfunction can mitigate patient harm. Previously, we described the lead impedance and non-physiologic signals as means of early detection of lead malfunctions. Similarly, most pulse generators have a series of internal system checks to produce faults codes which identify internal component issues sometimes before loss of function. Physician factors affecting outcomes include frequency of office follow-ups with device interrogation, use of remote follow-ups to follow the device, lead implant technique, and programming which rarely interacts with specific failures. Patient factors may include: the need for pacing; the presence of a spontaneous escape rhythm if pacing fails; the frequency of life threatening ventricular arrhythmia; and compliance of the patient with follow-ups which decreases the potential exposure time to a malfunction before detection and correction by a physician. Software issues can often be corrected by downloading the corrective action via a programmer, although a software issue may very rarely have potentially catastrophic patient impact, this type of issue can usually be corrected with minimal patient impact through a slightly longer office visit. If necessary, the whole pulse generator can be replaced.

Is There Under-Reporting of Device Malfunctions?

The accurate analysis of malfunction rates depends on physicians, hospitals and industry sales representatives reporting events, interrogating devices (even post mortem), and returning explanted devices for manufacturer analysis. Failure to report at any stage can result in rate estimates which are lower than the actual malfunction rate. Most malfunctions may produce evidence on pulse generator interrogation with a programmer, such as a fault code, which may be traced to a certain type of general failure mode, and return analysis that can further narrow the malfunction to a discrete component. However, if the malfunction results in patient death with no warning the rate estimates may be significantly lower than the actual rate of malfunction. The reasons include: that few devices are interrogated post mortem; few devices are explanted and returned to the manufacturer post mortem; and in many cases the patient's underlying health may have been poor with heart failure, so the death is not unexpected. Clinical events such as lead perforation or dislodgement tend to be under reported particularly if they occur after the implantation procedure. Pulse generator and lead malfunctions tend to be very well reported while the pulse generators are under warranty, the motivation being that the hospital and/or the patient may receive a partial reimbursement for costs of a device to replace the malfunctioning one. However, late in the product's life, post warranty expiration it is unknown how efficiently malfunctions are reported. Internal analysis of remote follow-up data using the in-home patient device communicators can provide a comparison between malfunctions detected by active reporting compared to passive detection from the communicator without patient or physician participation. In this subset of patients with communicators, significant differences were not observed in malfunction rates on leads when passive communication was compared to physician and patient reporting.

Is CIED Quality Improving?

In the early 2000s there were several publications suggesting that defibrillator malfunction rates were increasing [3]. However, it should be noted that those devices went through a period of rapid development from single chamber, to cardiac resynchronization (three chamber), and added numerous features. When malfunctions rates are normalized to component number, the malfunctions rates did not seem to have increased. However, since 2007 there has been a progressive decline in issues with pulse generators. Pacemaker leads also have not had any large recalls in the last decade, but there have been two large defibrillator lead failures. Thus, it appears that device quality in general has improved over the last decade. Defibrillator leads remain a question mark, particularly as younger primary prevention patients receive these devices and survive for longer time periods, it is unclear what percentage of leads will not only be malfunction free in 20 years, but also fully functional. As a consequence of this, there has been the recent development and approval of new leadless pacemakers and defibrillators, which eliminate the need for intracardiac leads which are subjected to high numbers of flex cycles.

Does a Malfunction of a Pulse Generator Mean Loss of Function?

Most pulse generators models may have rare malfunctions which lead to loss of pacing or shock therapy. However, in most products there are an equal number of malfunctions which are not associated with loss of pacing or shock therapy (Fig. 7.1). It is a common patient and physician misconception that all pulse generator malfunctions mean that the patient is at immediate risk of death, however death is very rarely caused by malfunction. Today's devices often will detect and warn of issues long before there is therapy loss. This is particularly the case with slow internal current leaks of batteries and capacitors. However, high voltage capacitors and batteries can rarely have sudden catastrophic failure, and thus accurate information from the manufacturer to physicians on these issues is important in mitigating risk. Sudden loss of device power or loss of integrated circuit function is particularly dangerous, as it may be associated with the loss of the warning systems. That is, many device systems have beepers or patient stimulators which warn the patient that there is a serious issue. In addition there may be remote communicators in the patient's home which provide device status to the treating physician. Sometimes when there is an abrupt and catastrophic loss of power, these warning systems no longer function, and thus, some time may pass before the issue is detected, exposing the patient to the risk of no therapy. There are some systems which can detect such loss of device function.

Conclusions

CIED malfunction rates have declined in the last decade. Although there have been defibrillator lead recalls involving large numbers of patients in these same years, it is important to remember that most of these leads still continue to function normally, and the leads which fail, usually have manifestations that permit detection before serious patient harm occurs. The pulse generators have increased in sophistication, thought a small numbers of malfunctions continue to occur, and physicians continue to learn about these. It is important to maintain regular patient and device follow-ups and encourage remote device follow-ups in order to maximize early detection of potential malfunctions, and hence minimize the risk of patient harm.

References

1. Swerdlow CD, Asirvatham SJ, Ellenbogen KA, Friedman PA. Troubleshooting implanted cardioverter defibrillator sensing problems I. Circ Arrhythm Electrophysiol. 2014;7:1237–61. doi:10.1161/CIRCEP.114.002344.
2. Doshi H, Reddy S, Root M, Sharma AD. Engineering aspects of pacemakers and leads. Chapter 30. In: Saksena S, Camm AJ, editors. Electrophysiologic disorders of the heart: expert consult. Elsevier/Saunders; 2012. isbn 1437702856, 9781437702859.
3. Maisel WH, Moynahan M, Zuckerman BD, Gross TP, Tovar OH, Tillman D-B, Schultz DB. Pacemaker and ICD generator malfunctions: analysis of food and drug administration annual reports. JAMA. 2006;295(16):1901–6. doi:10.1001/jama.295.16.1901.
4. Poole JE, Gleva MJ, Mela T, Chung MK, et al. for the REPLACE Registry Investigators. Complication rates associated with pacemaker or implantable cardioverter-defibrillator generator replacements and upgrade procedures: results from the REPLACE registry. Circulation. 2010;122:1553–61. doi:10.1161/CIRCULATIONAHA.110.976076.

Chapter 8
Psychological Effects of Device Recalls and Advisories in Patients with Implantable Cardioverter Defibrillators

Bianca D'Antono, Teresa Kus, and Audrey Charneux

Abstract Implantable cardioverter defibrillators (ICD) are subject to technical failures. The current chapter reviews the impact of the resulting public advisories on patient psychological welfare and quality of life.

Despite the paucity of research on the impact of ICD advisories, available data suggest that ICD advisories, involving either possible generator or lead malfunction, result in limited long-term adverse psychosocial effects in most patients. This appears particularly true in patients followed in supportive device clinics where provision of prompt information, counselling, and reassurance is provided by healthcare professionals. Individuals dependent on the ICD for pacing or requiring more intensive interventions (such as device replacement) following the advisory may be more vulnerable to increased distress, as may patients who have experienced inappropriate shocks. Additional counselling or psychological support in these patients may be required.

As research to date has relied mostly on small single-center observational ad hoc studies, more reliable information is required to confirm these impressions. Ideally, patient-reported outcomes would need to be routinely and repeatedly assessed and included within national registries.

Moreover, research on the psychosocial impact of advisories is consistent with other research in ICD patients, showing significant impairments in QoL and psychological status in many patients that persist for years, independently of advisories.

B. D'Antono, Ph.D. (✉)
Research Center, Montreal Heart Institute,
5000 Belanger Street, Montreal, QC H1T 1C8, Canada

Department of Psychology, Université de Montréal, Montreal, QC, Canada
e-mail: bianca.d.antono@umontreal.ca

T. Kus, M.D., Ph.D.
Cardiology Department, Hôpital du Sacré-Cœur de Montréal, Montreal, QC, Canada

Pharmacology and Physiology Department, Université de Montréal, Montreal, QC, Canada

A. Charneux, M.A.
Research Center, Montreal Heart Institute,
5000 Belanger Street, Montreal, QC H1T 1C8, Canada

© Springer International Publishing AG 2017

R. Proietti et al. (eds.), *Psychological, Emotional, Social and Cognitive Aspects of Implantable Cardiac Devices*, DOI 10.1007/978-3-319-55721-2_8

The psychosocial experiences of many patients are not adequately attended to, and this may contribute to a worse prognosis.

Information gleaned from research on this issue could facilitate physician-patient decision-making and lead to improved psychological support for patients whose devices are under advisory as well as those considering ICD therapy for the first time.

Keywords ICD • Advisory • Psychological distress • Depression • Anxiety • Depression • Quality of life

The implantable cardioverter defibrillator (ICD) has become the mainstay of therapy for the prevention of sudden death in patients with a history of ventricular arrhythmias, reducing overall mortality by 28% [1]. Implantation of this device is also recommended for the primary prevention of sudden death in patients at high risk of lethal ventricular arrhythmias. A benefit of 25–30% reduction of all-cause mortality has been noted in these cases [2].

Despite its life saving potential, a growing body of literature suggests that the costs of coping with a potentially life-threatening condition, in addition to the implantation of such a device and the possibility (0.4–2.3%) of procedure-related complications such as lead dislodgement, pneumothorax, infection and bleeding [3] and subsequent painful and sometimes inappropriate shock therapy may negatively impact patients' psychological health, as well as that of their partners [4–6]. Most notably, elevated rates of depression, anxiety, somatization, and phobic disorders have been reported, particularly among individuals receiving more frequent or intense shocks.

An additional challenge to patients' physical and psychological health can also result from the possibility that some devices do not perform as designed, either because of potential generator (battery) or lead (shock delivery system) failure. When such failures are observed in real life or through laboratory bench testing [7–10], device advisories may be issued to inform medical device users of the increased risk of device failure. Since 1997, several companies have been required to issue advisories for their ICDs, including Guidant [Indianapolis, IN, USA], St. Jude Medical [St. Paul, MN, USA], Medtronic [Minneapolis, MN, USA] and Sorin [France] for either generator malfunction involving unanticipated or rapid battery depletion [8, 9] or for lead malfunction due to internal wire fracture [7] or insulation breaks [10].

Device Advisory Categories

The FDA has categorized advisories for medical devices (which include ICD components) into three categories: Class 1, 2, and 3 [11]. Class 1 advisories refer to "dangerous or defective products with reasonable probability of causing serious health problems or death". Class 2 advisories involve "products that might cause a temporary health problem, or pose a slight threat of a serious nature". Class 3 advisories apply to "products that are unlikely to cause any adverse health reaction, but that violate Food and Drug Administration labeling or manufacturing regulation".

In the case of ICDs, three deficiencies typically justify the issue of advisories, and are for the most part of the Class 1 or Class 2 category. Prior to 2007, most advisories involved premature or sudden battery (generator) failure occurring in a small fraction of devices (.009–2.6% over a follow-up of 24 months) [12]. This could result in loss of function of the device and therefore failure to recognize ventricular arrhythmia and deliver therapy. These typically fell within Class 2 advisories. In the case of patients requiring bradycardia support, however, generator failure could have serious consequences such as syncope. Since 2007, more serious Class 1 advisories have been issued involving lead failure that could potentially cause patient harm and death [7, 10]. While a complete break in the high-voltage component of the lead could cause a failure of shock delivery in the case of a ventricular arrhythmia, a sense/pace component fracture would result in the detection of electrical noise which could be inappropriately diagnosed as ventricular arrhythmia requiring shock therapy. The patient could thus experience repeated shocks while fully conscious and in normal sinus rhythm. These inappropriate shocks delivered during normal rhythm could result in the induction of ventricular arrhythmias and cause death [13]. In one study of three implanting centers, 13% of Sprint Fidelis leads had failed at a 4-year follow-up [13]. Although no deaths occurred as a result of lead malfunction in this cohort of patients, inappropriate and repeated shocks were frequently reported prior to lead replacement. Since approximately 268,000 such leads have been implanted world-wide and the failure rate is expected to increase with time since implant, this type of dysfunction is of serious concern. This is all the more serious considering shock delivery is one of the most anxiety-provoking concerns for ICD patients [14, 15].

Medical Response to Device Advisories

When an advisory is issued, the affected model is recalled and all products not yet implanted are sent back to the responsible manufacturer. What should be done with the generators or leads that have already been implanted is subject to debate. The approach will vary from center to center and depend on the indication, whether the ICD was implanted as primary or secondary prevention. In the case of primary prevention, it will also depend on whether the device has already been called upon to treat ventricular arrhythmia. The decision will also be influenced by whether or not the patient is pacemaker dependent and requires bradycardia support.

The recent availability of home monitoring technologies that permit daily wireless battery and lead evaluation through cellular communication with a manufacturer-run website has revolutionized the approach to devices under advisory. However, in the case of early advisories, when home monitoring was not available and which mainly involved early or sudden battery depletion, an aggressive approach to replacement of the devices was adopted mainly in those treated for secondary prevention of ventricular arrhythmia or in those who were pacemaker dependent. Gould and Krahn [12] reported on complications associated with such generator replacement in 17 Canadian surveyed centers. Of 2915 devices, 18% were replaced. Major complications occurred in 5.6% of replacements, requiring re-operation for major hematoma or pocket infection and included two deaths from sepsis or concomitant lead extraction.

The approach to the more recent Class 1 advisories involving possible lead malfunction has also varied from center to center. However, the development of more sophisticated Lead Integrity Alert software and the introduction of intense follow-up with home monitoring technology has contributed to a more conservative approach with intervention occurring usually only in the case of demonstrated lead dysfunction or in pacemaker dependent patients. This avoids the published complication rate of 20% associated with prophylactic lead extraction and replacement or the 9% rate associated with lead abandonment and addition of a new lead [16]. A more recent publication [17] evaluating lead replacement in two high volume centers have reported lower major complication rates of slightly less than 2% for either the St Jude Riata lead or the Medtronic Sprint Fidelis lead, suggesting that a learning curve plays a significant role in the higher complication rates reported by smaller centers. This approach however leaves the patient with a potentially defective lead in anticipation for the first signs of lead dysfunction. With such a conservative approach, despite optimal lead integrity monitoring, Morrison et al. [13] reported that 38 of 85 Fidelis lead failures in their cohort of patients were associated with inappropriate shocks.

Psychological Impact of ICD Advisories

Given the potential life-threatening consequences of ICD malfunction and the increased media attention given to these advisories, being informed that one's ICD may be at risk of malfunction or requires replacement could contribute to increased psychological distress and impoverished quality of life in patients already vulnerable to psychopathology. Particularly worrisome has been the clinical observation that some patients have refused ICD implantation for primary or secondary prevention as a result of the negative publicity that advisories have received in the press. In light of such developments, Gibson et al. [18] have underlined the importance of increasing our understanding of the impact of device advisories on patients' experiences. Information gleaned from research on this issue could facilitate physician-patient decision-making and lead to improved psychological support for patients whose devices are under advisory as well as those considering ICD therapy for the first time.

As can be seen in Table 8.1, there is surprisingly little research on the impact of ICD advisories on patients' psychological functioning and quality of life. Most of the earlier research was performed on small samples of patients with ICDs. While more recent investigations have employed larger samples, only two investigations recruited from multiple sites, raising continued concerns regarding the generalizability of the findings. Moreover, this literature has produced conflicting results, which may reflect the heterogeneity of research (sample characteristics, measures, and study design) and clinical approaches used, as well as the type of advisory issued.

Nine of the twelve studies performed to date have been case control studies, in which investigators compared patients with an ICD under advisory (cases) with a group of patients with ICDs not under advisory (controls). The use of such a control group serves to better isolate the effects of the recall upon individuals who are otherwise experiencing the same challenges associated with their medical condition and treatment. Only five studies adopted a prospective or longitudinal design, which has unfortunately limited the acquisition of knowledge pertaining to the evolution of quality of life and psychological symptoms in patients with (or without) an ICD under advisory. In all but one study, data was obtained only after the issuance of the advisory. Most investigations evaluated psychological status months to years following the issuance of the advisory. As such, it is impossible to confirm that any elevations in distress are a result of the advisory. Similarly, lack of distress may be confounded by the elapse of time, which may have permitted a certain level of adaptation to occur. Despite these limitations, some understanding of patients' experiences can be gleaned from the literature, as described below.

Cuculi et al. [19] were among the first to investigate the psychological impact of ICD advisories. They compared 30 patients with an ICD under advisory to 25 patients with an ICD not under advisory. Cases were evaluated on the same day as the system control was performed on their ICD, shortly after the issuance of the advisory. The controls were evaluated during the same time period as cases, but no information was provided as to their manner of recruitment or testing. No significant differences between the two groups were observed on any of the composite scores and most of the subscales. However, patients in the control group reported significantly more obsessive-compulsive behaviour, hostility, and paranoid ideation. While counterintuitive, these differences may simply reflect the greater percentage of patients in the control group who had a personal or family history of sudden cardiac death, though this possibility was not examined by the authors of that study. Alternatively, the control patients who agreed to participate in the study may have been somewhat more distressed and eager to share their experiences compared to those who declined participation. As participation rates were not provided, it is impossible to know whether this represents a viable explanation.

Undavia et al. [20], for their part, compared the quality of life and symptoms of anxiety and depression in 61 patients whose ICD was under advisory with those of 43 control patients. No significant group differences emerged in their sample. Similarly, no significant increases in reported fear of shocks or death among patients with an ICD under recall were reported. Differences in patient assessment period and procedure may have contributed to reducing differences in psychological status between the two groups. Indeed, patients whose ICD was under advisory were evaluated by phone compared with controls who were evaluated at the clinic during a

Table 8.1 Summary of investigations on the psychosocial impact of ICD advisories

Authors/Country	Advisory	Sample details	Response rate	Study design
Sneed et al. (1994)	Cardiac Pacemakers Inc Ventak Models Failure within the generator	N = 31 advisory group (M_{age} = 61, 81% men) N = 21 caregivers (M_{age} = 62, 19% men)	100%	Prospective 1 month interval
Cuculi et al. (2006) Switzerland	Class I advisory Guidant Corporation	N = 30 advisory group (M_{age} = 62, 87% men) N = 25 controls (M_{age} = 60, 88% men)	Not available	Cross-sectional Case-control
van den Broek et al. (2006) Netherlands	Class II advisory Medtronic Battery depletion	N = 33 advisory group (M_{age} = 60, 98% men)	90%	Prospective Mean of 14.4 ± 4 months between assessments
Gibson et al. (2008) Virginia, United States	Class I and II advisories 35% Medtronic 23% St Jude Medical 42% Guidant	N = 31 advisory group (M_{age} = 63; 71% men) N = 50 controls (M_{age} = 63; 68% men)	89%	Cross-sectional Case-control
Undavia et al. (2008) NY, United States	Class I & II Advisories re: generators Companies touched by advisories not mentioned	N = 61 advisory group (M_{age} = 67; 70% men) N = 43 controls (M_{age} = 65; 65% men)	90%	Cross-sectional

Announcement	Time of psychological assessment after issuance of the advisory	Measures	Endpoint	Impact
Manufacturer sent out letters to physicians Patients were informed of the advisory at the next scheduled clinic visit Informed by same physician and nurse for consistency	Promptly after learning of the advisory & 1 month later	VAS	Confidence Fear Anger Depression Anxiety Helplessness Loss of control Uncertainty Confusion	• Increase in anxiety over the 1-month follow-up • Significant decrease in confidence of patients and caregivers • Caregivers had greater negative responses to recalls compared to patients, especially caregivers of patients who had received shocks
Information letter sent out about advisory notification and possible consequences	Shortly after the issuance of advisory (details not provided) Evaluation performed on same day as the system control for the device	BSI	Psychological distress	• Cases = controls in terms of psychological symptoms
Media (public report)	Before and after extra device evaluation <2 months	STAI	Anxiety	• Significant increase in proportion of advisory group to experience clinically significant levels of anxiety following public announcement compared to post-implantation (6.1% vs. 24.2%)
Patients had received a letter from their physician and were then seen in clinic	For 84% of advisory group, >4 months	PHQ SF-36 health survey	Emotional distress QoL	• No differences were found in symptoms of depression, anxiety, alcohol abuse, somatization, and QoL between advisory and control groups • When asked how felt about the advisory: 36% anxious, 13% sad, 13% angry, 23% frustrated
	M_{time} = 7.6 months	HADS Heart Disease Health-Related QoL (HRQL) Questionnaire Home questionnaire	Anxiety Depression QoL ICD-related concerns Trust toward the health-care system	• No difference in the QoL, nor in levels of anxiety and depression between cases and controls • No group difference in ICD-related concern • In both groups, there was a slightly reduced degree of trust toward the health-care industry • QoL was slightly worse overall among Class I versus Class II advisory groups

(continued)

Table 8.1 (continued)

Authors/Country	Advisory	Sample details	Response rate	Study design
Birnie et al. (2009) Ontario, Canada	Class II Advisory Medtronic Battery depletion	N = 86 advisory group (M_{age} = 68, 72% males) N = 94 controls (M_{age} = 65; 72% males)	Advisory group: 70.5% Controls: 70.1%	Cross-sectional Case-Control
Fisher et al. (2009) NY, USA	24% Medtronic, 52% Guidant/Boston scientific devices 24% St. Judes Medical devices Battery depletion	N = 100 advisory group (age not provided. 78% men)	27% of patients with ICDs under advisory at their clinic	Prospective
Keren et al. (2011) Ontario, Canada	Class 1 Advisory Medtronic Risk of lead fracture	N = 273 advisory group N = 249 advisory group without lead facture (M_{age} = 67, 84,7% men) N = 24 advisory group with lead fracture (M_{age} = 68, 83.2% men) N = 143 Control group (M_{age} = 61, 87.5% men)	Advisory group without fracture : 74% Advisory group with lead fracture: 92% Controls: 62%	Cross-sectional Case-control Significant group differences across several clinical and demographic variables
Pederson et al. (2011) Denmark	Class 1 Advisory Medtronic Risk of lead fracture	N = 207 advisory group Notified by letter (N = 74, M_{age} = 63, 89% men) Notified at clinic visit (N = 133, M_{age} = 62, 85% men) N = 510 controls (M_{age} = 64; 82% men)	Advisory group—% unknown Control group 84%	Cross-sectional Case-control
Heatherly et al. (2011) North Carolina, USA	Class 1 Advisory Medtronic Risk for lead fracture	N = 158 advisory group (M_{age} = 67, 74% men) N = 255 controls (M_{age} = 67, 71% men)	Advisory group: 92.8% Controls: 94%	Cross-sectional Case-control Multi-site

Announcement	Time of psychological assessment after issuance of the advisory	Measures	Endpoint	Impact
Media, followed by a call to receive a lecture on implications of the advisory (group format) and individual meeting with physician	M_{time} = 32 months after advisory	FPAS (by mail)	Device acceptance	• No evidence of reduced patient acceptance of devices in advisory group and control group
Media and physicians (roughly half and half)	Immediately after counselling regarding the advisory as well as 6 months later After counselling, provided a retrospective account of the worry experienced upon learning about the advisory as well as worry experiences following the session	Home worry scale	Level of worry	• After learning of the advisory, patients showed a moderate level of worry • Level of worry decreased significantly after counselling • Woman initially more worried than men, but not 6 months after counselling • Patients whose ICDs required replacement showed less effect of counselling and were significantly more worried than other patients
Immediately after advisory: one hour special information session at the clinic followed by individual session with device clinic specialist	13 months after advisory Completed via mail	HADS FPAS FSAS	Symptoms of anxiety and depression Device acceptance ICD shock-related anxiety	• Advisory group who did not experience a lead failure did not differ from control group on any of the measures of psychological functioning • Advisory group with lead fracture reported greater anxiety, fear of shocks, and poor device acceptance compared to group without lead fracture – appeared to be due to inappropriate shocks
By letter, calling patients in for an urgent clinical follow-up visit, or ad hoc during a routine clinical visit	Advisory group: 23–24 months after recall Control group: had completed the same questionnaires for a previous study (unknown whether within the same time frame)	HADS ICDC FPAS MLHFQ SF-36	Symptoms of anxiety and depression ICD related concerns Device acceptance Health-related QoL	• Advisory group did not differ significantly from controls on depression, anxiety, device acceptance, and health status • Advisory group reported fewer ICD concerns and better mental health status compared to controls
Letter from manufacturer notifying of the advisory Seen in clinic to adjust impedance monitoring; Told to contact clinic if audible alarm or shocks; Current risk estimates relayed; No other counselling provided	Most <18 months after initial advisory notification	ICDC	ICD-related concerns QoL	• Advisory group scored higher on ICD-related concerns compared to control group

(continued)

Table 8.1 (continued)

Authors/Country	Advisory	Sample details	Response rate	Study design
D`Antono et al. (2013) Quebec, Canada	Class 1 Advisory Medtronic ICD lead	N = 114 advisory group of which: N = 90 Self-surveillance (M_{age} = 65, 79% men) N = 24 CareLink weekly surveillance (M_{age} = 70, 79 % men) N = 46 case-matched controls (M_{age} = 69, 85% men)	86%	Prospective Longitudinal Case-control
Larsen et al. (2014) Denmark	Class 1 Advisory St Jude Medical Riata Risk of insulation defects in the lead	N = 256 advisory group (M_{age} = 68, 82 % men) N = 256 controls (M_{age} = 68, 82% men)	Advisory group: Baseline 86% 12-month 70% Controls: only one time point included	Prospective nationwide (5 centre) cohort study Case-control Case-matched controls

BDI-II Beck Depression Inventory II, *BSI* Brief Symptom Inventory, *FPAS* Florida Patient Acceptance Survey, *FSAS* Florida Shock Anxiety Scale, *GAD* Generalized Anxiety Disorder Questionnaire, *HADS* Hospital Anxiety and Depression Scale, *ICDC* ICD patient concerns questionnaire, *MLHFQ* Minnesota Living with Heart Failure Questionnaire, *PHQ* Patient-Health questionnaire, *STAI* State-Trait Anxiety Inventory, *VAS* visual analog scale

Announcement	Time of psychological assessment after issuance of the advisory	Measures	Endpoint	Impact
Met by a cardiologist who explained the need for and implications of the change in the surveillance system	<1.5 years after advisory notification but immediately before being told that the automatic lead surveillance system put in place had been inadequate in warning of impending failure; and 1 and 6 months after programming of lead monitoring was optimized	STAI BDI-II SF-36 Home questionnaire	Anxiety Depression QoL ICD-related concerns	• Advisory group = control group on anxiety level, depressive symptoms, and ICD-related concerns at baseline and F/U • At baseline, advisory group self-surveilling for alarm: greater limitation due to body pain vs. control • At baseline, Carelink advisory group—significantly more limitations in social functioning because of physical or emotional problems vs. other groups • Advisory group (Carelink and alarm) significantly less satisfied with ICD lead surveillance at follow-up than baseline • QoL impaired across subscales in all groups • Significant reduction of QoL related to body pain at final evaluation compared to first two evaluations • Symptoms of depression (31%) anxiety (48%) in ICD patients
First notified by letter, and provided with more details at the discretion of the physician during the first outpatient visit(no media coverage) No recommendation for psychological counselling	In advisory group: shortly after advisory issuance 12-month follow-up in advisory group	FPAS-12 ICDC PHQ-9 GAD-7 Single item VAS	Device acceptance ICD-related concerns Symptoms of depression Symptoms of anxiety (in advisory group only) Impact on well-being (in advisory group only)	At baseline, shortly following the advisory: • Slightly higher device-related concerns and greater general anxiety in advisory group • Women experienced more adverse effects as a result of the advisory At follow-up in the advisory group: • Slight improvement in device-related concerns

routine follow-up. Patients often experience transient increases in anxiety during clinical appointments, related among other factors, to fear of obtaining "bad news". This may have inflated distress in the control patients as compared to their usual levels. This is consistent with the fact that controls actually tended towards higher, not lower, anxiety scores compared to cases in this study ($p = 0.10$). Moreover, patients with ICDs under advisory were evaluated a mean of 7.6 months post issuance of the advisory which could have allowed patients sufficient time to adapt, in essence, reducing any advisory-related increases in distress.

Nonetheless, other investigations have since failed to observe significant group differences in quality of life [18], distress [21], fear of shocks [21] and device acceptance [21, 22] between advisory patients and controls. In the cross-sectional study by Birnie et al. [22], performed more than 2 years after the advisory, it is impossible to exclude the possibility that the advisory had increased distress in patients which they resolved by the time of testing. The authors also suggest that a response bias may have been introduced, as more anxious patients in the advisory group may have been more likely to refuse to participate compared to less anxious patients, though this could not be verified. If true, this could have reduced the probability that group differences could be observed. In a prospective study by our group ([23]; described later), ICD patients who dropped out over the 7-month follow-up period were indeed more likely to be depressed and anxious.

In contrast to the above investigations, two small prospective studies found evidence for increased anxiety in patients with an ICD under advisory [24, 25]. As part of a larger study on the psychological impact of ICD implantation, Van den Broek et al. [25] administered the State subscale of the State-Trait Anxiety Inventory (STAI) to 33 patients following device implantation as well as following the public advisory announcement (and extra device evaluation) for possible rapid battery depletion of Medtronic products. This evaluation took place a mean of 14 months following the baseline assessment, and within two months of the advisory announcement. A significant increase in the number of patients who reported clinically significant levels of anxiety (6.1% versus 24.2%) was noted following the advisory.

Furthermore, one of the largest cross-sectional studies performed to date reported greater ICD patient concerns in patients with an ICD under advisory ($N = 158$) versus those with an ICD not under advisory ($N = 255$) [26]. The ICD Patient Concerns Questionnaire (ICDC), used to measure "patients' overall perceptions of their device and quality of life, as well as device-specific concerns" was completed within 14 months of the advisory.

In another study that failed to find significant group differences in psychological distress and quality of life, patients with an ICD under advisory nonetheless reported negative emotions as a result of the recall: 36% of recall patients reported feeling anxious/nervous, 13% reported feeling sad, 13% reported feeling angry, and 23% reported feeling frustrated [18]. That these experiences did not lead to group differences in more general measures of psychological distress or quality of life is surprising. It is possible that increased distress observed in some patients may otherwise have been obscured by the use of group analyses, particularly in this small sample. Gibson et al. [18] further hypothesized that device advisories may specifically impact ICD-related distress rather than general distress, and lead to decreased confidence in their device while increasing other fears that may contribute to or exacerbate hypervigilance of somatic symptoms, avoidance, and catastrophic thinking. As mentioned by the authors, "although these concerns may not result in an identifiable psychiatric diagnosis, they may have an impact on behaviour and adjustment which is not captured by many assessment instruments".

Pedersen et al. [27], for their part, obtained mixed results. They compared 207 patients with an ICD under advisory to 510 controls on multiple general and ICD-specific questionnaires. Using a Bonferoni-adjusted clinical significance level of 0.0038, patients with a device under advisory did not differ from controls on mean scores of depression, anxiety, and health status. However, they reported *fewer* ICD concerns and *better* mental health than controls. Surprisingly, patients with an ICD under advisory also tended to show more device acceptance ($p = 0.023$) and vitality ($p = 0.016$). However, in a larger, more recent prospective nationwide cohort study pertaining to a different lead advisory, this same group obtained opposite results [28]. More specifically, patients whose ICD was under advisory reported significantly more device-related concerns (particularly concerns regarding shock therapy) as well as less device acceptance as compared to a contemporary control group matched for age, sex, and implant indication. There were no differences in symptoms of depression. However, on a one-item question regarding the impact of the advisory on well-being, women scored more than twice that of men. Whether this means that women have a greater difficulty coping with an ICD under advisory or, as the authors suggest, that they are more willing to report their distress compared to men is open to question. Furthermore, prospective analyses indicated that device-related concerns decreased over time, while other measures remained stable. These conflicting findings obtained by the same research team for two different lead advisories may reflect methodological differences across the two studies but may also represent the specific nature of the lead abnormalities involved in those investigations. In the case of Pederson et al. [27] which dealt with patients under the Medtronic Sprint Fidelis Lead Advisory, potential lead abnormalities could be well identified once a more sophisticated lead monitoring program and alarm system notification were downloaded into their ICD. The study by Larsen et al. [28] dealt with the Riata Lead Advisory. Defective functioning of the lead for this advisory was not always observable despite demonstration of inner lead externalization outside the outer isolation envelope through fluoroscopic or X-ray examination. Thus, management of this potentially defective device was challenging, and as suggested by the authors, may have contributed to reduced device acceptance and increased device-related concerns. Of course, no data was available on these measures prior to the advisory. It is thus impossible to conclude that this outcome was necessarily a result of the advisory.

ICD Advisory Category and Psychological Status

These conflicting results may reflect differences in the severity of the advisory issued. Only one study examined this issue. Undavia et al. [20] compared 43 patients subject to a Class I advisory (i.e., the most life threatening) to 18 patients with a Class II advisory on measures of anxiety, depression, and quality of life. There were no significant differences in symptoms of anxiety or depression. However, ICD patients under a class I advisory reported a slightly reduced quality of life across physical, social and emotional domains. While Class I advisory patients were significantly more likely to undergo defective component replacement, this did not appear to explain their impoverished quality of life compared to those subject to a Class 2 advisory.

ICD-Related Patient Characteristics and Distress Following an Advisory

In general, few differences in psychological profile emerged as a function of ICD-related patient characteristics. Whether the ICD had been implanted for primary versus secondary prevention did not lead to group differences in distress [20, 29]. Patients who experienced electrical storms (repeated shocks due to frequently recurring ventricular arrhythmias) or had a history of shock delivery tended to score lower on device acceptance and higher on ICD concerns [19, 22, 26], but this was true across both cases and controls. Similarly, patients with more dyspnea due to congestive heart failure (NYHA 2 versus NYHA 1) and lower ejection fraction tended to show greater distress across all groups [19]. On the other hand, Fisher et al. [29] did report that pace-dependent patients tended to be more worried following the advisory compared to others.

Learning About the Advisory

Patients usually first learn about the advisory from the media or their physician. However, in a study using vignettes to evaluate patient preferences for ICD recall strategies, patients seemed to prefer to learn about it from their physician [30]. Hearing first from the media had indeed increased distress in some patients in the study by van den Broek et al. [25]. On the other hand, others have not observed any differences in patient-reported outcomes according to mode of notification [29].

Pederson et al. [27] compared patients who were informed by letter calling them in for an urgent clinical follow-up visit to patients who were informed of the Medtronic Sprint Fidelis advisory during their next routinely scheduled follow-up clinical visit. In both cases, notification of the advisory was performed by physicians.

Using a very stringent significance level, the authors reported no difference in patient reported outcomes, other than a trend for patients who were notified at their routine follow-up visit of the advisory to report more ICD related concerns ($p = .035$) when tested nearly 2 years after the advisory issuance. No other trends were observed. According to the authors, the source (e.g., physician, manufacturer, news media, etc.) and type of information provided may be more important than the mode of debriefing in predicting patient-reported outcomes. At this stage, however, it is difficult to draw any firm conclusions regarding who should provide the information and when given the absence of large-scale well-designed studies [27].

Of note, however, Gibson et al. [18] reported that despite the fact that all advisory patients in their study had been informed of the advisory in writing and then in person by their physician, only 61% recalled learning of the advisory from their physician when questioned at a later date. This may suggest a need to verify patient understanding of the information they receive during the visit in which they are told of the advisory, and the need to repeat the information as needed in subsequent visits. As mentioned earlier, patients are frequently anxious when meeting their physicians, and this may decrease their attention and memory of the details provided. This may be all the more true when receiving news that threatens their well-being and that may lead to emotion-focused approaches such as denial as a means to cope with this information [31].

When Surveillance Methods for ICDs Under Advisory Do Not Work

As mentioned previously, it is frequently decided not to replace potentially defective ICDs but rather to follow the devices using stringent surveillance methods. However, these surveillance methods may occasionally fail to appropriately detect defective ICDs. For example, in the case of the Medtronic 6949 Lead Advisory, the surveillance method initially put in place had been found inadequate in detecting possible lead fractures [32]. We evaluated the psychological impact on 114 patients exposed to the dual stress of having an ICD that is at risk of malfunction and finding out that the surveillance method was inadequate [23]. We also examined the evolution of their psychological status over a 6-month period after downloading a new Lead Integrity Alert algorithm into their device. Patients with a Fidelis lead under advisory were evaluated in the clinic immediately before being informed of the suboptimal surveillance of their device (±1.5 years after the advisory) as well as 1 and 6 months later. Case-matched patients with ICDs not under advisory were recruited and tested within the same time frame. Measures of anxiety, depression, ICD-related concerns and quality of life were obtained. Patients with a lead under advisory did not differ significantly from case controls in their quality of life, nor in symptoms of anxiety or depression prior to notification. Nor did they differ on ICD-related concerns. These results are consistent with those of several other researchers mentioned earlier [18–22, 27], suggesting that while being subject to an advisory may increase distress acutely [25], it may not lead to sustained psychological difficulties beyond those already seen in patients with ICDs. Any additional distress caused by notification of suboptimal surveillance of their ICD appeared quickly coped with as reflected in the continued absence of group differences and lack of significant changes in anxiety and depression at the 1- and 6-month follow-ups.

Impact of Surveillance Methods Following an Advisory

The manner in which the surveillance is effected may also contribute to patient outcomes. Until recently, patients were generally responsible for self-testing their devices. For example, in the case of the Medtronic Marquis Advisory in which there could be early depletion of the battery, patients were advised to test their battery status weekly using a hand-held magnet. For the Medtronic Fidelis Lead Advisory, patients were informed that the device's surveillance system would sound an alarm should its parameters suggest possible lead fracture. They were requested to be mindful of their ICD in case such an alarm was emitted, and to contact the clinic immediately for evaluation if it did. However, in our study [23], 20% of patients could not hear the alarm in question, and thus were equipped with a different surveillance system, the Medtronic Carelink Network. A self-initiated interrogation of the device is performed weekly and transmitted from the patient's home to a central Medtronic server through the patient's telephone landline. The information is then transmitted to the pacemaker/defibrillator clinic personnel. If abnormal measurements are obtained, the arrhythmia service of the hospital is contacted immediately. We had hypothesized that self-monitoring might increase distress and dissatisfaction in advisory patients compared to Carelink or controls, serving as a constant reminder of the potential failure of their device and requiring considerable involvement on their part. This hypothesis was not supported by our results. However, given the small number of patients in the Carelink group, and their slightly more compromised health status compared to the Alarm group, it is possible that differences were underestimated. Additional research using a randomized approach to surveillance method allocation would be necessary to validate these findings. Nonetheless, the absence of greater distress in the Carelink monitoring group suggests that the increasing use of remote monitoring of ICDs may be psychologically safe.

When the ICD Actually Does Malfunction

In a large cross-sectional study, Keren et al. [21] compared the psychological functioning of patients with an ICD under advisory who had (N = 24) and had not (N = 249) actually experienced a lead malfunction against that of patients whose ICD was not under advisory. Symptoms of depression, anxiety, as well as device acceptance and fear of shock were evaluated via mail, on average 13 months after the advisory. Patients with an ICD under advisory who had not experienced a device malfunction did not differ from controls on any of the psychological measures. However, those patients who had experienced a lead fracture were more likely to suffer from adverse psychological morbidity compared to those who had not, and compared to controls. They were more anxious, more fearful of shocks from the device, and reported less device acceptance. This difference was particularly significant among those whose device malfunction resulted in inappropriate shocks.

Satisfaction with Care Following an Advisory

Device advisories may reduce the confidence patients have in their ICD [24, 27] or in their medical care in general. In their sample of patients, Undavia et al. [20] reported that patients subject to an ICD advisory experienced reduced trust in the health-care industry. It was similarly observed that patients experiencing an advisory showed a marked and prolonged reduction in satisfaction with the surveillance of their device [23]. Reductions in patient satisfaction can reduce patients' willingness to share pertinent information about their health status, as well as negatively impact doctor-patient relationships, clinical outcomes and adherence.

Clinical Implications and Recommendations

Ensuring good doctor-patient communication is critical to patient satisfaction with care. It involves developing a good interpersonal relationship with the patient, avoiding the use of medical jargon, exchanging information, and involving the patient in the decision-making process [33]. It facilitates diagnosis and patient understanding of the medical situation and treatment options. It permits better identification of patients' needs, perspectives, and expectations. In effect, it gives physicians the opportunity to respond to these needs in an appropriate and timely fashion. In turn, patients satisfied with their care are more likely to follow treatment recommendations and show improved physical and psychological health outcomes.

There is evidence from the investigations performed to date that prompt and better communication by health care professionals with patients subject to an ICD advisory may improve psychological outcomes. For example, Undavia et al. [20] reported that post recall management at their institution included psychological counselling by the attending physician and as needed, participation in ICD support groups to alleviate potential concerns relating to the advisory. These patients were generally satisfied with the manner in which their physicians had dealt with the advisory. The authors hypothesized that good physician-patient communication may have contributed to the fact that there were no group differences in levels of anxiety, depression or quality of life between patients with an ICD under advisory as compared to those without. While this is a likely explanation, other factors mentioned previously relating to methodology may have also contributed to the lack of group differences.

Nonetheless, separate research in this [23] and other institutions (e.g., [21, 22]) that have reported no sustained psychological consequences of ICD advisories have also typically offered rapid, structured and personalized counselling sessions by the medical staff to explain the pertinent facts relating to the advisories and the changes that were recommended. Such interventions likely mitigate the impact of advisories or related complications. In contrast, Heatherly et al. [26] who found greater device-specific concerns in patients with an ICD under advisory suggested that the lack of structured education and counselling about the advisory could have contributed to greater ICD concerns in these patients versus controls.

The benefits of a standardized nurse-driven counselling session on patients' worries following an ICD advisory were examined by Fisher et al. [29]. A hundred patients who were subject to an advisory on their ICD from 2005 to 2007 were seen in clinic to discuss the implications of their particular advisory. According to the authors, most of the counselling period involved "providing a sense of perspective or proportion of the risks" as many patients believed the risks of device failure to be high. Recommendations for handling their device were offered as suggested by the manufacturer. Patients were questioned as to their level of worry immediately following the counselling session and 6 months later. After the counselling session, they were also asked to provide a retrospective account of their level of worry when they first heard of the advisory. Results indicated a significant and enduring reduction in worry in advisory patients following educational information and counselling session. While significantly reduced, worry following counselling remained slightly higher among patients in whom recommendations involved replacement of the ICD. Interestingly it should be noted that the manner of evaluating worry post-counselling (10 cm visual analogue scale in person) and 6 months later (10-point numeric scale by telephone) in the current study were non-comparable, and may have over- or under-estimated the differences observed. Similarly, the level of worry at the time of finding out about the advisory was obtained retrospectively and could have been tainted by the effects of the counselling session that preceded it. Moreover, there was no "uncounseled" group, and as such, it is difficult to ascertain that the changes in worry were due to the counselling sessions. Despite these important methodological limitations, results are nonetheless concordant with other findings of minimal long-term effects of advisories on patients' psychological status in institutions where similar counselling interventions by medical staff were performed.

Available research thus strongly suggests that structured and prompt medical and/or psychological counselling be provided following advisories to improve patient distress, satisfaction, and quality of life. Keren et al. [21] add that concerns regarding the reliability of ICDs be addressed not only in patients affected by advisories but also in those considering de-novo implantation. The authors suggest that patients be informed from the onset that an advisory on some component of their ICD is possible, but that based on existing literature, the risks to their psychological or physical health of such advisories are likely to be very small, in comparison to the more significant benefits they are likely to obtain from the ICD.

Nonetheless, while a majority of individuals may adapt well to advisories in the long-term, others may be at increased risk for distress and may require additional support. This may be particularly true, for example, in individuals who are pace-dependent, who must undergo replacement of the ICD, or who have experienced inappropriate shocks as a result of a defective lead. Individuals in whom surveillance of the defective device is complicated (such as for the St Jude Medical Riata Advisory) may also be at greater risk for distress. In addition, women may be more greatly impacted by an ICD advisory, though this was examined in only one study. In fact, the research to date has been very male-dominant and greater effort is required to enhance our understanding of women's experiences with ICD advisories.

Similarly, there is but one study to our knowledge that examined the psychological impact of advisories on caregivers of patients with ICDs. Sneed et al. [24] have shown increased distress and decreased confidence in 20 caregivers that persisted for at least one month following the issuance of an advisory. It is necessary for health professionals to keep in mind that a patient's health status is never his alone but can significantly impact the psychological or physical welfare of his loved ones. Threats to his life become threats to their well-being. Given that difficulties in the capacity of caregivers to adapt to the patients' condition can impede the latter's' own adaptation and adherence to treatment recommendations [34], it is recommended that counselling and support be considered for family members following an advisory. Indeed, providing additional information to spouses has been shown to decrease their anxiety and distress [35]. Such interventions may in turn allow family members or other caregivers to be more supportive and encouraging of the patient. This is all the more important given research showing that cardiac patients that benefit from strong social support tend to adjust better, follow treatment recommendations more closely, recover sooner and survive longer than those with less social support [36–38].

Persistent Psychological Distress Among ICD Patients

While no prolonged psychological distress was observed as a result of ICD advisories (or the announcement of suboptimal surveillance following an ICD advisory) in the majority of the studies performed to date, results are nonetheless consistent with elevated distress and/or impoverished quality of life in ICD patients in general.

In research performed in our center, significant impairment on health-related quality of life was observed in both control and patients with an ICD subject to an advisory compared to population norms [23]. In addition, both groups showed elevated levels of psychological distress. Indeed, 23% reported mild to severe symptoms of depression while 48% of patients experienced anxiety. Undavia et al. [20], for their part, found 25% of patients with an ICD under advisory and 32% of controls to have clinically relevant levels of anxiety while depression was suggested in 17% of cases and 11% controls.

Previous studies have similarly reported rates of anxiety ranging from 8 to 63% and depressive symptoms from 5 to 41% following ICD implantation (for a review see [6]). As per our results in patients experiencing an advisory, symptoms of distress persist over extended periods of time in patients who have "simply" had an ICD implanted [39].

Impact of Psychological Morbidity on Cardiovascular Outcomes

Unfortunately, the prevalence and medical relevance of distress in these patients is frequently under-appreciated by health-care providers. The presence of even mild symptoms of anxiety or depression have been shown to predict poorer clinical outcomes in patients with ICDs [40, 41], heart failure [42–45] or a myocardial infarction [42, 46–48]. Moreover, distressed ICD patients tend to experience more ventricular arrhythmias that lead to shocks [49–51] and have an increased risk of mortality [52]. Thus, the very events (ventricular arrhythmias) that medical management is meant to prevent can be triggered by psychological distress that is not attended to or treated. This can be further compounded by reduced compliance to treatment recommendations often seen in distressed patients [42, 43, 53], which may lead to further medical complications.

Conversely, timely and appropriate management of patients' distress and ICD-related concerns can contribute to improved psychological outcomes [5]. Preliminary data also suggests that the risk of ventricular arrhythmias can be reduced by cognitive-behavioural therapy (CBT) or psychopharmacological intervention targeting distress. For example, in a small pilot study, Chevalier et al. [54] randomized seventy ICD patients to either a six-session group cognitive-behavioral stress-management intervention or to usual care. Patients in the CBT intervention tended to experience fewer ventricular arrhythmias 3-months following the intervention compared to controls. In addition, reductions in anxiety as a result of CBT were accompanied by improved measures of cardiac autonomic control, which may have served as the mechanism through which fewer patients experienced ventricular arrhythmias. In a small case study, five ICD patients with a panic disorder and depression, as well as frequent ICD shocks were treated with a selective serotonin reuptake inhibitor combined with a behavioural program. The latter consisted of psycho-education, management of panic attacks, and exposure therapy. At a 6-month follow-up, significant improvement was observed in psychiatric symptoms and only one patient had experienced a discharge of his ICD. Significant reductions were also observed in the number of premature ventricular beats, suggesting improved electrical stability of patients in the absence of any change in cardiac medication. Continued larger scale studies are obviously required but these preliminary results are encouraging.

The goal of any treatment is not only to help patients live longer, but to live more productive, healthier, happier lives. Psychological distress impedes such endeavors, and needs to be addressed as part of the overall treatment plan. In support of this, the American Heart Association [5] has recently emitted scientific statements recommending educational and psychological interventions in order to improve outcomes in patients with ICDs and their families.

However, health care professionals are often uncomfortable discussing emotional issues with patients or consider such discussions too time consuming. A national survey of ICD health care providers, for example, found that cardiologists and nurses were uncomfortable in managing anxiety in their patients [55]. Unfortunately, avoidance of such issues can lead to reduced opportunities for health professionals to reassure patients regarding concerns that may be excessive relative to reality, or to provide or refer patients to the psychological support they require. Alternatively, patients may become uncomfortable with reporting distress, which may also negatively impact their recovery as mentioned above.

Conclusion

Available data suggest that ICD advisories or notification of suboptimal ICD lead surveillance result in limited long-term adverse psychosocial effects in most patients. This appears truer in patients followed in supportive electrophysiology clinics where provision of prompt information, counselling, and reassurance provided by healthcare professionals may reduce patient distress and help them rapidly cope with these additional threats to their health [23]. Nonetheless, those dependent on the ICD for pacing or requiring more intensive interventions (such as device replacement) following the advisory may be more vulnerable to increased distress, as may women and those who have experienced inappropriate shocks. Additional counselling or psychological support in these patients may be required. As stated by Gibson et al. [18], "given the increase in device usage as well as the aging population, the likelihood of an increase in such recalls and potential distress is high, making the need for improved assessment and intervention a vital aspect of ICD therapy". Nonetheless, research to date has relied mostly on small single-center observational ad hoc studies. More reliable information on the impact of ICD advisories would be available if patient-reported outcomes were routinely and repeatedly assessed and included within national registries [27, 28]. Ideally, these assessments would begin prior to ICD implant to evaluate the changing dynamics of patient's experience over time.

Unfortunately, research on the psychosocial impact of advisories is consistent with other research in ICD patients, showing significant impairments in QoL and psychological status in some patients that persist for many years, independently of advisories. Clearly, the psychosocial experiences of many patients are not adequately attended to, and this may contribute to a worse prognosis. The routine assessment of depression and anxiety in patients, as well as the inclusion of or at least access to mental health professionals within electrophysiology clinics would permit rapid identification and treatment of distress in these patients.

References

1. Connolly SJ, Hallstrom AP, Cappato R, Schron EB, Kuck KH, Zipes DP, Greene HL, Boczor S, Domanski M, Follmann D, Gent M, Roberts RS. Meta-analysis of the implantable cardioverter defibrillator secondary prevention trials. AVID, CASH and CIDS studies. Antiarrhythmics vs Implantable Defibrillator study. Cardiac Arrest Study Hamburg. Canadian Implantable Defibrillator Study. Eur Heart J. 2000;21:2071–8.
2. Nanthakumar K, Epstein AE, Kay GN, Plumb VJ, Lee DS. Prophylactic implantable cardioverter-defibrillator therapy in patients with left ventricular systolic dysfunction: a pooled analysis of 10 primary prevention trials. J Am Coll Cardiol. 2004;44:2166–72.
3. Lee DS, Green LD, Liu PP, Dorian P, Newman DM, Grant FC, Tu JV, Alter DA. Effectiveness of implantable defibrillators for preventing arrhythmic events and death: a meta-analysis. J Am Coll Cardiol. 2003;41:1573–82.
4. De Ornelas Maia AC, Soares-Filho G, Pereira V, Nardi AE, Silva AC. Psychiatric disorders and quality of life in patients with implantable cardioverter defibrillators: a systematic review. Prim Care Companion CNS Disord. 2013;15
5. Dunbar SB, Dougherty CM, Sears SF, Carroll DL, Goldstein NE, Mark DB, Mcdaniel G, Pressler SJ, Schron E, Wang P, Zeigler VL, American Heart Association Council on Cardiovascular Nursing, C. O. C. C. and Council on Cardiovascular Disease in the Yong. Educational and psychological interventions to improve outcomes for recipients of implantable cardioverter defibrillators and their families: a scientific statement from the American Heart Association. Circulation. 2012;126:2146–72.
6. Magyar-Russell G, Thombs BD, Cai JX, Baveja T, Kuhl EA, Singh PP, Barroso MMB, Arthurs E, Roseman M, Amin N, Marine JE, Ziegelstein RC. The prevalence of anxiety and depression in adults with implantable cardioverter defibrillators: a systematic review. J Psychosom Res. 2011;71:223–31.
7. Kleemann T, Becker T, Doenges K, Vater M, Senges J, Schneider S, Saggau W, Weisse U, Seidl K. Annual rate of transvenous defibrillation lead defects in implantable cardioverter-defibrillators over a period of >10 years. Circulation. 2007;115:2474–80.
8. Maisel WH. Safety issues involving medical devices: implications of recent implantable cardioverter-defibrillator malfunctions. JAMA. 2005;294:2040–2.
9. Maisel WH, Moynahan M, Zuckerman BD, Gross TP, Tovar OH, Tillman DB, Schultz DB. Pacemaker and ICD generator malfunctions: analysis of Food and Drug Administration annual reports. JAMA. 2006;295:1901–6.
10. Vlay SC. Concerns about the Riata ST (St. Jude Medical) ICD lead. Pacing Clin Electrophysiol. 2008;31:1–2.
11. Sengupta J, Kendig AC, Goormastic M, Hwang ES, Ching EA, Chung R, Lindsay BD, Tchou PJ, Wilkoff BL, Niebauer MJ, Martin DO, Varma N, Wazni O, Saliba W, Kanj M, Bhargava M, Dresing T, Taigen T, Ingelmo C, Bassiouny M, Cronin EM, Wilsmore B, Rickard J, Chung MK. Implantable cardioverter-defibrillator FDA safety advisories: impact on patient mortality and morbidity. Heart Rhythm. 2012;9:1619–26.
12. Gould PA, Krahn AD. Complications associated with implantable cardioverter-defibrillator replacement in response to device advisories. JAMA. 2006;295:1907–11.
13. Morrison TB, Friedman PA, Kallinen LM, Hodge DO, Crusan D, Kumar K, Hayes DL, Rea RF, Hauser RG. Impact of implanted recalled Sprint Fidelis lead on patient mortality. J Am Coll Cardiol. 2011;58:278–83.
14. Hegel MT, Griegel LE, Black C, Goulden L, Ozahowski T. Anxiety and depression in patients receiving implanted cardioverter-defibrillators: a longitudinal investigation. Int J Psychiatry Med. 1997;27:57–69.
15. Pedersen SS, Van Domburg RT, Theuns DA, Jordaens L, Erdman RA. Concerns about the implantable cardioverter defibrillator: a determinant of anxiety and depressive symptoms independent of experienced shocks. Am Heart J. 2005;149:664–9.

16. Parkash R, Crystal E, Bashir J, Simpson C, Birnie D, Sterns L, Exner D, Thibault B, Connors S, Healey JS, Champagne J, Cameron D, Mangat I, Verma A, Wolfe K, Essebag V, Kus T, Ayala-Paredes F, Davies T, Sanatani S, Gow R, Coutu B, Sivakumaran S, Stephenson E, Krahn A. Complications associated with revision of Sprint Fidelis leads: report from the Canadian Heart Rhythm Society Device Advisory Committee. Circulation. 2010;121:2384–7.
17. El-Chami MF, Merchant FM, Levy M, Alam MB, Rattan R, Hoskins MH, Langberg JJ, Delurgio D, Lloyd MS, Leon AR, Saba S. Outcomes of Sprint Fidelis and Riata lead extraction: data from 2 high-volume centers. Heart Rhythm. 2015;12:1216–20.
18. Gibson DP, Kuntz KK, Levenson JL, Ellenbogen KA. Decision-making, emotional distress, and quality of life in patients affected by the recall of their implantable cardioverter defibrillator. Europace. 2008;10:540–4.
19. Cuculi F, Herzig W, Kobza R, Erne P. Psychological distress in patients with ICD recall. Pacing Clin Electrophysiol. 2006;29:1261–5.
20. Undavia M, Goldstein NE, Cohen P, Sinthawanarong K, Singson M, Bhutani D, Munson T, Gomes JA, Fischer A, Mehta D. Impact of implantable cardioverter-defibrillator recalls on patients' anxiety, depression, and quality of life. Pacing Clin Electrophysiol. 2008;31:1411–8.
21. Keren A, Sears SF, Nery P, Shaw J, Green MS, Lemery R, Gollob MH, Amyotte B, Birnie DH. Psychological adjustment in ICD patients living with advisory Fidelis leads. J Cardiovasc Electrophysiol. 2011;22:57–63.
22. Birnie DH, Sears SF, Green MS, Lemery R, Gollob MH, Amyotte B. No long-term psychological morbidity living with an implantable cardioverter defibrillator under advisory: the Medtronic Marquis experience. Europace. 2009;11:26–30.
23. D'Antono B, Goldfarb M, Solomon C, Sturmer M, Becker G, Essebag V, Hadjis T, Gizicki E, Gelais JS, Sas G, Cote MC, Kus T. Psychological impact of surveillance in patients with a defibrillator lead under advisory: a prospective evaluation. Pacing Clin Electrophysiol. 2013;36:221–30.
24. Sneed NV, Finch NJ, Leman RB. The impact of device recall on patients and family members of patients with automatic implantable cardioverter-defibrillators. Heart Lung. 1994;23:317–22.
25. Van Den Broek KC, Denollet J, Nyklicek I, Van Der Voort PH. Psychological reaction to potential malfunctioning of implantable defibrillators. Pacing Clin Electrophysiol. 2006;29:953–6.
26. Heatherly SJ, Simmons T, Fitzgerald DM, Mitchell M. Psychological effects of implantable cardioverter-defibrillator leads under advisory. Pacing Clin Electrophysiol. 2011;34:694–9.
27. Pedersen SS, Versteeg H, Nielsen JC, Mortensen PT, Johansen JB. Patient-reported outcomes in Danish implantable cardioverter defibrillator patients with a Sprint Fidelis lead advisory notification. Europace. 2011;13:1292–8.
28. Larsen JM, Riahi S, Johansen JB, Nielsen JC, Petersen HH, Haarbo J, Pedersen SS. The patient perspective on the Riata defibrillator lead advisory: a Danish nationwide study. Heart Rhythm. 2014;11:2148–55.
29. Fisher JD, Koulogiannis KP, Lewallen L, Katz D, Kim SG, Ferrick KJ, Gross JN, Krumerman AK, Johnston DR, Mercaldi BC. The psychological impact of implantable cardioverter-defibrillator recalls and the durable positive effects of counseling. Pacing Clin Electrophysiol. 2009;32:1012–6.
30. Stutts LA, Conti JB, Aranda JM Jr, Miles WM, Burkart TA, Sears SF. Patient evaluation of ICD recall communication strategies: a vignette study. Pacing Clin Electrophysiol. 2007;30:1105–11.
31. Shaw RE, Cohen F, Doyle B, Palesky J. The impact of denial and repressive style on information gain and rehabilitation outcomes in myocardial infarction patients. Psychosom Med. 1985;47:262–73.
32. Kallinen LM, Hauser RG, Lee KW, Almquist AK, Katsiyiannis WT, Tang CY, Melby DP, Gornick CC. Failure of impedance monitoring to prevent adverse clinical events caused by fracture of a recalled high-voltage implantable cardioverter-defibrillator lead. Heart Rhythm. 2008;5:775–9.

33. Ha JF, Longnecker N. Doctor-patient communication: a review. Ochsner J. 2010;10:38–43.
34. Molloy GJ, Perkins-Porras L, Strike PC, Steptoe A. Social networks and partner stress as predictors of adherence to medication, rehabilitation attendance, and quality of life following acute coronary syndrome. Health Psychol. 2008;27:52–8.
35. Broadbent E, Ellis CJ, Thomas J, Gamble G, Petrie KJ. Can an illness perception intervention reduce illness anxiety in spouses of myocardial infarction patients? A randomized controlled trial. J Psychosom Res. 2009;67:11–5.
36. Kaplan RM, Toshima MT. The functional effects of social relationships on chronic illnesses and disability. In: Sarason BR, Sarason IG, Pierce GR, editors. Social support: an interactional view. New York: Wiley; 1990.
37. Krantz DS, Deckel AW. Coping with coronary heart disease and stroke. In: Burish TG, Bradley LA, editors. Coping with chronic disease: research and applications. NewYork: Academic; 1983.
38. Lett HS, Blumenthal JA, Babyak MA, Strauman TJ, Robins C, Sherwood A. Social support and coronary heart disease: epidemiologic evidence and implications for treatment. Psychosom Med. 2005;67:869–78.
39. Suzuki T, Shiga T, Kuwahara K, Kobayashi S, Suzuki S, Nishimura K, Suzuki A, Ejima K, Manaka T, Shoda M, Ishigooka J, Kasanuki H, Hagiwara N. Prevalence and persistence of depression in patients with implantable cardioverter defibrillator: a 2-year longitudinal study. Pacing Clin Electrophysiol. 2010;33:1455–61.
40. Ladwig KH, Baumert J, Marten-Mittag B, Kolb C, Zrenner B, Schmitt C. Posttraumatic stress symptoms and predicted mortality in patients with implantable cardioverter-defibrillators results from the prospective living with an implanted cardioverter-defibrillator study. Arch Gen Psychiatry. 2008;65:1324–30.
41. Pedersen SS, Van Den Broek KC, Erdman RAM, Jordaens L, Theuns D. Pre-implantation implantable cardioverter defibrillator concerns and Type D personality increase the risk of mortality in patients with an implantable cardioverter defibrillator. Europace. 2010;12:1446–52.
42. Celano CM, Huffman JC. Depression and cardiac disease a review. Cardiol Rev. 2011;19:130–42.
43. Mcgrady A, Mcginnis R, Badenhop D, Bentle M, Rajput M. Effects of depression and anxiety on adherence to cardiac rehabilitation. J Cardiopulm Rehabil Prev. 2009;29:358–64.
44. Rutledge T, Reis VA, Linke SE, Greenberg BH, Mills PJ. Depression in heart failure—a meta-analytic review of prevalence, intervention effects, and associations with clinical outcomes. J Am Coll Cardiol. 2006;48:1527–37.
45. Shen BJ, Eisenberg SA, Maeda U, Farrell KA, Schwarz ER, Penedo FJ, Bauerlein EJ, Mallon S. Depression and anxiety predict decline in physical health functioning in patients with heart failure. Ann Behav Med. 2011;41:373–82.
46. Meijer A, Conradi HJ, Bos EH, Thombs BD, Van Melle KP, De Jonge P. Prognostic association of depression following myocardial infarction with mortality and cardiovascular events: a meta-analysis of 25 years of research. Gen Hosp Psychiatry. 2011;33:203–16.
47. Roest AM, Martens EJ, Denollet J, De Jonge P. Prognostic association of anxiety post myocardial infarction with mortality and new cardiac events: a meta-analysis. Psychosom Med. 2010;72:563–9.
48. Van Melle JP, De Jonge P, Spijkerman TA, Tijssen JGP, Ormel J, Van Veldhuisen DJ, Van Den Brink RHS, Van Den Berg MP. Prognostic association of depression following myocardial infarction with mortality and cardiovascular events: a meta-analysis. Psychosom Med. 2004;66:814–22.
49. Burg MM, Lampert R, Joska T, Batsford W, Jain D. Psychological traits and emotion-triggering of ICD shock-terminated arrhythmias. Psychosom Med. 2004;66:898–902.
50. Dunbar SB, Kimble LP, Jenkins LS, Hawthorne M, Dudley W, Slemmons M, Langberg JJ. Association of mood disturbance and arrhythmia events in patients after cardioverter defibrillator implantation. Depress Anxiety. 1999;9:163–8.

51. Whang W, Albert CM, Sears SF Jr, Lampert R, Conti JB, Wang PJ, Singh JP, Ruskin JN, Muller JE, Mittleman MA, Investigators TS. Depression as a predictor for appropriate shocks among patients with implantable cardioverter-defibrillators: results from the Triggers of Ventricular Arrhythmias (TOVA) study. J Am Coll Cardiol. 2005;45:1090–5.
52. Mastenbroek MH, Versteeg H, Jordaens L, Theuns DA, Pedersen SS. Ventricular tachyarrhythmias and mortality in patients with an implantable cardioverter defibrillator: impact of depression in the MIDAS cohort. Psychosom Med. 2014;76:58–65.
53. Ziegelstein RC, Fauerbach JA, Stevens SS, Romanelli J, Richter DP, Bush DE. Patients with depression are less likely to follow recommendations to reduce cardiac risk during recovery from a myocardial infarction. Arch Intern Med. 2000;160:1818–23.
54. Chevalier P, Cottraux J, Mollard E, Sai N, Brun S, Burri H, Restier L, Adeleine P. Prevention of implantable defibrillator shocks by cognitive behavioral therapy: a pilot trial. Am Heart J. 2006;151:191.
55. Sears SF, Todaro JF, Urizar G, Lewis TS, Sirois B, Wallace R, Sotile W, Curtis AB, Conti JB. Assessing the psychosocial impact of the ICD: a national survey of implantable cardioverter defibrillator health care providers. Pacing Clin Electrophysiol. 2000;23:939–45.

Chapter 9
ICD in Children and Youth

Abdullah Alabdulgader

Abstract The peculiarity of the pediatrics and adolescent age groups with the presence of congenital defects, genetic variance, developmental as well as puberty issues creates unique group of humans. This peculiarity of the pediatric and adolescent age groups can be easily explored when we discuss implanting defibrillator devices during this time of the human life. This chapter is devoted for Psychological, Emotional, Social and Cognitive Aspects of Implantable cardioverter Defibrillators in children and adolescents. The true impact of childhood ventricular fibrillation as well as milestones of professional care for this age group ICD candidates is discussed. Breaking the bad news-being an art by it self- has peculiarity in childhood and adolescent disease which was given concern in this chapter. Useful information and tips to be communicated to child, youth and families are given. Clear perspective of the important events of the child with ICD and reactions to it is given with emphasis to preserve normal life style as much as possible. Psychosocial Factors and Quality of Life in Children and adolescents with Implantable Cardioverter-Defibrillators are discussed. Although no longitudinal studies of psychosocial response over time for children and adolescents are available, focus in initial studies in children and young adults which illustrate higher levels of anxiety and lower quality of life scores in patients with implantable cardioverter–defibrillators has been given. The pediatric and adolescent age-specific concerns, together with the typical ICD patient concerns such as both inappropriate and appropriate shocks and physical activity restrictions were given concern. Reduced physical functioning and lower quality of life in adolescents and the importance of creating a positive emotional perspective is emphasized. Theoretical approaches to the psychosocial adjustment of ICD recipients in different age groups with discussion of general theories of psychological adjustment to the ICD has been discussed with some depth. We emphasize on the fact that psychoeducational plans and modules are the main theme in managing the psychosocial emotional and cognitive aspects of ICDs in children and adolescents. Up to date pharmacological treatment of PTSD in children and adolescents is mentioned. Finally recommendations for future research to improve

A. Alabdulgader, M.D., MRCP (UK), FRCP (Edin)
Prince Sultan Cardiac Centre, Hofuf, Alhasa 31982, Saudi Arabia
e-mail: kidsecho@yahoo.com

© Springer International Publishing AG 2017

R. Proietti et al. (eds.), *Psychological, Emotional, Social and Cognitive Aspects of Implantable Cardiac Devices*, DOI 10.1007/978-3-319-55721-2_9

psychological, emotional, social and cognitive aspects of Implantable Cardiac devices in children and adolescents are highlighted.

Keywords Implantable cardioverter defibrillators • Children and youth • Adolescents • Incidence of VF in children • Psychological • Emotional • Social and cognitive aspects • Breaking bad news • Quality of life (QOL) • Psychosocial adjustment • Psychoeducational interventions

Introduction

Until the first three decades of the last century childhood diseases were considered as part of general medicine. The peculiarity of the pediatrics age group with the presence of congenital defects, genetic variance, and developmental issues is the real demarcation line between childhood and adult medicine. Parallel to immature developing physiology of the pediatric age group is the psychological and developmental aspects which mandate special attention when discussing new therapeutic developments or practices related to this age group. It is one of the pillars of medicine nowadays, not to extrapolate adult practice to the pediatric age group as the child is not a miniature of the adult. The issues of guardianship, privacy, legal responsibility, and informed consent must always be considered in every pediatric procedure. In addition, pediatricians often have to treat the parents and sometimes, the family, rather than just the child. Not only medical issues but also legal affairs are of concern as the child in most jurisdictions, with certain exceptions, cannot make decisions for himself. This peculiarity of the pediatric age group can be easily explored when we discuss implanting defibrillator devices in a child. Apart from the implant surgery and its potential technical difficulties, psychosocial, emotional and cognitive aspects are of major and increasing concern. The paucity of medical literature in the field encourage us to devote this chapter to this purpose.

ICD Implants in Children and Youth

Indications for ICD implant in children and youth are usually different than those in adults. Congenital heart diseases as well as congenital heart surgery outcomes in the population dictate the increasing demand for ICD implantation in children and youth. Another important feature of pediatric ICD implants is the inability for children to consciously decide on ICD implantation. Another inherent feature of the ICD implant process is the relatively short time given to the caregiver to determine their choice, to either accept or reject the implant. Decision making in adult ICD implant has been investigated and suggested guidelines were published [1]. Some directions can be withdrawn from adult ICD guidelines but in general extrapolation is not applicable as the decision maker is not the patient him/herself. This difficulty, in the early stage before ICD implant, is the first psychological distress that children and their families have to face in the ICD time line. Knowledge of the actual impact of the situation should alleviate some of the distress of the child, adolescent, and family making them feel that they are part of a well-known community. Breaking the bad news of possible vulnerability of sudden death and introducing the choice of ICD implant is an art that needs to be practiced in a formal and professional approach.

It must be emphasized that PTSD in children and adolescent may display symptoms of PTSD which are not seen in adults, such as behavioral problems, developmental regression, physical symptoms and more generalized fears.

True Impact of the Problem (Incidence of VF in Children)

The Pediatric Advanced Life Support Task Force, International Liaison Committee on Resuscitation published into circulation (2003) an important advisory statement on the use of Automated External Defibrillators for Children [2]. They stated that ventricular fibrillation (VF) is an uncommon cause of out-of-hospital pediatric cardiac arrest in infants (first year of age), but its occurrence increases with age. Two studies reported VF as the initial rhythm in 19–24% of out-of-hospital pediatric cardiac arrests, if sudden infant death syndrome (SIDS) deaths were excluded [3, 4]. In studies that included SIDS victims, however, the frequency dropped to 6–10% [5–7]. The rationale for exclusion of SIDS patients was that SIDS is not amenable to treatment, so patients with SIDS should not be included in these studies for they may influence potential treatment strategies for cardiac arrest in children. Schwartz PJ et al., reported documented VF in a 3-month-old infant with SIDS who was subsequently diagnosed with prolonged QT syndrome [8]. Recent data suggest that VF is not a rare rhythm in pediatric arrest. This is encouraging because VF is the arrest arrhythmia associated with improved survival rate in most studies of children [3, 4, 9, 10]. For example, Mogayzel and colleagues reported that 5 of 29 children (17%) who presented VF in a prehospital setting survived with good neurological outcome versus only 2 of 128 (2%) who presented asystole/pulseless electrical activity (*P*_0.01) [3]. In-hospital studies of pediatric CPR also indicate that VF is not a rare rhythm among children in cardiac arrest. Two recent comprehensive studies reported the incidence of VF as the initial rhythm and the incidence of VF at some time during the arrest. Suominen et al., reported initial VF in 11% of children in cardiac arrest and VF in 20% of children some time during the arrest [11]. In a much larger study, cardiac arrest data submitted to the National Registry of CardioPulmonary Resuscitation revealed initial VF in 12% of children and VF in 25% of children some time during the pediatric arrest [12].

Child Has Been Diagnosed and Needs the Defibrillator; Breaking the Bad News

Breaking the bad news to parents and child is never easy [13]. It is the first psychological distress in the timeline of the story of the device. Neglecting its importance can create psychological stigma and life time consequences. In the past, we learned through experience, there has been little or no formal training in this important area. In the ICD community, all our patients are candidates of potential sudden death due to ventricular fibrillation or accelerated ventricular rhythm. Skillful medical personnel should focus on positive emotions enhancement based on facts. In case of a potential ICD implant, strong evidence of positive outcomes can assist the medical personnel in charge of breaking the bad news. This is because VF is the arrest arrhythmia associated with improved survival rate in most studies of children [2, 3, 8, 9]. Providing reassurance to palliate the bad news increases medical as well as social support in home, school, and community. Raising self-esteem by reminding the child and family of what they can do rather than cannot do should turn the mission of breaking bad news a successful experience. Breaking bad news can be divided into three phases:

(a) Preparation Phase
(b) Breaking the news Phase
(c) Follow-up Phase

Written documentation should be done for all steps.

(a)—Preparation Phase

The medical personnel should feel competent for the mission. He or she should give time and attention to the child and family. Short tempered and busy personnel *must not* deal with this mission. A special prepared room, ideally a quiet and comfortable one should be available for this purpose. Audiovisual aids should ideally be available in this room to display the device and procedure information, in addition to interviews with children and parents, focus on positive conceptual emotional building towards the device as a safeguard of life. Reviewing patient record before the interview to obtain background knowledge of the child and family should help build trust and confidence from the child's and family's perspective. To ensure a successful interview, special consideration should be given to the child's developmental age and to family cultural values and attitudes.

(b)—Breaking the News Phase

This is the critical phase where the interviewer should appear competent, but in the same time emotional and compassionate. The interviewer should know in-advance what the family already knowns. Introduction of the news should be gradual, not abrupt, and at the same time honest. It is a fine art to be concise in telling the truth yet avoiding lies. Simple language not medical jargon should be used. Classically, a successful interviewer should use as many emotional and peaceful words as possible. Conveying in a balanced way facts about the success of science in aborting VF, should be done smartly. If parents ask directly about the probability of their child's death, the interviewer should refer to medical literature figures with optimism. After covering the important points, the interviewer should terminate the interview with a smile and thanking the family for their time. This phase, in our experience, should take 15–25 min. Longer interviews are not advised.

(c)—Follow-up Phase

Child and family must be seen a short time after breaking the news, preferably 1–3 days. The follow-up is suitable to strengthen the trust and the previously established rapport with the child and family. Awaiting results may be given at this time. Date for ICD implant might be given. This phase should continue after ICD implant as psychosocial, emotional and cognitive support for life.

Accepting ICD Implant and Thereafter

Diagnosing heart problem in a child can create fear, disappointment and sometimes guilty-feelings for parents. It is not unusual for parents to interpret their child's rhythm disorder as God's punishment for something they or one of them did in the past. Proper explanations and skillful communication and timely behavioral management can give satisfying results and minimize the psychosocial and emotional distress.

Useful Information To Be Communicated to Child and Family

1. *The ICD is an intelligent and loyal device*:
   An ICD is not a cure, but can be viewed as a safety device that protects the child from the risk of lethal heart rhythms. Previous research has indicated that ICDs significantly reduce the risk of sudden cardiac death in patients at risk [14]. It is capable of performing strict monitoring and do accurate reading of all rhythm types. Fatal arrhythmias can be detected and managed immediately either by rapid pace or delivering a shock. It is reassuring to be able to tell the family and child that the ICD is an intelligent and loyal device. A CPR certified person should always be available to reassure children and adolescents with an ICD.
2. *Open heart surgery is not needed*:
   In a cardiac patient the word "surgery" does not always mean open heart surgery. The ICD is typically placed in the upper left chest, without interfering directly with the heart. It has sensing wires that attached to the walls of the right ventricle. The child will likely have the ICD throughout his or her lifetime and will need the battery changed every 5–7 years. It requires monitoring by a

cardiologist, typically every 3–6 months, which can be done painlessly with a telemonitoring system from home or in the cardiologist's office.

3. *It is natural to through frequent device related questions*
At first, it may feel like the family has many questions that they don't even know where to begin. Some important questions that might be asked may mainly be related to the child and his future. The child as an index case in the family, will increase parents' worries about future children as well as the child's future off-springs. Other frequently asked questions are device precautions, genetic screening, the need for additional medicine, insurance coverage and level of activity, all of which are related directly or indirectly to the child and family's Quality of Life (QOL).
4. *Emotional related issues*
Usually, children candidates for ICD implant are not seriously ill, but they are under the threat of a fatal rhythm disorder that can terminate their life in a few seconds. This fact is well understood by the cardiologist but most of the times not by the parents. Confronting them with this bad news is always shocking. It is best to encourage the parents to talk openly with their child [13]. If the parents ask the doctor not to discuss things with their child, he/she should make it clear that if the child asks questions, he will give them honest answers. Children think in more concrete terms than adults, and may not have grasped the finality and irreversibility of death, a developmental understanding is usually achieved when the child is eight. However, there is also growing recognition that even young children who face death personally may have a better understanding than often assumed. Adolescents need more explanations and patience. Adolescents are also more resistant to ICD implant but emphasis should be conveyed in a balanced approach that with the ICD they are protected in the best way medical science has to offer. Recorded material with referral to specialized websites that expose children and adolescents to the science of ICD devices as well as the experience of others is optimal.

   The child may benefit from focusing on a survivorship mentality that emphasizes being committed to living long and well, regardless of occasional medical intrusions [15]. A strong community of family and friends can support this approach [16]. If anxiety, depression, or emotional distress becomes a problem, mental health professionals should be involved to offer support and guidance.
5. *The device is a new life experience to maintain good QOL:*
Young ICD patients are adaptive and often courageous. Although an ICD can undoubtedly save a life, living with one can be challenging. Parents who find their children withdrawing from their favorite activities or interests can help them by encouraging the child's participation in normal life activities and discouraging avoidance [15]. Parents often believe that their children have a lower quality of life than the children actually report [17].

   Keeping an open dialogue with the child about his or her reaction to having an ICD will help the child to feel better and at the same time keep the cardiologist informed about the child's ability to cope with new or ongoing stressors [4].

Research has also shown that females can experience unique challenges related to social role maintenance, femininity, sexuality, and caretaking abilities [18]. QOL of children with ICDs is going to be discussed further in Sect. 2.5 of this chapter.

6. *The normal and the exaggerated reactions towards the device: when to ask for help?*
   How children deal with stress depends on age, developmental level, temperament, and family situations. Anxiety is the most common psychological symptom experienced by ICD recipients, and therefore, they may experience a greater need for affirmation from friends and family [19]. Signs that a youngster is having difficulties adjusting includes school absences, social isolation, or avoidance behaviors. Family and counseling therapy can be helpful for patients and their loved ones when coping difficulties are observed [17].

   It is always wise and productive for cardiologist and parents alike, to speak to the children in a way tailored to their maturity level, health literacy, needs, and readiness to understand their cardiac condition. Children exhibit an increased readiness to learn at key points in development [15]. This maturity guarded communication and care is the best way to differentiate between normal and abnormal reactions. Teachable moments should be caught intelligently in order to provide education and counseling at the child's developmental level. As they grow older, children can be encouraged to take an active role in the next developmental level by speaking for themselves, managing their condition and participating in taking medication, and interacting with their pediatric cardiologist at appointments. It is important to make sure that the child's and adolescent's reaction is normal for age and expected maturity level before asking for specialized help.
7. *Medications and related conditions*
   As children mature, they should become progressively more independent and informed about managing their medications, medical visits, and any necessary lifestyle modifications. Commonly, ICD children will be prescribed medications such as beta blockers to lower the chances for arrhythmia and therefore, decrease the chance of a shock from the ICD. These medications may cause fatigue until the child gets used to them; however, those medications are imperative to the child's treatment plan [20]. Taking the medication at night before bed can help with these side effects and the child will adjust to a normal energy level over time.

   Viral illnesses are common in the pediatric age group especially infants and toddlers. The manifestations of viral illnesses should not be confused with the side effects of antiarrhythmic medications, like skin rashes and arthralgia.

   Avoiding dehydration is also important because it can precipitate electrolytes disorders and consequently, arrhythmias. Therefore, it is important to be in close contact with the child's pediatrician if the child is experiencing vomiting or diarrhea. Empowering the child to manage these issues, without being fearful or overprotective, nonetheless watchful is the balance for which parents should strive [15].

8. *Careful transition to adulthood:*
   In middle to late adolescence, conversations about vocations and careers, pregnancy, and long-term goals are appropriate and helpful to empower children to manage their own health. The transition to an adult cardiologist should be a gradual process that involves the child, parents, and pediatrician. It is during middle to late adolescence that many pediatric patients move to adult cardiologists but also have the most difficulty adhering to medication [18]. We emphasize the importance of life time presence of congenital cardiologist care for ICD individuals with either operated or native congenital heart disease. The peculiarity of congenital heart disease hemodynamics especially ventricular volume and/or pressure overload and the propensity of this to ventricular arrhythmias mandate the presence of congenital cardiologist for life-long care of children and adolescents with ICD and Congenital Heart Disease.

The First Shock and Thereafter

When the child receives the first shock a new stage, and experience begins. The experience of an ICD shock is the most unique (and worst) aspect of living with an ICD. The first shock—although discomforting and unpleasant, should be emphasized to both child and parents as a positive and constructive experience. I used to tell my pediatric patient and family that this little uncomfortable experience is an announcement of successful abortion of sudden death and signifies new and renewable life for the youngster. Parents will learn that touching the child during the shock is harmless. Successful planning, management, and response to an ICD shock will allow each member of the family to be prepared and respond optimally. Figure 9.1 strategic plans in the ICD patients time line.

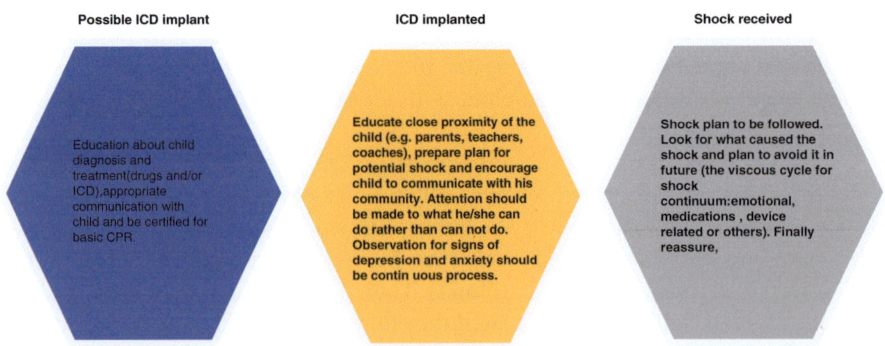

Fig. 9.1 Strategic plans in the ICD patients time line

The child will adapt to life with an ICD and cope with the anticipation of an arrhythmia or shock. It is expected that he or she will experience some level of emotional stress and it is important to provide open, honest, and age-appropriate information, in order to acquire the necessary tools for adaptation. The child must be provided with a sense of safety by keeping life at home as coherent as possible. Parental withdrawal can cause the child feelings of insecurity, sadness, and guilt. Parents should not be afraid to communicate and express their feelings of sadness or worry to their child. They should treat their child as normally as possible within the limits of his or her illness [8]. The child's community neighbors, teachers, coaches, relatives, and friends also plays an important role in giving a sense of security and safety to the child. Each social contact functions as an important advocate, and should receive the same information as provided to the child. A child-friendly medical alert bracelet and contact information can offer both the child and parent, peace of mind in case of emergency. Figure 9.2 depicts actions for parents across three situations.

Self-esteem can be optimized by building positive emotions and acceptance for the ICD and its aspects. Carolina Dimsdale et al. [15], gave a smart suggestion, giving a friendly name to the device. This friendly name should create successful incorporation of the device in the child's life. Names like "*my safeguard*" or "*my soldier*" are capable of creating implicit and explicit positive perspectives and attitudes towards the defibrillator.

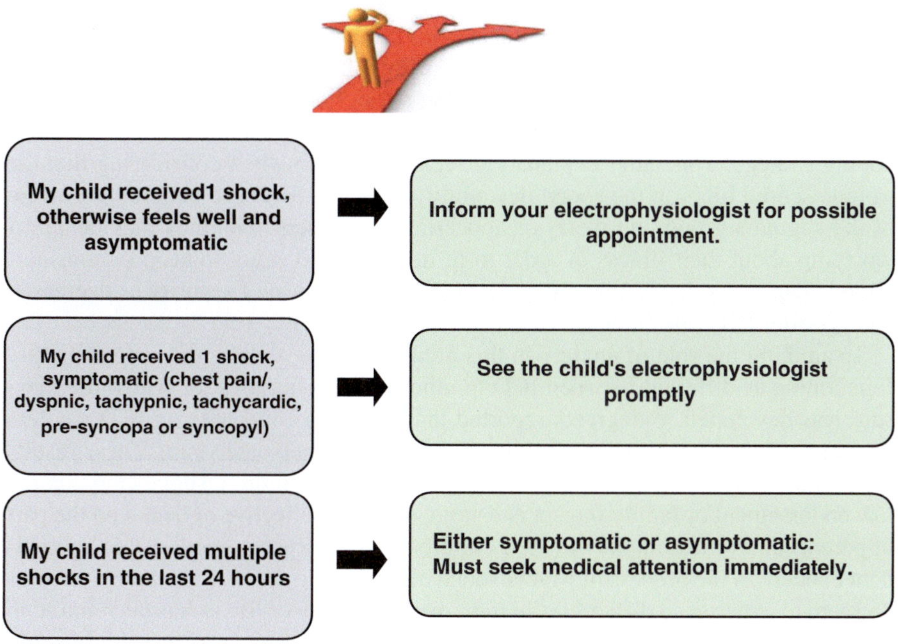

Fig. 9.2 Parents decision making when shock(s) received

Psychosocial Factors and Quality of Life in Children and Adolescents with Implantable Cardioverter-Defibrillators

Although, the findings of adult investigations cannot be extrapolated to children, the prevalence of anxiety and depressive symptoms among adult-patients with implantable cardioverter-defibrillators (ICDs) [21–34], who arguably have greater intellectual, developmental, and emotional resources than their pediatric counterparts, suggests the need to examine these symptoms in children who have received ICD implants. David Ray DeMaso et al., in a founding study in the field, using parent and patient self-report, examined the psychosocial functioning and quality of life of children and adolescents with ICDs [19]. The study specifically investigated anxiety, depression, family functioning, and quality of life in pediatric patients with ICDs.

They were able to answer many questions concerning the psychosocial factors, and quality of life in children and adolescents who received ICDs. Previously, the adjustments of pediatric patients after implantation were not examined, leaving health-care providers with little alternative than to extrapolate the conflicting research findings from adults with ICDs and apply them to the pediatric age group. This extrapolation definitely leads to errors because the assumption that the two groups are comparable is wrong. This study was able to shed light on some of the ways in which adolescents with ICDs appear to adjust similarly to their adult counterparts, as well as some of the important ways in which their adjustment may differ. Contrary to the adult morbidity rates [21, 22], only 2 of 20 subjects met depression criteria whereas no subject met clinical criteria for anxiety. Levels of worry/oversensitivity were low, perhaps a reflection of how having a pediatric heart disease specifically affects this aspect of anxiety. We strongly support the authors' assumption that the low occurrence of worry and anxiety could be a reflection of a denial-coping strategy. This latter explanation seems plausible when considering that the sample scored high on the social desirability subscale. Because patients are aware of the stigma surrounding worry or appearing overly sensitive, they may denial of worrying about their illness in order to fit in socially. A point to keep in consideration is that, these low ratings may actually reflect a sense of security or decreased anxiety after ICD placement.

Examining the role of anxiety in this population, the authors did not see family functioning as different between ICD families and the families for which the measure was developed. Caregivers reported that having a child with an ICD has less impact on their family/social relations, and less direct personal strain. These results parallel the absence of findings of anxiety within their children, suggesting that the low endorsement of family impact and strain could be reflective of denial on the part of parents and/or less anxiety in their children. In our experience, denial is a prominent concern in the process of psychosocial evaluation in families. Pediatric patients do seem to experience difficulties in their overall quality of life as has been found in previous studies [26–28, 33]. Parents perceived that their children have significantly lower physical functioning, social-physical roles, and general health perceptions than a normative sample. In contrast, there was no significant difference in overall psychosocial functioning between youngsters with ICDs and the normative sample. Despite this lack of difference, it is worth noting that the domains of social emotional/behavioral role, self-esteem, and the emotional impact of a child's health on the caretaker were all significantly lower than the normal sample. Sample size is this study's major limitation. The author concluded that pediatric patients with ICDs appear to experience significantly lower physical functioning in their quality of life than healthy youngsters. However, most do not appear to experience clinical levels of depression or anxiety, although they may experience a greater need for social acceptance. They do not appear to experience lower psychosocial functioning, although there may be vulnerabilities in their social/behavioral roles and self-esteem. Illness severity does not appear to be indicative of psychosocial functioning, whereas feelings of anxiety and depression, as well as family functioning show strong ties to their quality of life.

Quality of life is a generic term describing *interdependent functions outcome of biological, psychological, and social status*. QoL is difficult to evaluate in the pediatric age group. ICD shock is clearly the primary culprit when patients describe a decrease in quality of life, and coping with both inappropriate and appropriate shocks remains the most significant psychosocial challenge for the ICD populations [25]. Sears SF and Conti JB reported that younger age and greater frequency of ICD firings were the two most commonly reported ICD specific risk factors for psychological distress [35, 36]. Younger patients (ages 50 years and/or younger) may experience greater problems because of increased lifestyle disruption and distressing social comparisons [34]. In addition to adjusting to the risk of potentially life threatening arrhythmias, young patients must deal with the presence of the ICD device, the likely experience of life saving shock, and the social and lifestyle ramifications of the ICD. Not surprisingly, the ICD can present significant psychological difficulties for some young patients. *Returning to a full life is the hallmark feature of quality of life*. Comprehensive, interdisciplinary care plans, such as those reported by Fitchest and colleagues [37], demonstrate that an exercise and stress management programme is a safe and valuable addition for ICD patients and results in reduced anxiety and improved exercise capacity.

Richard J. Czosek et al., in a recent study, evaluated the effects of implanted cardiac rhythm devices on the QOL of pediatric and adolescent patients [38]. Using pediatric generic and cardiac specific measurement tools. The reported QOL scores of this study demonstrated that devices significantly impacted patient-and-parent-proxy. Key drivers of QOL scores included patient-and-parent specific self-perception and behavioral variables, Congenital Heart Disease (CHD), and the presence of an ICD system as opposed to a pacing system. Several studies have highlighted the issues surrounding the management of devices in pediatric populations [39–42]. Major demarcating differences between pediatric age group and adults are: underlying cardiac disease processes, patient size, and peer related social structures. In this group, the presence of concomitant CHD was relatively high, especially in the pacemaker group, in which nearly 60% of patients had associated CHD. Similarly, the high rate of device-related complications in both device groups added additional concerns to an already high-risk group of patients. Despite these morbidities, overall measurements of self-perception, as well as emotional and behavior functioning in both device groups were similar to previously reported measures in healthy pediatric populations [43]. Despite this, the effects of the devices on individual patients within these groups led to significant differences in PedsQL QOL scores compared with healthy populations and PCQLI scores in patients with mild forms of CHD, such as isolated Bicuspid Aortic Valve (BAV). Similar to data from pediatric ICD studies by Demaso et al. [19], the presence of an ICD was correlated with lower QOL scores in both patients and their parent-proxy. In total, the ICD group had lower PedsQL QOL scores compared with the healthy group and lower PCQLI scores compared with patients with isolated BAV. Furthermore, in terms of disease impact subscale scores, ICD patients have scores significantly lower than patients with TOF and similar to patients with Fontan physiology. Although the precise mechanisms behind lower QOL scores in ICD systems cannot be elucidated in this retrospective analysis, several potential causes include larger device generator, underlying disease mechanisms, and the potential for device shock. In addition to device type, this study also underscores the synergistic detrimental effects of CHD on the QOL of patients with devices. Not surprisingly, the long-term comorbidities associated with CHD had significant additive effects associated with lower QOL, placing this vulnerable population at increased risk. This effect was most evident in the pacemaker group. Although pacemaker patients without CHD had lower PedsQL QOL scores compared with healthy controls, their PCQLI scores were comparable with patients with mild forms of CHD, such as isolated BAV. In the presence of CHD, pacemaker patients had significantly lower scores compared with the BAV group, comparable with patients with TOF and Fontan physiology. In this pediatric cohort, there was a high rate of device shocks, and nearly 50% were inappropriate. In the total ICD group, authors were surprised to find that a history of any prior ICD shock was not associated with lower QOL scores. Smaller patients sample may contribute to this finding. There were significant differences in the effects of self-perception and behavioral issues between patient and parent-proxy assessments of QOL. Although patient assessments were driven primarily by issues surrounding self-perception, parent-proxy QOL assessments were driven by behavioral issues. These differences are not unique to patients with devices, and similar findings have been demonstrated in other pediatric groups with chronic illness [44–46]. These findings suggest that although patients are aware of their own self-perception, they are unaware of the outward manifestations of their behavior. In direct contrast, parents are more aware of the effects on their child's behavior but less able to perceive the effects of their children's own self-perception. *They concluded that Patient-and-parent-proxy–reported QOL is significantly affected by the presence of cardiac rhythm devices and is worsened in those patients with CHD and ICD systems as opposed to pacing systems. These findings should encourage us to consider the negative impact of devices, particularly ICDs on pediatric patients and to develop strategies to mitigate these effects.*

A scientific statement from the American Heart Association, *endorsed by the Heart Rhythm Society and the American Association of Critical-Care Nurses*

(*Circulation* 2012) [47] in their state of science statement, they emphasize the burden of the psychosocial distress created by the underlying arrhythmia and its potential treatments in patients and family members that is underappreciated by clinical care teams. They are in agreement with our general feeling about the difficulties and entanglement of cardiac disease and device-related concerns. The majority of ICD patients and families may adjust to the ICD, but optimal care pathways may require additional psychosocial attention to all ICD patients and particularly those experiencing psychosocial distress. This state-of-the-science report was developed on the basis of an analysis and critique of existing science to (1) describe the psychological and quality-of-life outcomes after receipt of an ICD and define related factors, such as patient characteristics; (2) describe the concerns and educational/informational needs of ICD patients and their family members; (3) outline the evidence that supports interventions for improving educational and psychological outcomes for ICD patients; (4) provide recommendations for clinical approaches that improve patient outcomes; and (5) identify priorities for future research in this area. The ultimate goal of this statement was to improve the precision of identification and care of psychosocial distress in ICD patients to maximize the derived benefit of the ICD.

Although figures until 2012 suggest that pediatric ICD recipients constitute less than 1% of the total ICD population [48], the authors of the statement believe that pediatric patients must be included in any discussion about the educational and psychological needs of ICD recipients because of factors that distinguish them from their adult counterparts. First, in contrast to adults, the diseases that result in a need for ICD implantation in the pediatric population are much more heterogeneous. Second, clinical issues or complications associated with ICD placement in the pediatric age group are more frequent than those seen in adults, including the fact that children will have to live with their ICDs for a much longer period of time. The ICD is used for both primary and secondary prevention of SCA in children and adolescents [49]; however, the types of disease that prompt ICD placement in pediatric patients differ from those of adults. These types generally fall into one of the following categories: Congenital heart disease, including but not limited to Tetralogy of Fallot (TOF), Dextro-transposition of the Great Arteries (D-TGA), and Aortic Stenosis (AS) [50]; cardiomyopathy, including dilated [51, 52] hypertrophic [51–53] and arrhythmogenic right ventricular dysplasia [54] forms; or ion channel abnormalities such as the congenital form of long-QT syndrome [55] Brugada syndrome [56] and catecholaminergic polymorphic ventricular tachycardia [56]. The diverse indications for ICD placement create a heterogeneous population with varied disease and treatment histories. The psychosocial outcomes in pediatric and adolescent ICD patients and their caregivers have not been well studied. An examination including 9 years of data (1997–2006) from a national registry database [57] revealed a significant increase in the number of pediatric ICD implantations per year, which translated to a threefold increase during this time frame. Other important findings included a decrease in the number of patients receiving a device for secondary prevention and a decrease in the age of pediatric patients receiving ICDs (from 13.6 to 12.2 years). Interestingly, the percentage of children less than 5 years of age receiving ICDs increased, and the complication rate decreased over time. The pediatric ICD population has unique issues, including growth and development, high likelihood of prior cardiac surgery, complex cardiovascular anatomy, high incidence of supraventricular arrhythmias, and a high incidence of ICD discharges. However, research on the psychosocial needs, outcomes, and associated factors in pediatric patients with ICDs is in its infancy, and many studies have had small sample sizes. The incidence of inappropriate shocks in pediatric patients has been reported to be in the range of 21–47%, and in a number of patients, the shocks were caused by supraventricular tachycardia, lead and device complications, and T-wave oversensing [49, 58, 59]. No difference in the incidence of device discharges in patients with single-versus-dual-chamber devices was noted. Patients 12 years of age or less had more appropriate shocks than those 13–18 years old [59]. In a study of 28 patients, Celiker and colleagues [60] concluded that the high incidence of shocks, whether appropriate or inappropriate, interfered with QOL in their sample, although the measure of QOL was unclear. Lead or device complications are not rare in the pediatric population, and the incidence of lead fractures has been found to be higher in the pediatric population than in adults, possibly because of growth-related issues, increased physical activity in children, and device location [61, 62]. Lead-specific complications in the pediatric population range from 7 to 50% at a median follow-up of 2 years, with the highest incidence being in the younger, smaller patients [40, 63]. No studies of device recall or lead issues in relation to psychosocial outcomes in pediatric and adolescent ICD patients were found. The limited literature about the psychosocial aspects of having an ICD in the pediatric age group has, until recently, been largely descriptive and not inclusive of QOL issues. Early exploratory studies about the effects of ICD placement in the young suggested adjustment-related difficulties [37, 64] as well as concerns about peer rejection, device explosion, depression, and suicidal ideation [65]. In a small qualitative pilot study of adolescents aged 12–19 years in 1995, when ICDs were first used as a treatment option in the pediatric age group, participants reported being anxious about the device and described life with an ICD as "being on a roller coaster" [66]. Themes that emerged from this study included the need for normalcy, parental over-protectiveness, adjustment time, and concerns about the future. In a subsequent qualitative study with 14 adolescents with ICDs (nine males and five females, mean age 16 years), the researchers concluded that having an ICD was described as "almost normal" [67]. The participants experienced social isolation, transient depression, being shocked, fear of and anxiety associated with being shocked, problems associated with activity restrictions, and trying to live a normal life in the midst of dealing with a chronic heart condition. The inability to participate in full-contact organized sports was particularly burdensome to those who had genetically determined diseases that put them at increased risk for SCA [67]. Stefanelli et al. [68], reported that 3 of 27 pediatric patients who had received repeated shocks experienced anxiety that persisted for more than 1 month, and school phobias and PTSD requiring antidepressants, anxiolytics, and ongoing psychiatric therapy were also experienced by some. DeMaso et al. [69], sought to determine whether anxiety, depression, family functioning, and QOL were related to cardiac illness severity in children with ICDs. Patient/parent dyads (n = 20) participated in this quantitative study. ICD patients aged 9–19 years (mean age 14.8 years) appeared to experience lower physical functioning as a component of their QOL than did their healthy peers [69]. Parents of the participants reported significantly lower physical functioning in their children than in the normative population (using the US normative sample mean). The study participants overall did not experience clinical levels of depression; however, two did meet depression criteria. Participants scored significantly lower on worry/oversensitivity and higher on the social desirability measures than the normative sample. There were no differences in any of the measures among those who had or had not received shocks. There were no correlations between illness severity (Defibrillator Severity Index) and psychosocial functioning; however, there were strong associations between QOL and feelings of anxiety and depression, as well as family functioning. Half of the participants indicated that their biggest worry was receiving a shock [69]. In a Polish study of 45 ICD recipients aged 14–29 years designed to identify both clinical and psychological problems associated with living with an ICD [70], 84.4% of the participants reported anxiety associated with ICD discharge that subsequently led to self-imposed activity restrictions, with 29% refusing to accept limitations. Other findings included difficulty accepting the ICD or the disease that necessitated its placement, non acceptance of the ICD, negative perceptions of follow-up visits, noncompliance, refusal to accept limitations, denial of disease existence, and thoughts of having the device removed. The largest psychosocial functioning and QOL study to date of pediatric ICD patients was a survey of patient/parent dyads (n = 60) from six major medical centers in the United States by a pioneer in the field Sears SF et al. [17]. The age of the ICD recipients ranged from 8 to 18 years, and the sample was primarily white. There were 25 girls and 35 boys, and 48.3% had experienced one or more shocks. Parents were primarily mothers (75%). Similar to subjects in the study by De Maso et al. [69], the ICD recipients had significantly lower scores on both psychosocial and physical dimensions of QOL than the norms of healthy children. Compared with children with other chronic illnesses, the ICD recipients had significantly lower scores on the psychosocial health dimension but not the physical dimension. Parents also scored their children significantly lower on the psychosocial and physical dimensions of QOL than the norms of parents with healthy children and scored them lower on both dimensions than the children themselves. With respect to medical severity, those patients with greater medical severity reported significantly lower psychosocial and physical scores. There were no significant differences in any of the QOL variables based on having received a shock. Sex differences manifested in that the girls reported significantly lower QOL scores in the psychosocial and physical domains and were more likely to avoid places than boys; however, 84.7% of the entire sample reported avoidance behaviors after ICD implantation [17].

These results suggest that clinical attention for young ICD patients likely needs to include activity expectations and recommendations to prevent the common occurrence of avoidance behaviors. A recent report of 30 pediatric ICD patients in the Netherlands (mean age 16.3 years, mean duration 3.6 years) showed greater psychological problems in those who were younger and those with shocks [71].

In summary, few data are available to fully understand the psychosocial impact of the ICD on pediatric and adolescent ICD recipients, and no longitudinal studies of psychosocial response over time are available. Initial studies in children and young adults have identified higher levels of anxiety and lower quality of life scores in patients with implantable cardioverter–defibrillators. Anxiety is highly prevalent in young patients with ICDs but the higher rates can be attributed to medical disease severity and age at implantation rather than type of device. Patients with pacemakers have depression and anxiety but at lower rates.

The existing data about psychosocial functioning of young children and young adults with ICDs suggest that they encounter more physical and psychosocial challenges than same-aged peers but are quite similar to other young people with chronic disease. Collectively, these age-specific concerns, together with the typical ICD patient concerns such as both inappropriate and appropriate shocks and physical activity restrictions, remain targets of clinical and research attention.

Adolescents with Implantable Cardioverter Defibrillators

Compared to older ICD recipients, adolescents share adults common physical and technical ICD problems but have their own psychosocial and developmental aspects. Adolescence is a unique stage of life between childhood and adulthood with all the difficulties of transition. Adding ICD to this life stage deserve special discussion.

Compared to older ICD recipients, young patients face decades of life with the device and the long-term impact and implications are important to consider. Until recently the use of ICDs in young patients was rare comprising less than 1% of ICD patients (under 21 years of age) [72]. As there are little data available about young people with ICDs, the psychosocial impact of having the device as an adolescent is largely unknown. As we emphasize earlier, it would be inappropriate to extrapolate the results from research on older patients to younger recipients. We always incorporate pediatric age group in adolescent discussion, as it is the immediate developmental stage before adolescence. It is very important also to note that the indication for ICDs implant in pediatric and adolescent age groups can be different from the indication in adults. For example, in younger patients, ICDs are more often used as a preventative measure of sudden death in genetic diseases [56]. There can also be more complications associated with the device in younger populations, which may result in more surgery, increased time spent in the hospital, and increased risk of infection at the wound site [73]. Adolescence is also a time of potential conflict, confusion, and stress marked by physical, emotional, and psychosocial changes [67]. A potentially life-threatening diagnosis and the challenge of coping with an ICD may exacerbate this already difficult period in adolescents' lives and may challenge young people in establishing identity, intimacy, and autonomy. Young ICD patients are a "unique subset" who face challenges specific to their age and stage of development [34]. By identifying the challenges that adolescents have to face, a greater understanding of their experiences can be developed which will in turn inform clinical practice and encourage further research.

Theoretically, the ICD medical community investigating adolescents' psychosocial impact of ICD identified fear of being shocked by the device, activity restrictions, and feeling different from peers as the most significant psychosocial issues which may distress adolescents.

To prioritize those issues and others, expert consensus from experienced pediatric dysrhythmia clinicians was obtained by Zeigler et al. [74]. A three-round electronic Delphi study was conducted. A multidisciplinary purposive sample was drawn from two international organizations of pediatric and young adult cardiovascular caregivers who specialize in rhythm disturbances in this patient population. The top ten psychosocial issues identified by the panel included, in order of importance: fear of being shocked, sports participation/activity restrictions, feeling different from peers/peer acceptance, depression, adjustment problems, fear of death, medication noncompliance, acting out, body change/weight gain, and issues related to planning for adulthood.

Most research has been quantitative using clinical measures or self-report questionnaires with only a small number of studies using interviews to explore opinions and attitudes related to psychosocial issues of ICD implantation. Poor psychosocial adjustment measured by increased levels of anxiety and depression has been shown in younger ICD recipients [34, 75]. Perceived decrease in quality of life has been shown in both adolescent ICD patients [56] and their parents [69]. A recent study of 14 adolescents with ICDs used in-depth interviews to explore their experiences of living with the device [67]. The overall theme that emerged from this study was that adolescents felt "almost normal," with the concept of normality and perceptions of their previous existence altered by ICD implantation so that life was "not quite ever the same again". Although the adolescents were conscious of the challenges both the device and their diagnoses presented, learning to acknowledge their strengths, minimize their limitations, and/or recognize the benefit of the device assisted them in moving forward with their lives. Belinda Rahman et al., took a crucial step to qualitatively explore the experiences of young people with ICDs, and their parents [76]. Their study, building on this previous research concerning young people and ICDs, sought to document and explore in detail their experience of living with the device. The study also aimed at exploring the experience of the parents of these adolescents to better understand the impact of ICD implantation on the primary caregiver. They used qualitative methods due to the limited knowledge that currently exists about young people's experiences of ICDs. Phenomenology through in-depth study of individual experiences, aims to identify both the meaning and common features of a particular experience or event, prioritizing the personal, subjective perspective [77]. Thus, the use of qualitative methods in this study facilitated understanding the impact of the ICD on adolescents and their parents by providing an opportunity for these individuals to express their personal accounts. A unique finding from this study was the differences that exist between parental perceptions and adolescent perceptions. Parents felt that their children were "normal," whereas adolescents described being "not normal" or "different." In this study, the adolescent participants described how once they received an ICD, life had changed irreversibly: "the concept of normal disappeared when ICD placement was required".

In the current study, adolescents perceived physical and other restrictions as not only limiting them in what they *used* to do, but also preventing them from doing what their peers and other "normal" people were currently able to do. It was this comparison to life before their ICD and the life of their peers currently that created the feeling of being different. *We may express this new feeling after ICD implant as the adolescent who feels normal but for the new situation.*

Also, unique to this study was the sense of greater independence that the ICD provided to two adolescent participants. This is in contrast to the loss of independence described by adults with ICDs, which may be due to the restrictions the device imposes on driving and work life that in fact remove independence in adults with ICDs [78, 79].

For the adolescent participants in Belinda Rahman et al. study [76], physical restrictions were seen as the most significant aspect of living with an ICD and the most challenging to adjust to. Unlike the restrictions in this sample of adolescents, physical restrictions in adults with ICDs are often self-imposed [79]. Adult ICD patients are reluctant to resume previous activities such as routine exercise for fear of triggering an ICD shock, which therefore leads to a self-imposed restricted lifestyle [78]. Reduced physical functioning has been described as a factor associated with increased psychological distress in adults with an ICD [80]. Lower levels of physical functioning have also been associated with a reduced quality of life in children with ICDs [56]. *Evidence from these studies suggests it is important for adolescents to maintain their involvement in recreational activities as much as possible, particularly as quality of life is strongly influenced by the ability of the ICD patient to resume a "pre-ICD lifestyle"* [78].

The main benefit associated with the ICD was the reassurance and peace of mind that it provided for the adolescents as well as their parents, mostly through the knowledge that it was a protective, life-saving device. We usually tell adolescents and parents that "*the ICD is an intelligent and loyal device*". It seems they like the description. Sense of relief and reassurance was reflected in a study of children with ICDs for long QT syndrome, where both the young people and their parents felt that the sense of security provided by the ICD far outweighed the negative experiences [81]. Adults with ICDs have described relief and a sense of gratitude that "the device was keeping them alive." [79] Adolescent ICD patients have also described the security and "freedom from danger" as an important benefit of having the device [67].

Concern and anxiety surrounding the expectation and experience of an ICD shock is well documented [67, 79]. Although the parents in Belinda Rahman et al. study [76] reflected anxiety, some parents acknowledged that the shock could potentially be a life-saving event. A similar attitude has previously been described; four children who received inappropriate shocks felt the discomfort of the experience was outweighed by the sense of security provided by the ICD, and none of the participants regretted the decision to have the device implanted based on the discomfort associated with the shocks [81].

Creation of a positive emotional perspective, experiencing device shock as a herald of new life, is in our opinion, a very important step towards healthy psychosocial outcomes including minimizing anxiety and other negative feelings. Negative emotions like anger tend to increase T-Wave Alternance (TWA) and altered ventricular repolarization predicts future ventricular arrhythmias in adult patients with ICDs [82]. As the mechanism of VF is the same in all age groups, we can deduce with confidence that interrupting the cycle of negative emotion shock continuum in children and adolescents-should minimize the psychological distress and its ramifications in this important age group.

Theoretical Approaches to the Psychosocial Adjustment of ICD Recipients; General Theories of Psychological Adjustment to the ICD

Samuel F. Sears, Jr., Ph.D. is a true father and international pioneer and expert in the psychological care and quality of life outcomes of ICD patients. He has published over 100 articles and chapters in medical literature on the psychological aspects of cardiology. It is very hard to write about the psychological aspects of ICDs without making explicit reference to him. In one of his earliest publications, he and his colleagues review the data related to psychosocial adjustment of young ICD recipients, postulate theories to explain potential adjustment difficulties to ICD therapy experienced by younger recipients, and suggest clinical management techniques for addressing the unique psychosocial concerns of young ICD recipients [34]. Of particular importance is their discussion of how general theories can help describe the psychological adjustment to the ICD.

Three theories that hold heuristic value in explaining the adjustment of ICD recipients across age groups were discussed [37]. First, the *Classical Conditioning Theory* can be used to explain how repeated shocks given by the ICD may be paired with previously neutral environmental or behavioral stimuli, resulting in conditioned responses including anxiety or fear [83]. Second, the *Learned Helplessness Theory* can be used to explain how ICD recipients who feels as if they have no control over the necessary defibrillation discharges may develop feelings of hopelessness and depression about their current and future health status [84]. Sears et al. [37] proposed a third theory, the *Cognitive Appraisal Theory of ICD Activity*, as a model for how some ICD recipients seek greater perceived cognitive control by interpreting the activity or inactivity of the device as an indicator of their level of current cardiac functioning. Recipients use the firings of the device as a "sickness scoreboard," believing that when the device fires they are becoming sicker and when it does not fire that their health is improving.

Age-Specific Theories of Adjustment

To address familial role issues and other stressors that would be obscured if young ICD recipients were considered as one group, the authors again divided the group into those 18 and younger (children/adolescents) and those 19–50 years of age (adults) [34].

Children and Adolescents

No comprehensive theory of adjustment specific to children who have received an ICD has been published. To fill this void, they found it useful to draw material from the literature on children with chronic illnesses. While a ventricular arrhythmia is an event rather than a chronic illness, it is a life-threatening condition that must be monitored and treated for the life of the patient. Therefore, analogies to children with chronic illness can be made. Wallander and Thompson [85] asserted that the wide range of special psychosocial adjustment challenges faced by children with a chronic illness put them at "increased risk for mental health and adjustment problems". In their *disability stress-coping model*, Wallander and Varni [86] proposed three categories of **risk factors** that may contribute to the maladjustment of children with a chronic illness:

1. Disease and disability parameters include factors like type of diagnosis the child has received, the level of physical and behavioral impairment caused by the condition, the visibility of the condition, and if cognitive functioning is impaired by the condition.
2. Functional dependence in activities of daily living. In other words, can the child walk, talk, eat, dress, etc., without assistance?
3. Psychosocial stressors include disability problems, major life-events, and daily hassles.

According to the disability-stress-coping model, when children experience increased stress associated with their condition that may be related to disability parameters or functional dependence, these condition related stressors increase the effects of daily life stressors already experienced by children and psychosocial adjustment problems develop.

Furthermore, the disability stress-coping model postulates that adjustment is influenced by **resistance factors**. These factors fall under three categories:

1. Personal factors such as problem-solving abilities, temperament, and motivation.
2. Social-ecological factors including familial resources and social support.
3. Stress processing abilities such as coping strategies and cognitive appraisals.

The researchers postulate that if the child has an adequate number of resistance factors he or she may be less vulnerable to psychosocial adjustment disorders [86].

Clinical experience with children who have ICDs suggests many applications for the theory of Wallander and Varni. For example, perceived physical limitations may make going to school especially stressful for young ICD recipients. Also, the inability to predict when the device might discharge and the fear of the discharges may compound the stress of interacting with peers and lead to increased social anxiety. Finally, resistance factors, like a strong family support system, may facilitate adjustment to the real and perceived limitations of young ICD recipients.

A second model of adjustment was extended by Thompson et al. [87] who proposed a *transactional-stress-coping model* based on an ecological systems approach to understanding stress and coping in children with chronic illnesses. The model focuses on the transactions between biomedical, developmental, and psychosocial systems and how familial and extrafamilial systems affect illness outcomes. Furthermore, Thompson hypothesized that the adaptational processes of the child and other family members, specifically the mother, are the key factors that affect the child's psychosocial adjustment [87]. Adaptational processes are described as expectations about self-esteem, the child's health focus of control, how caregivers appraise stress, familial functioning, and methods of coping for the child and the caregivers. Adaptational processes are thought to affect the adjustment of the chronically ill child above and beyond medical and demographic variables [88]. Appropriate adaptational processes may be seen as similar to the resistance factors described by Wallander and Varni [86], the disability-stress-coping model; the more appropriate the processes, the less vulnerable a child is to maladjustment.

Young Adults

The adjustment of young adult ICD recipients may be explained by *the social comparison theory*, which hypothesizes that when no objective standard is available for a person to test their abilities directly, they compare themselves to others [89]. Early research on the social comparison theory and coping with major medical problems indicated that individuals suffering from major illnesses may not seek or be given information they can use to understand their illness or modify its outcome; this makes an objective self-evaluation improbable. They may suffer from lowered self-esteem if they see themselves as victims or they are perceived by others to be victims. Finally, they may experience distress that cannot be controlled or mediated by problem-focused coping, thereby increasing their feelings of helplessness [90]. The social comparison theory also asserts that individuals compare themselves to groups of people or other individuals to whom they feel similar. The relatively small number of adults aged 19–50 years with ICDs may result in a lack of communication between individuals in this age group. This lack of communication with other young ICD recipients may lead to comparisons with other people in their age group who do not have ICDs or related heart arrhythmia concerns (i.e., individuals who are working, active, and physically fit). These comparisons may result in lowered self-esteem and unrealistic self-evaluations and consequent adjustment difficulties.

Psychoeducational Interventions for Children and Adolescents with ICD

Due to the fact that children and adolescents with ICD are a new population for the medical community, medical literature investigating their psychosocial aspects is relatively rare and accordingly the treatment plans publications for this group of patients is scarce. In most situations psychological distress is related to the impact of the primary disease. Familial as well as social factors are also strong contributors to the outcomes. According to the present literature, Post-Traumatic Stress Disorder

(PTSD) in children and adolescents with ICDs seems to be a rare event. Accordingly, intervention plans are mostly non-pharmacological. Psychoeducational plans and modules are the main theme in managing the psychosocial and emotional aspects of ICDs in children and adolescents. Even in adult ICD population the use of medications is exceptional and mostly limited to some PTSD patients.

Psychoeducation, which is widely attributed to the American researcher C.M. Anderson who developed it in the 1980's in the context of the treatment of schizophrenia, is the corner stone in treatment of psychosocial distress in ICD patients of all age groups. Psychosocial interventions are effective for adults with cardiac devices and could potentially impact adolescents' adjustment to these devices. Mindfulness Based Stress Reduction (MBSR) is a structured psychoeducational program that includes meditation, yoga, and group support has been studied extensively among adults. Vicki A. Freedenberg examined the feasibility of the MBSR program for adolescents with ICDs and pacemakers, a population previously unexamined in the research literature. Anxiety frequency decreased from baseline to post-intervention (Fisher's exact test $p = .024$), and 90% of participants reported decreased anxiety scores post-intervention. Coping skills related negatively to anxiety ($r = -.65$, $p = .04$) and depression ($r = -.88$, $p = .001$). Post-intervention, the group independently formed their own Facebook group and requested to continue meeting monthly. Although generalizability is limited due to the small sample size, this successful pilot study paves the way for larger studies to examine the efficacy of MBSR interventions in adolescents with high-risk cardiac diagnoses [91].

As with other developments in pediatric medicine, clinicians using CBT with children initially had to extrapolate findings with adults, and based on their experience adapt the results appropriately so that they could be applicable to children.

Particular adaptations that therapists make when working with children have to do with pacing the content and speed of therapy at a level appropriate for the child, bearing in mind the younger child's limitations in metacognition and ineptitude in labeling feelings. With younger children, the therapist is likely to be more active and will make use of a higher proportion of behavioral rather than cognitive techniques.

Although with adults much of the work in CBT, especially with patients with neurotic disorders, is concerned with correcting maladaptive and dysfunctional distortions of thinking, with children more attention is given to deficits in social skills or interpersonal problem-solving. Training in social skills and problem-solving is an important part of interventions not only for children with conduct disorder, attention-deficit hyperactivity disorder (ADHD) or empathy disorders but also for children with anxiety, a major psychological complaint in children and adolescents with ICD. Applications of CBT to particular disorders is well described in Graham's *Cognitive–Behavior Therapy for Children and Families* [92], which should be recommended reading for child and adolescent psychiatrists.

Over the past two decades, 15 adult studies have tested the effects of psychological or psychoeducational interventions (mainly CBT) on outcomes of anxiety, depression, ICD shocks, QOL, and symptoms in people who have an ICD [85, 93–103]. The majority of interventions directed towards improving psychosocial functioning have included patients who received an ICD for secondary prevention of Sudden Cardiac Death (SCA). In two studies, there was no definition of the exact patient population, and five studies included both primary and secondary prevention patients; however, no differences were noted in psychosocial outcomes by ICD implantation indication. In general, the sample sizes have ranged from 8 to 246 subjects, with 8 studies having a total sample size of less than 100 subjects. The majority of the studies used a randomized trial format, with two using a sample of convenience [51, 56]; two-studies were cross-sectional comparisons [54, 55] and one used a crossover design [37]. The outcomes of the interventions were measured from 3 to 12 months after the intervention, with long-term benefits of psychosocial interventions noted in five studies at 12 months [93, 98, 99, 103, 104]. More than two-thirds of the interventions tested were based on a cognitive behavioral therapy (CBT) framework. The length of CBT interventions ranged from 4 to 12 sessions, with the majority including six sessions. CBT interventions have demonstrated significant effects on anxiety, depression, and ICD concerns. Education and psychosocial support interventions have ranged from 2 to 8 sessions using a group or telephone mode of delivery. These interventions demonstrated significant improvements with regards to patient concerns, anxiety, and knowledge. Stress management interventions demonstrate significant effects on anxiety and have ranged from 6 to 11 hourly sessions.

Anxiety and depression in children and adolescents involves cognitive deficit. Cognitive–behavioral therapy for anxious children can be built around a formulation of the problem in cognitive and behavioral terms. The level of sophistication of the child may determine the degree to which adult-type cognitive strategies can be used. For children and less sophisticated adolescents, Wood & Harrington have produced a comprehensible manual of their Depression Treatment Programme. This includes useful charts and is supplemented by a videotape for clinicians. It can be used by child mental health professionals with minimal additional training.

Pharmacological Treatment of PTSD in Children and Adolescents

It must be underlined that the true incidence of children and adolescents with ICDs diagnosed to have PTDS is not known.

Supported by pre-clinical and clinical studies that demonstrate dysregulated CNS noradrenergic functioning and PFC underfunctioning, adrenergic medications are increasingly being used in the treatment of trauma in children. Centrally acting a2-agonists including guanfacine, guanfacine extended release (GXR), and clonidine appear effective in diminishing the intensity of trauma induced hyperarousal symptoms, including impaired concentration, poor impulse control, hypervigilance, nightmares and insomnia, and exaggerated startle response in children and adolescents. Although there are no controlled trials of these agents in pediatric PTSD, case reports and open trials suggest that clonidine may reduce flashbacks and traumatic repetitive play in children and that guanfacine may reduce trauma-induced nightmares [105, 106]. Presently, there are no reports of clonidine extended release use in pediatric PTSD. An open label study of GXR suggests effectiveness for symptoms of traumatic stress and PTSD in children [107]. In an 8-week open-label design, and using an average GXR daily dose of 1.19 mg ± 0.35 mg and an average weight adjusted daily dose of 0.03 mg/kg ± 0.01 mg/kg significant improvement was found in re-experiencing, avoidant, and overarousal rating scale child trauma symptoms. Of study completers, 71% met a priori criteria for response. This open-label study suggests that the a2A-adrenoceptor agonist GXR may have therapeutic effects in the treatment of PTSD symptoms in traumatically stressed children and adolescents and that the effective dose may be lower than that found for ADHD [107]. The a1-antagonist, prazosin, has been shown to be effective in treating PTSD in controlled trials of adult subjects. At present, the data on the use of prazosin for symptoms of traumatic stress in the pediatric years is limited to open case reports, generally describing use in adolescents [108–111]. There is one case report of successful treatment of a 7-year-old child with PTSD using 1 mg of prazosin [112]. Case reports suggest that in daily doses between 1 mg and 4 mg prazosin appears helpful in reducing trauma nightmares in adolescents and possibly in children with PTSD. Although prazosin is used in doses up to 15 mg/day to treat pediatric hypertension, these case reports suggest possible PTSD effectiveness at lower doses. However, conclusions on the suggested efficacy of prazosin for symptoms of PTSD and traumatic stress await data from more controlled clinical trials.

It is especially important to assay and develop treatments for childhood PTSD, because it can have such far-reaching effects. The epidemiology of pediatric trauma exposure reveals that outcomes vary, from resilience to psychopathology, and early death. Influencing outcomes are child specific factors such as antecedent mental health vulnerabilities, family factors such as intact caregiving relationships that serve to buffer stress, and characteristics of the trauma such as proximity, presence of injury, chronicity, and characteristics of the agent (natural disaster versus caregiver inflicted). When psychopathology is an outcome, comorbidity is the rule. The sequelae of childhood traumatic stress include a range of possible outcomes encompassing persistence of posttraumatic symptoms, alterations in developmental trajectories with subsequent impairment in emotional and behavioral control, learning disabilities, persistent aggression and/or violence which increases the risk for juvenile justice involvement, substance abuse, and early death [113–115]. The presence of ICDs in this age group acts like a persistent stimulus for abnormal behavior, thus, there is an imperative need for effective treatments children with ICDs diagnosed with PTSD.

Recommendations for Future Research

Implanting ICD in all age groups is a recent development in the management of fatal arrhythmia, creating a breakthrough in the trajectory of arrhythmia treatment history. Relative paucity of literature of psychosocial aspects in children and adolescents with ICDs is creating enormous potential for research in this field. Areas to be investigated in the future to optimize outcomes for children and adolescents with ICDs are the following:

1. Identifying *risk factors for ICD recipients* in order to minimize or abort risk of psychological distress after implantation, in order to promote increased physical exertion and engagement in life. Establishment of risk stratification peculiar for pediatric and adolescent disease should be priority. Special emphasis should be devoted to Congenital Heart Disease (CHD) and channelopathies.
2. *Education and psychological support* before and after implant: In addition to CBT, what other psychoeducational interventions are effective in reducing or preventing adverse psychological responses. Translation of the effective methods of competent psychoeducational interventions into practice for children, adolescents and families alike.
3. *ICD technological improvements* to facilitate patient and family experience with shock; like accurately anticipating shocks with friendly alarms that alert the ICD patient before the possible shock. Important indicators for possible shock anticipation, that we suggest, are detecting potassium level and micro T wave Alternans (micro TWA). The time between alarm and potential shock can be used to abort the shock with patient related or hospital based procedures. Remote intervention based therapies in this context is a priority.
4. *Information* from media, technology holders and industry directed to patients and their family members to *improve QOL* outcomes and measures to minimize patient and family distress in case of *device or lead recall.*
5. The effect of *ICD shocks on sympathovagal regulation* and physical functioning; the role of *cardiac coherence* training to minimize anxiety and negative emotions in children and adolescents with ICDs.
6. *Evaluating specific programming and patient character data* from existing databases to establish strategies aimed at reducing inappropriate shocks their deleterious effects.
7. *Exercise and physical activity*: what interventions promote safe unmonitored exercise and physical activity for children and adolescents (home-based, walking, gym)? What are the psychosocial outcomes of these interventions? How can family members be involved in promoting physical activity interventions? What are optimal exercise testing protocols to prescribe and promote exercise in ICD patients? What information, educational content, and formats regarding exercise and physical activity can be considered optimal for standard use in clinical practice? What other outcomes of exercise interventions can be expected in addition to oxygen consumption and oxygen uptake outcomes? Rehabilitation.
8. *The cognitive impairment* level in ICD children and adolescents especially those with frequent shocks.
9. The true incidence and required management plans of *Post-Traumatic Stress Disorder* (PTSD) in pediatric and adolescent population with ICD.

References

1. Garrett A, Hazelton SSF, Ford J, Cahill J, Nekkanti R, Deantonio H, Ottoboni L, Norton L, Wang P. Decisional balance among potential implantable cardioverter defibrillator recipients: development of the ICD-Decision Analysis Scale (ICD-DAS). Pacing Clin Electrophysiol. 2014;37:63–72.
2. Samson RA, Berg RA, Bingham R. Members of the PALS task force :use of automated external defibrillators for children: an update, an advisory statement from the pediatric advanced life support task force, International Liaison Committee on Resuscitation Writing Group. Circulation. 2003;107:3250–5.
3. Mogayzel C, Quan L, Graves JR, et al. Out-of-hospital ventricular fibrillation in children and adolescents: causes and outcomes. Ann Emerg Med. 1995;25:484–91.
4. Hickey RW, Cohen DM, Strausbaugh S, et al. Pediatric patients requiring CPR in the pre hospital setting. Ann Emerg Med. 1995;25:495–501.2.
5. Eisenberg M, Bergner L, Hallstrom A. Epidemiology of cardiac arrest and resuscitation in children. Ann Emerg Med. 1983;12:672–4.
6. Sirbaugh PE, Pepe PE, Shook JE, et al. A prospective population-based study of the demographics, epidemiology, management and outcome of out-of-hospital pediatric cardiopulmonary arrest. Ann Emerg Med. 1999;33:174–84.
7. Young KD, Seidel JS. Pediatric cardiopulmonary resuscitation: a collective review. Ann Emerg Med. 1999;33:195–205.
8. Schwartz PJ, Priori SG, Dumaine R, et al. A molecular link between the sudden infant death syndrome and the long-QT syndrome. N Engl J Med. 2000;343:262–7.
9. Losek JD, Hennes H, Glaeser PW, et al. Prehospital counter shock treatment of pediatric asystole. Am J Emerg Med. 1980;7:571–5.
10. Quan L, Wentz KR, Gore EJ, et al. Outcome and predictors of outcome in pediatric submersion victims receiving prehospital care in King County Washington. Pediatrics. 1990;86:586–93.
11. Suominen P, Olkkola KT, Voipio V, et al. Utstein style reporting of in-hospital pediatric cardiopulmonary resuscitation. Resuscitation. 2000;45:17–25.
12. Nadkarni VM, Berg RA, Kaye W, et al. Survival outcome for in-hospital pulseless cardiac arrest reported to the National Registry of CPR is better for children than adults. Crit Care Med. 2003;31:A14.
13. Billson A, Tyrrell J. How to break bad news: current. Pediatrics. 2003;13:284–7.
14. Sreeram N, Trieschmann U, de Haan E. Device therapy in children: current indications. Indian Pacing Electrophysiol J. 2008;8:S92–S104.
15. Dimsdale C, Dimsdale A, Ford J, Shea JB, Sears SF. My child needs or has an implantable cardioverter-defibrillator: what should i do? Circulation. 2012;126:e244–7.
16. Ittenbach RF, Cassedy AE, Marino BS, Spicer RL, Drotar D. Adherence to treatment among children with cardiac disease. Cardiol Young. 2009;19:545–51.
17. Sears SF, Hazelton AG, St. Amant J, Matchett M, Kovacs A, Vazquez LD, Fairbrother D, Redfearn S, Hanisch D, Dubin A, Cannon BC, Fishbach P, Kanter R, Bryant RM. Quality of life in pediatric patients with implantable cardioverter defibrillators. Am J Cardiol. 2011;107:1023–7.
18. Sable C, Foster E, Uzark K, Bjornsen K, Canobbio J, Connolly HM, Graham TP, Curvitz MZ, Kovacs A, Meadows AK, Reid GJ, Reiss JG, Rosenbaum KN, Sagerman PH, Saidi A, Schonberg R, Shah S, Tong E, Williams RG. Best practices in managing transition to adulthood for adolescents with congenital heart disease: the transition process and medical and psychosocial issues: a Scientific Statement from the American Heart Association. Circulation. 2011;123:1454–85.
19. DeMaso DR. Pediatric heart disease. In: Brown RT, editor. Handbook of pediatric psychology in school settings. Mahwah: Lawrence Erlbaum Associates; 2004. p. 283–98.
20. Ko D, Herbert P, Coffey C, Sedrakyan A, Curtis J, Krumholtz H. Beta-blocker therapy and symptoms of depression, fatigue, and sexual dysfunction. JAMA. 2002;288:351–7.

21. Burke JL, Hallas CN, Clark-Carter D, White D, Connelly D. The psychosocial impact of the implantable cardioverter-defibrillator: a meta-analytic review. Br J Health Psychol. 2003;8:165–78.
22. Morris PL, Badger J, Chmielewski C, Berger E, Goldberg RJ. Psychiatric morbidity following implantation of the automatic implantable cardioverter defibrillator. Psychosomatics. 1991;32:58–64.
23. Cooper DK, Luceri RM, Thurer RJ, Myerburg MJ. The impact of the automatic implantable cardioverter defibrillator on quality of life. Clin Prog Electrophysiol Pacing. 1986;4:306–9.
24. Heller SS, Ormont MA, Lidagoster L, Sciacca RR, Steinberg JS. Psychosocial outcome after ICD implantation: a current perspective. Pacing Clin Electrophysiol. 1998;21:1207–15.
25. Sears SF, Conti JB. Understanding implantable cardioverter defibrillator shocks and storms: medical and psychological considerations for research and clinical care. Clin Cardiol. 2003;26:107–11.
26. Vitale MB, Funk M. Quality of life in younger persons with an implantable cardioverter defibrillator. Dimens Crit Care Nurs. 1995;14:100–11.
27. Irvine J, Dorian P, Baker B, O'Brien BJ, Roberts R, Gent M, Newman D, Connolly SJ. Quality of life in the Canadian Implantable Defibrillator Study (CIDS). Am Heart J. 2002;144:282–9.
28. McCready MJ, Exner DV. Quality of life and psychological impact of implantable cardioverter defibrillators: focus on randomized controlled trial data. Card Electrophysiol Rev. 2003;7:63–70.
29. Vlay SC, Olson LC, Fricchione GL, Friedman R. Anxiety and anger in patients with ventricular tachyarrhythmias: responses after automatic internal cardioverter defibrillator implantation. Pacing Clin Electrophysiol. 1989;12:366–73.
30. Pycha C, Gulledge AD, Hutzler J, Kadri N, Maloney J. Psychological responses to the implantable defibrillator: preliminary observations. Psychosomatics. 1986;27:841–5.
31. Bainger EM, Fernsler JI. Perceived quality of life before and after implantation of an internal cardioverter defibrillator. Am J Crit Care. 1995;4:36–43.
32. Sears SF, Todaro JF, Urizar G, Lewis TS, Sirois B, Wallace R, Sotile W, Curtis AB, Conti JB. Assessing the psychosocial impact of the ICD: a national survey of implantable cardioverter defibrillator health care providers. Pacing Clin Electrophysiol. 2000;23:931–3.
33. Dubin AM, Batsford WP, Lewis RJ, Rosenfeld LE. Quality-of-life in patients receiving implantable cardioverter defibrillators at or before age 40. Pacing Clin Electrophysiol. 1996;19:1555–9.
34. Sears SF, Burns JL, Handberg E, Sotile WM, Conti JB. Young at heart: understanding the unique psychosocial adjustment of young implantable cardioverter defibrillator recipients. Pacing Clin Electrophysiol. 2001;24:1113–7.
35. Sears SF, Conti JB. Implantable cardioverter-defibrillators for children and young adolescents: mortality benefit confirmed—what's next? Heart. 2004;90(3):241–2.
36. Sears SF, Todaro JF, Saia TL, et al. Examining the psychosocial impact of implantable cardioverter defibrillators: a literature review. Clin Cardiol. 1999;22:481–9.
37. Fitchet A, Doherty PJ, Bundy C, et al. Comprehensive cardiac rehabilitation programme for implantable cardioverter defibrillator patients: a randomized controlled trial. Heart. 2003;89:155–60.
38. Czosek RJ, Bonney WJ, Cassedy A, Mah DY, Tanel RE, Imundo JR, Singh AK, Cohen MI, Miyake CY, Fawley K, Marino BS. Impact of cardiac devices on the quality of life in pediatric patients. Circ Arrhythm Electrophysiol. 2012;5:1064–72.
39. Czosek RJ, Meganathan K, Anderson JB, Knilans TK, Marino BS, Heaton PC. Cardiac rhythm devices in the pediatric population: utilization and complications. Heart Rhythm. 2012;9:199–208.
40. Alexander ME, Cecchin F, Walsh EP, Triedman JK, Bevilacqua LM, Berul CI. Implications of implantable cardioverter defibrillator therapy in congenital heart disease and pediatrics. J Cardiovasc Electrophysiol. 2004;15:72–6.
41. Berul CI, Van Hare GF, Kertesz NJ, Dubin AM, Cecchin F, Collins KK, Cannon BC, Alexander ME, Triedman JK, Walsh EP, Friedman RA. Results of a multicenter retrospec-

tive implantable cardioverter-defibrillator registry of pediatric and congenital heart disease patients. J Am Coll Cardiol. 2008;51:1685–91.
42. Fortescue EB, Berul CI, Cecchin F, Walsh EP, Triedman JK, Alexander ME. Patient, procedural, and hardware factors associated with pacemaker lead failures in pediatrics and congenital heart disease. Heart Rhythm. 2004;1:150–9.
43. Harter S. Manual for the self-perception profile for children. 1985:1–25.
44. Buyan N, Türkmen MA, Bilge I, Baskin E, Haberal M, Bilginer Y, Mir S, Emre S, Akman S, Ozkaya O, Fidan K, Alpay H, Kavukcu S, Sever L, Ozçakar ZB, Dogrucan N. Quality of life in children with chronic kidney disease (with child and parent assessments). Pediatr Nephrol. 2010;25:1487–96.
45. Theunissen NC, Vogels TG, Koopman HM, Verrips GH, Zwinderman KA, Verloove-Vanhorick SP, Wit JM. The proxy problem: child report versus parent report in health-related quality of life research. Qual Life Res. 1998;7:387–97.
46. White-Koning M, Arnaud C, Dickinson HO, Thyen U, Beckung E, Fauconnier J, McManus V, Michelsen SI, Parkes J, Parkinson K, Schirripa G, Colver A. Determinants of child-parent agreement in quality-of-life reports: a European study of children with cerebral palsy. Pediatrics. 2007;120:e804–14.
47. Dunbar SB, Dougherty CM, Sears SF, Carroll DL, Goldstein NE, Mark DB, McDaniel G, Pressler SJ, Schron E, Wang P, Zeigler VL. A scientific statement from the American Heart Association, *Endorsed by the Heart Rhythm Society and the American Association of Critical-Care Nurses*, on behalf of the American Heart Association Council on Cardiovascular Nursing, Council on Clinical Cardiology, and Council on Cardiovascular Disease in the young educational and psychological interventions to improve, outcomes for recipients of implantable cardioverter defibrillators and their families. Circulation. 2012;126:2146–72.
48. Epstein AE, Dimarco JP, Ellenbogen KA, Estes NA III, Freedman RA, Gettes LS, Gillinov AM, Gregoratos G, Hammill SC, Hayes DL, Hlatky MA, Newby LK, Page RL, Schoenfeld MH, Silka MJ, Stevenson LW, Sweeney MO. ACC/AHA/HRS 2008 guidelines for device-based therapy of cardiac rhythm abnormalities: executive summary: a report of the American College of Cardiology/American Heart Association Task Force on Practice Guidelines (Writing Committee to Revise the ACC/AHA/NASPE 2002 Guideline Update for Implantation of Cardiac Pacemakers and Antiarrhythmia Devices) [published correction appears in *Circulation.* 2009;120:e33]. Circulation. 2008;117:2820–40.
49. Berul CI. Implantable cardioverter defibrillator criteria for primary and secondary prevention of pediatric sudden cardiac death. Pacing Clin Electrophysiol. 2009;32(suppl 2):S67–70.
50. Walsh EP. Practical aspects of implantable defibrillator therapy in patients with congenital heart disease. Pacing Clin Electrophysiol. 2008;31(suppl 1):S38–40.
51. Chatrath R, Porter CB, Ackerman MJ. Role of transvenous implantable cardioverter-defibrillators in preventing sudden cardiac death in children, adolescents, and young adults. Mayo Clin Proc. 2002;77:226–31.
52. Pass R, Liberman L, Spotnitz H, Lamberti JJ, Hordof AJ. Implantable cardioverter defibrillators in children and adolescents: a reassessment of indications. J Am Coll Cardiol. 2003;41(Suppl A):482A.
53. Almquist AK, Montgomery JV, Haas TS, Maron BJ. Cardioverter defibrillator implantation in high-risk patients with hypertrophic cardiomyopathy. Heart Rhythm. 2005;2:814–9.
54. Roquin A, Bomma CS, Nasir K, Tandri H, Tichnell C, James C, Rutberg J, Crosson J, Spevak PJ, Berger RD, Halperin HR, Calkins H. Implantable cardioverter-defibrillators in patients with arrhythmogenic right ventricular dysplasia/cardiomyopathy. J Am Coll Cardiol. 2004;43:1843–52.
55. Schwartz P, Spazzolini C, Priori S, Crotti L, Vicentini A, Landolina M, Gasparini M, Wilde AA, Knops RE, Denjoy I, Toivonen L, Mönnig G, Al-Fayyadh M, Jordaens L, Borggrefe M, Holmgren C, Brugada P, De Roy L, Hohnloser SH, Brink PA. Who are the long-QT syndrome patients who receive an implantable cardioverter-defibrillator and what happens to them? Data from the European long-QT Syndrome Implantable Cardioverter-Defibrillator (LQTS ICD) Registry. Circulation. 2010;122:1272–82.

56. Costa R, Da Silva KR, Mendonca RC, Nishioka SA, F SS, Tamaki WT, Crevelari ES, LFP M, Filho MM. Incidence of shock and quality of life in young patients with implantable cardioverter defibrillator. Arq Bras Cardiol. 2007;88:258–64.
57. Burns KM, Evans F, Kaltman JR. Pediatric ICD utilization in the United States from 1997 to 2006. Heart Rhythm. 2011;8:23–8.
58. Korte T, Köditz H, Niehaus M, Paul T, Tebbenjohanns J. High incidence of appropriate and inappropriate ICD therapies in children and adolescents with implantable cardioverter defibrillator. Pacing Clin Electrophysiol. 2004;27:924–32.
59. Heersche JHM, Blom NA, van de Heuvel F, Blank C, Reimer AG, Clur S-A, Witsenburg M, ten Harkel ADJ. Implantable cardioverter defibrillator therapy for prevention of sudden cardiac death in children in the Netherlands. Pacing Clin Electrophysiol. 2010;33:179–85.
60. Celiker A, Olgun H, Karagoz T, Özer S, Özkutlu S, Alehan D. Midterm experience with implantable cardioverter-defibrillators in children and young adults. Europace. 2010;12:1732–8.
61. Tomaske M, Bauersfeld U. Experience with implantable cardioverter defibrillator therapy in grown-ups with congenital heart disease. Pacing Clin Electrophysiol. 2008;31(suppl 1):S35–7.
62. Link MS, Hill SL, Cliff DL, Swygman CA, Foote CB, Homoud MK, Wang PJ, Estes NA 3rd, Berul CI. Comparison of frequency of complications of implantable cardioverter-defibrillators in children versus adults. Am J Cardiol. 1999;83:263–6, A5–A6.
63. Shah MJ. Implantable cardioverter defibrillator-related complications in the pediatric population. Pacing Clin Electrophysiol. 2009;32(Suppl 2):S71–4.
64. Sears SF, Shea JB, Conti JB. How to respond to an implantable cardioverter-defibrillator shock. Circulation. 2005;111:e380–2.
65. Wilson WR, Greer GE, Grubb BP. Implantable cardioverter defibrillators in children: a single-institutional experience. Ann Thorac Surg. 1998;65:775–8.
66. Zeigler VL, Corbett K, Lewis A, Gillette P. Implantable cardioverter defibrillators. In: Zeigler V, Gillette P, editors. Practical management of pediatric cardiac arrhythmias. Armonk: Futura; 2001. p. 359–409.
67. Zeigler VL, Nelms T. Almost normal: experiences of adolescents with implantable cardioverter defibrillators. J Spec Pediatr Nurs. 2009;14:142–51.
68. Stefanelli CB, Bradley DJ, Leroy S, Dick M 2nd, Serwer GA, Fischbach PS. Implantable cardioverter defibrillator therapy for life-threatening arrhythmias in young patients. J Interv Card Electrophysiol. 2002;6:235–44.
69. DeMaso DR, Lauretti A, Spieth L, Van Der Feen JR, Jay KS, Gauvreau K, Walsh EP, Berul CI. Psychosocial factors and quality of life in children and adolescents with implantable cardioverter-defibrillators. Am J Cardiol. 2004;93:582–7.
70. Wójcicka M, Lewandowski M, Smolis-Bak E, Szwed H. Psychological and clinical problems in young adults with implantable cardioverter defibrillators. Kardiol Pol. 2008;66:1050–8.
71. Koopman H, Vrijmoet-Wiersma C, Langius J, van den Heuvel F, Clur S, Blank C, Blom N, ten Harkel A. Psychological functioning and disease related quality of life in pediatric patients with an implantable cardioverter defibrillator. Pediatr Cardiol. 2012;33:569–75.
72. Blom NA. Implantable cardioverter-defibrillators in children. Pacing Clin Electrophysiol. 2008;24:32–4.
73. Sears SF, Amant JB, Zeigler V. Psychosocial considerations for children and young adolescents with implantable cardioverter defibrillators: an update. Pacing Clin Electrophysiol. 2009;32:80–2.
74. Zeigler VL, Decker-Walters B. Determining psychosocial research priorities for adolescents with implantable cardioverter defibrillators using Delphi methodology. J Cardiovasc Nurs. 2010;25(5):398–404.
75. Eicken A, Kolb C, Lange S, Brodherr-Heberlein S, Zrenner B, Schreiber C, Hess J. Implantable cardioverter defibrillator (ICD) in children. Int J Cardiol. 2006;107:30–5.
76. Rahman B, Macciocca I, Sahhar M, Kamberi S, Connell V, Duncan RE. Adolescents with implantable cardioverter defibrillators: a patient and parent perspective. Pacing Clin Electrophysiol. 2011;35:62–72.

77. Starks H, Trinidad SB. Choose your method: a comparison of phenomenology, discourse analysis, and grounded theory. Qual Health Res. 2007;17:1372–80.
78. Shea JB. Quality of life issues in patients with implantable cardioverter defibrillators: driving, occupation, and recreation. AACN Adv Crit Care. 2004;15:478–89.
79. Tagney J, James JE, Albarran JW. Exploring the patient's experiences of learning to live with an implantable cardioverter defibrillator (ICD) from one UK centre: a qualitative study. Eur J Cardiovasc Nurs. 2003;2:195–203.
80. Dunbar SB. Psychosocial issues of patients with implantable cardioverter defibrillators. Am J Crit Care. 2005;14:294–303.
81. Goel AK, Berger S, Pelech A, Dhala A. Implantable cardioverter defibrillator therapy in children with long QT syndrome. Pediatr Cardiol. 2004;25:370–8.
82. Lampert R, Shusterman V, Burg M, McPherson C, Batsford W, Goldberg A, Soufer R. Anger-induced T-wave alternans predicts future ventricular arrhythmias in patients with implantable cardioverter-defibrillators. J Am Coll Cardiol. 2009;53(9):774–8. doi:10.1016/j.jacc.2008.10.053.
83. Wolpe J, Plaud J. Pavlov's contributions to behavior therapy: the obvious and not so obvious. Am Psychologist. 1997;52:966–72.
84. Peterson C, Seligman M. Explanatory style and illness. J Pers. 1987;55:237–65.
85. Dougherty CM, Lewis FM, Thompson EA, Baer JD, Kim W. Short-term efficacy of a telephone intervention by expert nurses after an implantable cardioverter defibrillator. Pacing Clin Electrophysiol. 2004;27:1594–602.
86. Wallander JL, Varni JW. Adjustment in children with chronic physical disorders: programmatic research on a disability-stress—coping model. In: La Greca AM, Siegel LJ, Wallander JL, Walker CE, editors. Stress and coping in child health. New York: Guilford; 1992. p. 279–97.
87. Thompson RJ, Gustafson KE, George LK, et al. Psychological adjustment of children with cystic fibrosis: the role of child cognitive processes and maternal adjustment. J Pediatr Psychology. 1992;17:741–55.
88. Wallander JL, Thompson RJ. Psychosocial adjustment of children with chronic physical conditions. In: Roberts MC, editor. Handbook of pediatric psychology. 2nd ed. New York: Guilford; 1995. p. 124–41.
89. Festinger L. A theory of social comparison processes. Hum Relations. 1954;7:117–40.
90. Affleck G, Tennen H, Pfeiffer C, et al. Appraisals of control and predictability in adapting to chronic illness. J Pers Soc Psychol. 1987;53:273–9.
91. Freedenberg VA, Thomas SA, Friedmann E. A pilot study of a mindfulness based stress reduction program in adolescents with implantable cardioverter defibrillators or pacemakers. Pediatr Cardiol. 2015;36(4):786–95.
92. Graham P. Cognitive behavior therapy for children and families. Cambridge: Cambridge University Press; 1998.
93. Irvine J, Firestone J, Ong L, Cribbie R, Dorian P, Harris L, Ritvo P, Katz J, Newman D, Cameron D, Johnson S, Bilanovic A, Hill A, O'Donnell S, Sears S Jr. A randomized controlled trial of cognitive behavior therapy tailored to psychological adaptation to an implantable cardioverter defibrillator. Psychosom Med. 2011;73:226–33.
94. Sneed NV, Finch NJ, Michel Y. The effect of psychosocial nursing intervention on the mood state of patients with implantable cardioverter defibrillators and their caregivers. Prog Cardiovasc Nurs. 1997;12:4–14.
95. Kohn CS, Petrucci RJ, Baessler C, Soto DM, Movsowitz C. The effect of psychological intervention on patients' long-term adjustment to the ICD: a prospective study. Pacing Clin Electrophysiol. 2000;23:450–6.
96. Carlsson E, Olsson SB, Hertervig E. The role of the nurse in enhancing quality of life in patients with an implantable cardioverter-defibrillator: the Swedish experience. Prog Cardiovasc Nurs. 2002;17:18–25.
97. Frizelle DJ, Lewin RJP, Kaye G, Hargreaves C, Hasney K, Beaumont N, Moniz-Cook E. Cognitive-behavioural rehabilitation programme for patients with an implanted cardioverter defibrillator: a pilot study. Br J Health Psychol. 2004;9:381–92.

98. Dougherty CM, Thompson EA, Lewis FM. Long-term outcomes of a telephone intervention after an ICD. Pacing Clin Electrophysiol. 2005;28:1157–67.
99. Chevalier P, Cottraux J, Mollard E, Sai N, Brun S, Burri H, Restier L, Adeleine P. Prevention of implantable defibrillator shocks by cognitive behavioral therapy: a pilot trial. Am Heart J. 2006;151:191.
100. Sears SF, Sowell LDV, Kuhl EA, Kovacs AH, Serber ER, Handberg E, Kneipp SM, Zineh I, Conti JB. The ICD shock and stress management program: a randomized trial of psychosocial treatment to optimize quality of life in ICD patients. Pacing Clin Electrophysiol. 2007;30:858–64.
101. Smeulders ESTF, van Haastregt JCM, Dijkman-Domanska BK, van Hoef EFM, van Eijk JTM, Kempen GIJM. Nurse- and peer-led self management programme for patients with an implantable cardioverter defibrillator: a feasibility study. BMC Nurs. 2007;6:6.
102. Lewin RJ, Coulton S, Frizelle DJ, Kaye G, Cox H. A brief cognitive behavioral preimplantation and rehabilitation programme for patients receiving an implantable cardioverter-defibrillator improves physical health and reduces psychological morbidity and unplanned readmissions. Heart. 2009;95:63–9.
103. Dunbar SB, Langberg JJ, Reilly CM, Viswanathan B, McCarty F, Culler SD, O'Brien MC, Weintraub WS. Effect of a psychoeducational intervention on depression, anxiety, and health resource use in implantable cardioverter defibrillator patients. Pacing Clin Electrophysiol. 2009;32:1259–71.
104. Crössmann A, Schulz SM, Kühlkamp V, Ritter O, Neuser H, Schumacher B, Bauer W, Pauli P. A randomized controlled trial of secondary prevention of anxiety and distress in a German sample of patients with an implantable cardioverter defibrillator. Psychosom Med. 2010;72:434–41.
105. Harmon RJ, Riggs PD. Clonidine for posttraumatic stress disorder in preschool children. J Am Acad Child Adolesc Psychiatry. 1996;35:1247–9.
106. Horrigan JP. Guanfacine for PTSD nightmares. J Am Acad Child Adolesc Psychiatry. 1996;35:975–6.
107. Connor DF, Grasso DJ, Slivinsky MD, Pearson GS, Banga A. An open label study of guanfacine extended release for traumatic stress related symptoms in children and adolescents. J Child Adolesc Psychopharmacol. 2013;23:244–51.
108. Brkanac Z, Pastor JF, Storck M. Prazosin in PTSD [Case reports e Letter]. J Am Acad Child Adolesc Psychiatry. 2003;42:384–5.
109. Fraleigh LA, Hendratta VD, Ford JD, Connor DF. Prazosin for the treatment of posttraumatic stress disorder-related nightmares in an adolescent male. J Child Adolesc Psychopharmacol. 2009;19:475–6.
110. Oluwabusi OO, Sedky K, Bennett DS. Prazosin treatment of nightmares and sleep disturbances associated with posttraumatic stress disorder: two adolescent cases (Case Reports). J Child Adolesc Psychopharmacol. 2012;22:399–402.
111. Strawn JR, Delbello MP, Geracioti TD. Prazosin treatment of an adolescent with posttraumatic stress disorder (Case Reports Letter). J Child Adolesc Psychopharmacol. 2009;19:599–600.
112. Strawn JR, Keeshin BR. Successful treatment of posttraumatic stress disorder with prazosin in a young child. Ann Pharmacother. 2011;45:1590–1.
113. Deans KJ, Thackeray J, Askegard-Giesmann JR, Earley E, Groner JI, Minneci PC. Mortality increases with recurrent episodes of nonaccidental trauma in children. J Trauma Acute Care Surg. 2013;75:161–5.
114. Stoddard FJJ. Outcomes of traumatic exposure. Child Adolesc Psychiatr Clin N Am. 2014;23:243–56.
115. Subica AM, Claypoole KH, Wylie AM. PTSD'S mediation of the relationships between trauma, depression, substance abuse, mental health, and physical health in individuals with severe mental illness: evaluating a comprehensive model. Schizophr Res. 2012;136:104–9.

Chapter 10
Psycho-educational Support Interventions for Patients with an Implantable Cardioverter Defibrillator

Giada Pietrabissa, Francesco Borgia, Gian Mauro Manzoni, Riccardo Proietti, Luca Alessandro Gondoni, Mariella Montano, Ferruccio Nibbio, Anna Maria Titon, Gian Andrea Bertone, and Gianluca Castelnuovo

Abstract The implantable cardioverter defibrillator (ICD) has established superiority in reducing mortality for survivors of cardiac arrest or patients at high risk of sudden death. However, because of the nature of their spontaneous, chronic, and potentiality life-treating condition, patients with an ICD are at risk of developing mild to serious psychological distress. Critical events, such as ICD shocks or ICD recalls may occur, significantly altering the course of individuals' psychosocial adjustment; a number of studies from different countries demonstrate that patients with an ICD that experience higher emotional difficulties undergo a greater incidence of shock therapy.

G. Pietrabissa (✉) • G. Castelnuovo
Psychology Research Laboratory, Ospedale San Giuseppe, IRCCS Istituto Auxologico Italiano, Oggebbio (VCO), Italy

Department of Psychology, Università Cattolica del Sacro Cuore, Milan, Italy
e-mail: giada.pietrabissa@unicatt.it

F. Borgia
Department of Psychology, Università Cattolica del Sacro Cuore, Milan, Italy

G.M. Manzoni
Psychology Research Laboratory, Ospedale San Giuseppe, IRCCS Istituto Auxologico Italiano, Oggebbio (VCO), Italy

Faculty of Psychology, eCampus University, Novedrate, Como, Italy

R. Proietti
Department of Cardiology, Ospedale Luigi Sacco, Milan, Italy

Cardiac Center, Morriston Hospital, University of Swansea, Swansea, UK

L.A. Gondoni • F. Nibbio • A.M. Titon • G.A. Bertone
Division of Cardiological Rehabilitation, Ospedale San Giuseppe, IRCCS Istituto Auxologico Italiano, Oggebbio (VCO), Italy

M. Montano
Department of Cardiology, Ospedale Castelli, Verbania, Italy

© Springer International Publishing AG 2017

R. Proietti et al. (eds.), *Psychological, Emotional, Social and Cognitive Aspects of Implantable Cardiac Devices*, DOI 10.1007/978-3-319-55721-2_10

A proper biopsychosocial assessment and conceptualization of the needs of patients with an ICD, and the delivery of tailored interventions is, therefore, mandatory for ensuring optimal clinical care.

Brief education sessions are effective in reducing concerns among patients with mild levels of psychosocial distress, and a continuum of treatment strategies is available as the recipients' severity of psychological distress and associated maladaptive behavior grows, spanning in ICD support groups, individual consultations using cognitive behavioral techniques and pharmacotherapy.

Yet, while short-term positive outcomes are usually achieved, applicable and effective long-term management of psychological symptoms secondary to ICD implantation is still a challenge for healthcare providers, and the high degree of heterogeneity in content and methodology across studies has made it difficult to formulate broad conclusions on the feasibility and effectiveness of existing interventions. Further research producing valid and reliable data needs to be undertaken in order to maximize positive patient outcomes.

Keywords Implantable cardioverter defibrillator • Psychological distress • Biopsychosocial assessment • Psycho-educational intervention

Introduction

Clinical trials data consistently demonstrate that ICD implantation markedly improves survival in persons at high risk of Sudden Cardiac Death (SCD), and that the majority of patients with an ICD experience a desirable Quality of Life (QoL) and a high acceptance rate [1]. However, whereas somatic symptoms seem to have little or no influence on QoL [2, 3], 30–40% of patients with an ICD report mild to serious psychological distress because of the nature of their spontaneous, chronic, and potentiality life-treating condition [4]. Specifically, as activation of the device is unpredictable and sometimes painful, both meta-analysis and individual trials indicate that patients who experienced ICD shock to achieve cardioversion or defibrillation are more likely to show impaired QoL [5–8] and to engage in avoidance patterns [9, 10]. Behavioral limitations, in fact, may be prescribed, but are more often due to perceived inability and individuals' erroneous association of the shock to those everyday life activities that take place/occur during shock (i.e., showering, gardening, working situations, driving, sexual activity and, particularly, physical exercise), even when there is no inherent connection [1]. Patients with an ICD may also fear that the device will suddenly stop functioning or operate incorrectly and therefore experience constant psychological distress [11].

Especially, r*ecipients younger* than 50 years at implantation, female patients and those with poor social support are more prone to experience adjustment difficulties to the ICD than their device-baring counterpart [12].

Distressed personality (type-D personality), the tendency to experience negative affectivity paired with social inhibition, is another risk marker for poor QoL in patients with an ICD [13]; and the severity of the disease, the presence of comorbidities, as well as a poor understanding of the therapy may furthermore make patients with and ICD more vulnerable to a number of psychological issues, such as anxiety, depression and anger [3, 14, 15].

Anxiety is a common problem for those implanted with a biomedical technology device, to the point that the term shock anxiety has been coined to indicate the particular fear and anticipation of shock that is unique to this patient population. Shock anxiety may be experienced in isolation or within the context of psychological disorders, independently from having received a shock [4]. The presence of anxiety has been documented in 13–38% of device recipients across multiple studies [4], and it may exist on a continuum from normalized fear, generalized anxiety, panic disorder, to Post Traumatic Stress Disorder (PTSD) [10].

Notably, anxiety symptoms increase avoidance behavior, fear of increasing autonomic arousal, sleep disturbances, sexual dysfunction, irritability, and difficulty concentrating [16]. Similarly, 24–46% of patients express ICD-related depression, most likely as a response to perceived physical and mental disabilities associated with daily life activities [6]. The incidence of anger is also higher in the ICD population than in the general population or other disease populations [17].

The main psychological theories explaining the appearance of distress among patients with an ICD are classical conditioning, operant conditioning, cognitive distortions and learned helplessness. *Classical conditioning* can be observed when recipients develop anxiety or fear (unconditioned response) that causes them to avoid the activity they were doing when a discharge occurred (unconditioned stimulus) [18], including those actions that patients once enjoyed; and the employment of consequences (or lack thereof) to modify the occurrence of the behavior contribute to maintaining avoidance patterns over time (*operant conditioning*). Patients implanted with a biomedical technology device may also overestimate the negative consequences of an ICD discharge or overgeneralize its occurrence; studies show that catastrophic cognitions about future events [19] are important determinants of psychological problems among patients with an ICD as well as prospective predictors of the occurrence of subsequent arrhythmias and shocks [20]. By definition, c*ognitive distortion* refers to biased ways of thinking and perceiving reality. Individuals' thoughts and emotions are structured in a negative and inflexible way, this results in errors of interpretation related to personal performance and judgment of external situations [21, 22]. Cognitive reactions include making faulty conclusions that the ICD is actually harmful, instead of life-saving and that physical exertion will cause the ICD to discharge, this leads to learned helplessness. The theory of l*earned helplessness* suggests that psychological distress stems from the patients' perceived inability to handle situations that are believed inescapable and uncontrollable [23, 24] and it is thought to be one of the main underlying causes of depression [25].

Despite the fact that the manifestation of emotional distress has been generally attributed to ICD shocks, in reality, concerns about shock, rather than the shock itself, as well as psychosocial adjustment difficulties that are typical of those living with this particular biomedical technology (i.e., distressful changes in body image due to implantation, worries about scars, poor body satisfaction) need to be carefully investigated and promptly addressed [4].

In fact, recent research demonstrates that patients who reveal *device acceptance*, that is “the psychological accommodation and understanding of the advantages and disadvantages of the device, the recommendation of the device to others, and the derivation of benefit in terms of biomedical, psychological, and social functioning” (p. 385) [26] have better QoL [27].

It is crucial for mental health providers to normalize recipients’ reaction to an abnormal event (ICD implantation or shock) and to articulate a clear treatment plan for recovery that may involve specific ICD- psychological interventions.

Assessment and Treatment for Patients with an ICD in Routine Clinical Practice

A proper biopsychosocial assessment of patients with an ICD and conceptualization of their needs is mandatory for ensuring effective clinical care, since it allows the implementation of tailored intervention [28]. Firstly, medical factors such as, device indication, history of device therapies, cardiac disease severity/prognosis, surgical history, neurological deficits related to hypoxia, and comorbid diseases must be considered.

Moving onto the psychosocial field, anxiety, depression, QoL, psychiatric history, risk for self-harm, coping skills, social support strengths and deficits, financial distress, as well as general and health literacy represent common domains to explore. Healthy behaviors, related to tobacco, alcohol and drug use, physical activity level, medication observance, eating habits, and monitoring of medical parameters (i.e., blood pressure, weight) that frequently influence both medical and psychosocial outcomes also maximizes identification of potential difficulties [29] and recognition of behavioral change strategies to enhance adherence to therapy and to help patients living with the device. Routine clinical assessment for patients with and ICD is summarized in Table 10.1.

Assessment Tools

Both generic and specific tools are available to measure psychological distress and adjustment in patients with an ICD, with particular attention to the level of anxiety and depression experienced by the individuals, as well as to their QoL. Table 10.2 provides a summary of the main measures of psychological concerns that are available [29].

Individuals should be screened for emotional distress before and after the device is implanted. Potential patients must be well informed about the ICD, a sincere conversation about the risk of death, focused on positive risk (i.e., ICD is superior to medication in terms of saving lives) and increased QoL associated with the device, should be carried out by cardiologists through *supportive communication* that conveys empathy and shows respect for the person. To provide information and

Table 10.1 Clinical-based psychosocial assessment strategies (adapted from [1])

• *Risk factors* analysis	Socio-demographic	– Age < 50
		– Female gender
		– Unemployment
		– Ethnicity
	ICD-related	– ICD size
		– >5 Defibrillations (appropriate or inappropriate)
		– Negative cognitive appraisal of ICD discharge
		– Operation under anesthesia
		– Previous resuscitation
		– Comorbidities
		– Premorbid psychiatric diagnosis
		– Lifestyle measures
		– Time for implant
		– Inappropriate patients education
	Psycho-social	– Type-D personality
		– Negative coping strategy
		– Poor social support
		– Hyper-protective family
• *Risk behavior* reported, such as avoidance of physical exertion, sex or recreational activities		
• *Behavioral/clinical observations* indicating poor psychosocial functioning (i.e., tearfulness, display of distress, hopelessness, anger, catastrophizing, symptoms of hypervigilance, significant family discord, etc.)		
• *Critical event experience* that may have changed how patients see themselves or the device, including poor implant experience or multiple shock experience, device recall, and end-of-life concerns		
• *Existence of* any *referral source* with some familiarity with the psychosocial issues common in patients with an ICD (i.e., clinical health psychologist, consulting psychiatrist, clinical social worker)		
• *Brief diagnostic interview questions* that would confirm the presence of psychological impairments (i.e., depressed mood, anxiety, PTSD, anhedonia, suicidal ideation, device regret or device discontinuation)		
• Use of *diagnostic questionnaires* for further evaluation		

opportunities for patients to verbalize fear or concerns related to the device not only enhances the patient-physician communication, but it also empowers and induces confidence in the person, as well as sets the stage for the ultimate outcome, which is the individuals' perception of greater safety because of the ICD (i.e., patient acceptance) [1]. To this aim Eads et al. [30] suggested seven principles of rehabilitation which medical professionals must be skilled in effectively communicating in routine clinical practice [30]: (1) *Defining the problem* asking patients about their specific concerns about having an ICD; (2) *Providing information* answering individuals' doubts or questions about the ICD; (3) *Creating team support* by reassuring patients with an ICD and producing an expectation of participation on the treatment team; (4) *Normalizing fears* as a normal reaction to ICD implantation, (5) *Eliciting emotional release* giving patients the opportunity to discuss troublesome issues;

Table 10.2 Assessment tools for measuring psychological distress in patients with ICD (adapted from [29])

Measure	Concept measured	Subscales	No. of items
Device-specific measures			
Florida Patient Acceptance Scale	Device acceptance	Return to function, device-related distress, body image concerns	18
Florida Shock Anxiety Scale	Device-specific anxiety	Consequence of shock, trigger of shock	10
ICD Concerns Questionnaire	Device-related concerns	Device-specific concerns, perceived limitations	20
Brodsky ICD Questionnaire	Device-related concerns	Embarrassment, suffering, worry, fear, wishes, experience, effect on significant other, changes in lifestyle	46
The Implanted Device Adjustment Scale	Adjustment to an implanted device	Fear/anxiety, attitude, preparation, and body awareness	22
Generic measures			
Cardiac Anxiety Questionnaire	Disease-specific anxiety	Fear, avoidance, heart-focused attention	18
Hospital Anxiety and Depression Scale	Depression and anxiety in non-psychiatric medical settings	Anxiety, depression	14
Beck Anxiety Inventory	Anxiety	N/A	21
State-Trait Anxiety Inventory	Anxiety	State anxiety, trait anxiety	40
Beck Depression Inventory II	Depression	N/A	21
Patient Health Questionnaire	Depression	N/A	9
Brief Symptom Inventory-18	Psychological distress	Somatization, depression, anxiety	18
Impact of Event Scale—Revised	PTSD	Avoidance, hyperarousal, intrusion	22
PTSD Checklist	PTSD	N/A	17
Mishel Uncertainty in Illness Scale	Uncertainty related to symptom, diagnosis, treatment, relationship with caregivers, and planning for the future	Multi-attributed ambiguity, unpredictability	30
The Control Attitude Scale	Perceived control on heart disease (for patients and their family members)	N/A	4
Quality of Life Index—Cardiac version	QOL in terms of satisfaction and importance with respect to various aspects of life	Health and functioning, social and economic aspects, psychological and spiritual status, family and relationships	36

Table 10.2 (continued)

Measure	Concept measured	Subscales	No. of items
Medical Outcomes Study (MOS) 36-Item Short Form Health Survey	Health status	Vitality, physical functioning, bodily pain, general health perceptions, physical role functioning, emotional role functioning, social role functioning, mental health	36
Profile of Mood States	Mood state	Tension-anxiety, depression-dejection, anger-hostility, fatigue-inertia, vigor-activity, confusion-bewilderment	65
Impact of Events Scale—revised	Post-trauma phenomena	Intrusion, avoidance, hyperarousal	22

(6) *Instilling hope* that the physical discomfort and emotional distress patients are experiencing will likely diminish with time and (7) *Encouraging* patients *to take action*, thus to enhance their self-care abilities and self-efficacy.

Clinic-Based Therapeutic Intervention for Patients with and ICD

To properly detect and manage psychosocial issues in ICD clinics, cardiology practitioners should refer to the "four A's checklist" [24]: Ask, Advise, Assist, and Arrange referral. Specifically, research shows that the primary components of patient education, relaxation/stress management training, and group social support provide benefits by increasing health and psychosocial outcomes (Table 10.3).

Brief education sessions have proven effectiveness in reducing patients' initial concerns or post-ICD discharge distress among individuals with mild levels of psychosocial distress, but they may not be appropriate for those recipients suffering from severe psychological distress [31]. Physicians should, therefore, arrange a consultation with a mental health specialist [24] that will assess patients for clinical distress.

A continuum of treatment strategies is available for patients with an ICD experiencing psychosocial difficulties, spanning in *ICD support groups*, and *individual consultations* using *cognitive behavioral techniques*. *Support groups* can serve as an adjunctive intervention and are especially useful for those individuals with poor social support or families experiencing high levels of distress. Through education, social support, and vicarious learning, group participation provides an opportunity for normalization of fears and mobilization of coping resources [32]. However, as the severity of psychological distress and associated maladaptive behavior grows, the need for *individualized psychosocial interventions* increases accordingly. These may include individualized relaxation training, cognitive restructuring, and

Table 10.3 Clinic-based psychosocial care components (adapted from [1])

Patient-specific information component	Clinical task
Patient education	Provide information on proper device functioning, strengths and weaknesses of living with an ICD, and stress the importance of clinic and remote monitoring
Psychosocial information	– Acknowledge challenges of living with a cardiac disease, and reassure patients that they will be able to cope well;
	– Assistance/support will be available if/when needed;
	– Highlight that patient and family outlook involving a positive and hopeful future is reasonable and health promoting
Identify and support physical activities	Short-term follow-up
	Help patient and family: 1. Recognize the importance of returning to appropriate activity level to prevent activity avoidance; 2. Understand the patients' expectation of return to activity
	Long-term follow-up
	Health care team should: – Assess for signs of emotional distress or avoidance of activity – Seek cardiac rehabilitation referral for support in return to activity
Discuss clinic plan to communicate and manage a ICD recalls	
Discuss a standard for managing future ICD shock	– If you get a single shock and feel fine, please call the clinic and schedule appointment or remote monitor transmission
	– If you get a single shock and experience problematic symptoms (i.e., chest pain, dizziness, coughing, weakness), seek emergency medical attention
	– If you get two or more shocks in 24 h period, seek emergency care
Offer reassurance for end-of-life concerns	

systematic desensitization. Specifically, the latter provides patients with skills to manage physiological arousal and distressing thought patterns associated with the ICD [33]. *Pharmacologic* approaches are also appropriate for patients with excessive levels of fear, anxiety, or depression [30].

Patients with an ICD may also express difficulties in reporting emotional problems because of embarrassment, lack of insight, or the nature of their symptoms. They may also present symptoms that do not meet specific diagnostic criteria, but that still impair their QoL and functioning.

Cognitive and Behavioural Techniques

CBT-Based Psychoeducational Intervention

Brief cognitive-behavioral interventions focused on subclinical specific behavioral or psychological symptoms may help to address mild mood impairments, treatment adherence problems, reduced health, risk behaviors, and given the uniqueness of the

Table 10.4 Brief CBT interventions for common psychological symptoms in ICD patients (adapted from [34])

Behavioral or psychological symptoms	CBT intervention
Medication nonadherence	Motivation interviewing and problem-solving techniques
Tobacco use or substance abuse	– Motivational interviewing
	– Provide referral for tobacco cessation or substance abuse counseling
Poor knowledge about ICD and ICD shock	– Review established benefit of ICD
	– Verbally prepare patient and family to respond to ICD shock(s) and provide them handout on the topic
Concerns about sexual activity with an ICD	– Verbally confirm safety of sexual activity with patient
	– Provide patient handout on sexual activity in ICD patients
Concerns about ICD device recall	– Verbally prepare patient to respond to a device recall and provide him/her handout on the topic
	– Review low probability of device malfunction and extensive monitoring of device reliability
Family expresses questions or concerns about patient's ICD	– Acknowledge, normalize, and discuss the relatively increased stress in ICD partners and families
	– Verbally prepare patient and family to cope with an ICD and provide them handout on the topic
Mild, intermittent depressive symptoms	Behavioral activation. Provide referral for further psychological treatment, if indicated
Weight management	– Promote goal setting as a strategy to make changes in daily food consumption
	– Provide referral to nutritionist (if available)
	– Prescribe an exercise program or referral to CR
Physical inactivity	– Review eventual activity restrictions
	– Promote goal setting as a strategy to increases in daily physical activity
	– Encourage use of personal activity trackers like Fitbit

challenges faced by both patients with an ICD and their family, increase ICD device knowledge and acceptance [11, 34]. This type of single-session intervention is particularly helpful within a hospital setting where professional consultations need to be short term and goal oriented (Table 10.4).

Traditional Cognitive-Behavioral Interventions with Stress Management Techniques

Studies indicate that Cognitive Behavioral Therapy (CBT) and stress management frameworks are particularly well-suited for ICD-related adjustment issues [11, 35], since they provide tailored intervention strategies aimed at addressing common cognitive, affective, and behavioral difficulties experienced by patients with an ICD. This form of psychotherapy is effective not only in managing stress and symptoms related to anxiety, and minimizing catastrophic thoughts related to depressive symptoms in patients with an ICD, but also in reducing the number of arrhythmias that result in ICD discharges [36].

The CBT protocol comprises four to six sessions and has four key components: (1) patient education, (2) relaxation/stress management training, (3) cognitive reframing techniques, and (4) promotion of social support. The first component focuses on increasing the patient's knowledge about both the device and the likelihood of ICD shocks, thus reducing the uncertainty and ambiguity that perpetuates shock-related anxiety and equipping recipients with the information needed to understand and discuss their medical condition, thus increasing their self-efficacy and QoL [37]. The second component of the CBT-driven intervention for patients with an ICD aims to help recipients identify and increase distress tolerance, and to address the psychological and physical rigors of living with cardiac disease and an ICD; and standard procedures that promote a state of deep relaxation [38] such as *yoga* techniques [39], *diaphragmatic breathing, progressive muscle relaxation exercises* and *self-hypnosis* may be introduced, practiced in session, and assigned as homework.

In presence of patients exhibiting a traumatic response to ICD shock, professionals might also consider the use of *mindfulness-based cognitive strategies* [40] and *Eye Movement Desensitization and Reprocessing (EMDR) therapy* [41].

Since CBT is based on the assumption that emotional and behavioral problems arise as a result of distorted or dysfunctional manners with which patients perceive events, which influence the persons' sociability and behavior [11], the third phase of treatment makes use of cognitive reframing techniques to help patients with an ICD to identify and reframe inaccurate cognitions related to the ICD or shocks [42]. It is not uncommon, in fact, that patients with an ICD might interpret electrical discharges as a sign of device malfunctioning. Some people may also associate social activities, physical effort, and sex with the occurrence of electric shocks, thus deliberately avoiding such behaviors [10]. Finally, social support is promoted.

Patients with an ICD are further helped to cope with events and emotions that trigger their desire to engage in problematic behaviors [35] by: (a) establishing weekly goals to enable them to return to normal daily life activities; (b) forming groups to facilitate the sharing of coping strategies, feelings, experiences, and the provision of emotional support from people in similar circumstances; and (c) structuring a set of daily exercises compatible with their physical condition [35]. Evidence shows that CBT strategies also prepare patients with an ICD for future run-ins with shock and cardiac dysfunction, and that CBT is a more effective treatment for PTSD symptoms than pharmacologic therapy or even their combination [43].

Despite being considered the gold standard in the treatment of chronic conditions, evidence of the beneficial effects of CBT-based psychosocial interventions in patients with an ICD is only short-term and further research able to overcome the methodological limitations of past studies aimed at assessing its effectiveness needs to be undertaken to refine the data collected so far.

ICD Support Groups

The rapid acceleration of the use of the ICD over the past decade led health care practitioners to the development of adjunctive treatments aimed at supporting the health literacy and adjustment of patients and their families, and the most common approach by medical treatment centers has been the initiation of ICD support groups. They can take many forms, ranging from provider-led question and answer groups or didactic classes, to patient-led groups that encourage emotional expression or peer-to-peer support [29].

The active ingredients of support groups consist on the universality of the concerns of patients and the sharing of information and strategies for aiding in adaptation and encouraging psychological adjustment after receiving an ICD [44]. Lifestyle and family role changes, fear of shocks and limitations of daily life activity, battery and device failure, etc. are some of the main issues of concern that commonly arise from storytelling of ICD patients [24]. Even though the efficacy and effectiveness of ICD support groups has not been adequately investigated, they likely activate the known benefits of group interventions, such as universality of concerns, generation of hope, information sharing, and acquisition of coping skills via vicarious learning [29].

Cardiac Rehabilitation and Exercise Training

The main goal in the rehabilitation of ICD patients is to guarantee professional care during the transition period between acute therapy and ambulatory care, and to prevent re-hospitalizations. The beneficial effects of secondary prevention on the physiological and psychosocial functioning of cardiac patients are generally well-established [45].

However, the ICD has major implications on the physical and emotional status of the patients, and the referral to CR centers of patients with an ICD is usually negatively influenced by fear of inappropriate shock delivery during exercise [46]. Since negative emotions among patients with an ICD might be the cause rather than the result of arrhythmia, and that psychological distress might increase the risk of shock [47] and mortality [48], this particular patient population should receive special attention as their needs differ from those of ordinary heart patients. A comprehensive CR program including control of coronary risk factors, psycho-educational interventions and individualized exercise programs is, therefore, greatly recommended for restoring physical function and improving QoL [49].

Physical activity and exercise has a substantial role in enabling patients with an ICD to take control of their condition, and enhancing their ability to perform everyday activities (25). Sport participation is allowed at least 6 months after ICD implantation or after the most recent arrhythmic episode, in order to reduce the risk of inappropriate shock related to sinus tachycardia induced by exercise [9]. During

Table 10.5 ICD: type of exercise (adapted from [9])

Modes	Goals
Aerobic	
Large muscle activity	• Increase functional capacity and ability to perform daily life activity
	• Increase self-efficacy
Strength	
Circuit training	• Increase ability to perform leisure, occupational, and daily life activities
	• Increase muscle strength and endurance
Flexibility	
Upper and lower body range of motion activity	

CR, exercise training is performed safely, under careful supervision and according to the patient medical condition, thus permitting patients to overcome personal limits without adverse effects, and therefore increase their psychological and physical outcomes [50]. The cut-off heart rate for the ICD patient needs to be appropriately set by exercise testing and 24-h Holter monitoring [9].

The mode of exercise required must be similar to daily activity, in order to gain the most from exercise sessions and maintain the effect over years (Table 10.5).

However, the benefits of CR in increasing adherence to treatment recommendations among patients with an ICD are not yet established, and maintenance of physical activity in *daily life* still appears challenging. A long-term approach to exercise is essential to ensure greater benefits among recipients. Hospital follow-up visits and/or remote patient monitoring via telemedicine and mHealth (see Chap. 11) *is thus recommended in order to maintain and improve* health outcomes among patients with an ICD.

End of Life Intervention

The last stage in the treatment of patients with an ICD is a conversation regarding the deactivation of the device. The majority of implanted patients are not aware that the shock therapy can be deprogrammed and that the deactivation of the ICD allows for a more comfortable death [51]. Concerns associated with the device at the end of life include, the belief that the ICD will deliver painful shocks during the dying process, as well as ethical concerns related to turning off such a device. The basic principles of medical ethics (Autonomy, Beneficence, Non-maleficence, and Justice) must be kept in mind by healthcare professionals, since potentially conflicting at the end of life [52].

A frank discussion of ICD therapy, including the option of deactivation, must be conducted with potential recipients pre-implantation in order to ensure informed consent and address eventual doubts and concerns. A simple approach for physicians to assess patients with an ICD is to ask whether they have documented the circumstances, if any, in which they would want their ICD turned off, so as to prevent subsequent uncertainty [53]. Professionals can also advise the patients that “if at some future date, you decide you no longer want the device, it can easily be disabled”, awareness of their control over the deactivation option is empowering for patients, and at the same time provides an opportunity to contemplate their wishes. Importantly, health care providers should use an organized approach that identifies palliative needs, thus ensuring that the care plan is in alignment with patient and family preferences and goals [54].

Pharmacological Interventions

Since ICD shock is associated with adverse psychological outcomes within 30 days following the event [55], cardiologists often start psychiatric mental health medications. Patients may benefit from pharmacological intervention, but studies focusing on the cardiovascular side effects of psychotropic treatments on patients with an ICD suggest that certain classes of medications should be avoided. Physicians should, therefore, be aware of the cardiovascular risks associated with various psychotropic medications and consider their giving in conjunction with other form of psychological treatment [34].

Conclusion

Empirical data supports the feasibility and efficacy of various treatment modalities to improve the emotional well-being and to reduce device-specific distress in patients living with an ICD and their families [20]. Providers should be equipped with the knowledge to recognize symptoms of psychological difficulties among recipients, so as to provide them with information about the device, and to deliver evidence-based care in a brief consultation and longer-term clinical settings. Specifically, treatments involving cognitive-behavioral interventions and exercise training have demonstrated efficacy in improving patients’ psychological and cardiovascular health [27]. Evidence of the benefits of psychological intervention in ICD patients is most convincing for symptoms of anxiety and exercise capacity [27], but the effect of these treatments on depressive symptoms, heart rate variability, and shocks are weaker ([36, 56]). These research findings, however, should be viewed in the context of their studies, characterized by small sample sizes, high heterogeneity of participants as well as large variability in their methodological quality, and further research is warranted to increase the generalizability of research findings, in order to provide optimal care [57]. Specific attention should also be given to the choice of instruments used to evaluate the effect of the different interventions [27].

Moreover, to date, there is a lack of trials aimed at testing partner-focused interventions [58]. In fact, to ensure positive outcomes in the immediate post-ICD implantation period after returning home, clinical psychosocial attention must also be given to the patients' support network [59], especially spouses [60]. Since the intimate partners' experience may influence that of the recovering patient [61], it is of great importance in the healthcare context to properly assess their physical and mental health and to equipt spouses to provide effective social support [62]. Also, while short-term positive outcomes are usually achieved, to ensure effectiveness of evidence-based interventions in the long-term mental health providers need to fully understand the complex array of medical, psychological, and social factors that lead to the development and maintenance of psychological distress in patients with an ICD. In this regard, a web-based intervention may be worth considering, as it is accessible and can reach underserved populations [63]. Moreover, the impact of psychological interventions on health care utilization and the cost-effectiveness of the intervention is poorly understood in this population and should be the focus of future investigations.

References

1. Sears SF, Matchett M, Conti JB. Effective management of ICD patient psychosocial issues and patient critical events. [Meta-analysis research support, non-U.S. Gov't review]. J Cardiovasc Electrophysiol. 2009;20(11):1297–304. doi:10.1111/j.1540-8167.2009.01526.x.
2. Exner DV, Schron E, Yao Q. Defibrillator shocks and self-perceived quality of life in the antiarrhythmics versus implantable defibrillators (AVID) trial. J Am Coll Cardiol. 2000;35(Suppl A): 153a.
3. Godemann F, Butter C, Lampe F, Linden M, Werner S, Behrens S. Determinants of the quality of life (QoL) in patients with an implantable cardioverter/defibrillator (ICD). Qual Life Res. 2004;13(2):411–6.
4. Sears SF, Matchett M, Vazquez LD, Conti JB. Innovations in psychosocial care for implantable cardioverter defibrillator patients. In: Allan R, Fisher J, editors. Heart and mind: the practice of cardiac psychology. 2nd ed. Washington, DC: American Psychological Association; 2012. p. 524.
5. Francis J, Johnson B, Niehaus M. Quality of life in patients with implantable cardioverter defibrillators. Indian Pacing Electrophysiol J. 2006;6(3):173–81.
6. Kamphius HCM, de Leeuw JRJ, Derksen R, Hauer RNW, Winnubst JAM. Implantable cardioverter defibrillator recipients: quality of life in recipients with and without ICD shock delivery. A prospective study. Europace. 2003;5:381–9.
7. Mark DB, Anstrom KJ, Sun JL, Clapp-Channing NE, Tsiatis AA, Davidson-Ray L, Lee KL, Bardy GH. Quality of life with defibrillator therapy or amiodarone in heart failure. [Comparative study multicenter study randomized controlled trial research support, N.I.H., Extramural research support, non-U.S. Gov't]. N Engl J Med. 2008;359(10):999–1008. doi:10.1056/NEJMoa0706719.
8. Schron EB, Exner DV, Yao Q, Jenkins LS, Steinberg JS, Cook JR, Kutalek SP, Friedman PL, Bubien RS, Page RL, Powell J. Quality of life in the antiarrhythmics versus implantable defibrillators trial: impact of therapy and influence of adverse symptoms and defibrillator shocks. [Clinical trial comparative study multicenter study randomized controlled trial research support, non-U.S. Gov't research support, U.S. Gov't, P.H.S.]. Circulation. 2002;105(5):589–94.

9. Hussein NA, Thomas MA. Rehabilitation of patients with implantable cardioverter/defibrillator: a literature review [Review]. Acta Cardiol. 2008;63(2):249–57. doi:10.2143/AC.63.2.2029535.
10. Sears SF Jr, Todaro JF, Lewis TS, Sotile W, Conti JB. Examining the psychosocial impact of implantable cardioverter defibrillators: a literature review. [Meta-analysis research support, non-U.S. Gov't]. Clin Cardiol. 1999;22(7):481–9.
11. Maia AC, Braga AA, Soares-Filho G, Pereira V, Nardi AE, Silva AC. Efficacy of cognitive behavioral therapy in reducing psychiatric symptoms in patients with implantable cardioverter defibrillator: an integrative review. [Evaluation studies research support, non-U.S. Gov't review]. Braz J Med Biol Res. 2014;47(4):265–72. doi:10.1590/1414-431X20133418.
12. Sears SF, Burns JL, Handberg E. Young at heart: understanding the unique psychosocial adjustment of young implantable cardioverter defibrillators recipients. Pacing Clin Electrophysiol. 2001;24:1113–7.
13. Denollet J, Tekle FB, Pedersen SS, van der Voort PH, Alings M, van den Broek KC. Prognostic importance of distressed (Type D) personality and shocks in patients with an implantable cardioverter defibrillator. [Multicenter study research support, non-U.S. Gov't]. Int J Cardiol. 2013;167(6):2705–9. doi:10.1016/j.ijcard.2012.06.114.
14. Tsuyoshi S, Tsuyoshi S, Katsuji N. Psychological distress in patients with an implantable cardioverter defibrillator. J Arrhythm. 2013;29(6):310–3.
15. Undavia M, Goldstein NE, Cohen P, Sinthawanarong K, Singson M, Bhutani D, Munson T, Gomes JA, Fischer A, Mehta D. Impact of implantable cardioverter-defibrillator recalls on patients' anxiety, depression, and quality of life. [Research support, N.I.H., Extramural research support, non-U.S. Gov't]. Pacing Clin Electrophysiol. 2008;31(11):1411–8. doi:10.1111/j.1540-8159.2008.01204.x.
16. Metoyer PA. The importance of psychological support for the implantable cardioverter defibrillator patient. EP Lab Digest. 2005; 5(10). http://www.eplabdigest.com/article/4744.
17. Lampert R. Anger and ventricular arrhythmias. [Case reports review]. Curr Opin Cardiol. 2010;25(1):46–52. doi:10.1097/HCO.0b013e32833358e8.
18. Beck JS. Cognitive therapy: basics and beyond. New York: Guilford Press; 1995.
19. Pauli P, Wiedemann G, Dengler W, Blaumann-Benninghoff G, Kuhlkamp V. Anxiety in patients with an automatic implantable cardioverter defibrillator: what differentiates them from panic patients? [Comparative study research support, non-U.S. Gov't]. Psychosom Med. 1999;61(1):69–76.
20. Dunbar SB, Kimble LP, Jenkins LS, Hawthorne M, Dudley W, Slemmons M, Langberg JJ. Association of mood disturbance and arrhythmia events in patients after cardioverter defibrillator implantation. [Comparative study research support, U.S. Gov't, P.H.S.]. Depress Anxiety. 1999;9(4):163–8.
21. Frizelle DJ, Lewin RJ, Kaye G, Hargreaves C, Hasney K, Beaumont N, Moniz-Cook E. Cognitive-behavioural rehabilitation programme for patients with an implanted cardioverter defibrillator: a pilot study. [Clinical trial randomized controlled trial]. Br J Health Psychol. 2004;9(Pt 3):381–92. doi:10.1348/1359107041557039.
22. Irvine J, Firestone J, Ong L, Cribbie R, Dorian P, Harris L, Ritvo P, Katz J, Newman D, Cameron D, Johnson S, Bilanovic A, Hill A, O'Donnell S, Sears S Jr. A randomized controlled trial of cognitive behavior therapy tailored to psychological adaptation to an implantable cardioverter defibrillator. [Comparative study multicenter study randomized controlled trial research Support, non-U.S. Gov't]. Psychosom Med. 2011;73(3):226–33. doi:10.1097/PSY.0b013e31820afc63.
23. Range BP, Marlatt GA. Cognitive-behavioral therapy for alcohol and drug use disorders. Rev Bras Psiquiatr. 2008;30(2):S88–95.
24. Sears SF Jr, Conti JB. Quality of life and psychological functioning of icd patients. [Review]. Heart. 2002;87(5):488–93.
25. Vollmayr B, Gass P. Learned helplessness: unique features and translational value of a cognitive depression model. [Research support, non-U.S. Gov't review]. Cell Tissue Res. 2013;354(1):171–8. doi:10.1007/s00441-013-1654-2.

26. Burns JL, Serber ER, Keim S, Sears SF. Measuring patient acceptance of implantable cardiac device therapy: initial psychometric investigation of the Florida Patient Acceptance Survey. [Comparative study research support, non-U.S. Gov't]. J Cardiovasc Electrophysiol. 2005;16(4):384–90. doi:10.1046/j.1540-8167.2005.40134.x.
27. Pedersen SS, Spindler H, Johansen JB, Mortensen PT, Sears SF. Correlates of patient acceptance of the cardioverter defibrillator: cross-validation of the Florida Patient Acceptance Survey in Danish patients. [Research support, non-U.S. Gov't validation studies]. Pacing Clin Electrophysiol. 2008;31(9):1168–77. doi:10.1111/j.1540-8159.2008.01158.x.
28. Kirian K, Sears SF, DeAntonio H. Sudden cardiac arrest: a biopsychosocial approach to patient management of ventricular fibrillation and implantable cardioverter defibrillators. In: Dornelas EA, editor. Stress proof the heart. New York: Springer; 2012. p. 25–43.
29. Whited A, Sears SF, Cahill J, Chelu MG. Psychological consultation for patients with implantable cardioverter defibrillator: confounding challenges of cardiac disease, technology, and the patient experience. In: Alvarenga ME, Byrne D, editors. Handbook of psychocardiology. Singapore: Springer; 2016. p. 1–16.
30. Eads AS, Sears SF Jr, Sotile WM, Conti JB. Supportive communication with implantable cardioverter defibrillator patients: seven principles to facilitate psychosocial adjustment. [Review]. J Cardpulm Rehabil. 2000;20(2):109–14.
31. Sotile WM, Sears SF. You can make a difference: brief psychosocial interventions for ICD patients and their families. Medtronic, Incorporated. 1999.
32. Badger JM, Morris PLP. Observations of a support group for automatic implantable cardioverter-defibrillator recipients and their spouses. Heart Lung. 1989;18:238–43.
33. Sears SF Jr, Conti JB, Curtis AB, Saia TL, Foote R, Wen F. Affective distress and implantable cardioverter defibrillators: cases for psychological and behavioral interventions. [Case reports review]. Pacing Clin Electrophysiol. 1999;22(12):1831–4.
34. Rosman L, Whited A, Ford JH, Nekkanti R, Cahill J, Sears SF. Adding psychological intervention to high-tech care for patients with implantable cardioverter defibrillators. In: Byrne ME, Alvarenga D, editors. Handbook of psychocardiology. Singapore: Springer Science + Business Media; 2016. p. 1–16.
35. Smith LC, Fogel D, Friedman S. Cognitive-behavioral treatment of panic disorder with agoraphobia triggered by AICD implant activity. [Case reports research support, non-U.S. Gov't research support, U.S. Gov't, P.H.S.]. Psychosomatics. 1998;39(5):474–7. doi:10.1016/S0033-3182(98)71311-8.
36. Kohn CS, Petrucci RJ, Baessler C, Soto DM, Movsowitz C. The effect of psychological intervention on patients' long-term adjustment to the ICD: a prospective study. [Clinical trial comparative Study randomized controlled trial research support, non-U.S. Gov't]. Pacing Clin Electrophysiol. 2000;23(4 Pt 1):450–6.
37. Powell VB, Abreu N, Oliveira IR, Sudak D. Cognitive-behavioral therapy for depression. [Research support, non-U.S. Gov't review]. Rev Bras Psiquiatr. 2008;30(Suppl 2):s73–80.
38. Habibovic M, Burg MM, Pedersen SS. Behavioral interventions in patients with an implantable cardioverter defibrillator: lessons learned and where to go from here? [Research support, N.I.H., Extramural research support, non-U.S. Gov't review]. Pacing Clin Electrophysiol. 2013;36(5):578–90. doi:10.1111/pace.12108.
39. Toise SC, Sears SF, Schoenfeld MH, Blitzer ML, Marieb MA, Drury JH, Slade MD, Donohue TJ. Psychosocial and cardiac outcomes of yoga for ICD patients: a randomized clinical control trial. [Randomized controlled trial research support, N.I.H., Extramural research support, non--U.S. Gov't]. Pacing Clin Electrophysiol. 2014;37(1):48–62. doi:10.1111/pace.12252.
40. Salmoirago-Blotcher E, Crawford S, Carmody J, Rosenthal L, Ockene I. Characteristics of dispositional mindfulness in patients with severe cardiac disease. J Evid Based Complementary Altern Med. 2011;16(3):218–25. doi:10.1177/2156587211405525.
41. Engelhard IM, van den Hout MA, Janssen WC, van der Beek J. Eye movements reduce vividness and emotionality of "flashforwards". [Research support, non-U.S. Gov't]. Behav Res Ther. 2010;48(5):442–7. doi:10.1016/j.brat.2010.01.003.

42. Lewin RJ, Coulton S, Frizelle DJ, Kaye G, Cox H. A brief cognitive behavioural preimplantation and rehabilitation programme for patients receiving an implantable cardioverter-defibrillator improves physical health and reduces psychological morbidity and unplanned readmissions. [Multicenter study randomized controlled trial research support, non-U.S. Gov't]. Heart. 2009;95(1):63–9. doi:10.1136/hrt.2007.129890.
43. Ansari S, Arbabi M. Cognitive behavioral therapy (CBT) in a patient with implantable cardioverter defibrillator (ICD) and posttraumatic stress disorder (PTSD). Iran J Psychiatry. 2014;9(3):181–3.
44. DeBasio N, Rodenhausen N. The group experience: meeting the psychological needs of patients with ventricular tachycardia. Heart Lung. 1984;13(6):597–602.
45. Ades PA. Cardiac rehabilitation and secondary prevention of coronary heart disease. [Research support, non-U.S. Gov't research support, U.S. Gov't, P.H.S. review]. N Engl J Med. 2001;345(12):892–902. doi:10.1056/NEJMra001529.
46. Vanhees L, Kornaat M, Defoor J, Aufdemkampe G, Schepers D, Stevens A, Van Exel H, Van Den Beld J, Heidbüchel H, Fagard R. Effect of exercise training in patients with an implantable cardioverter defibrillator. Eur Heart J. 2004;25:1120–6.
47. Steinberg JS, Arshad A, Kowalski M, Kukar A, Suma V, Vloka M, Ehlert F, Herweg B, Donnelly J, Philip J, Reed G, Rozanski A. Increased incidence of life-threatening ventricular arrhythmias in implantable defibrillator patients after the World Trade Center attack. [Comparative study evaluation studies]. J Am Coll Cardiol. 2004;44(6):1261–4. doi:10.1016/j.jacc.2004.06.032.
48. Ladwig KH, Baumert J, Marten-Mittag B, Kolb C, Zrenner B, Schmitt C. Posttraumatic stress symptoms and predicted mortality in patients with implantable cardioverter-defibrillators: results from the prospective living with an implanted cardioverter-defibrillator study. [Research support, non-U.S. Gov't]. Arch Gen Psychiatry. 2008;65(11):1324–30. doi:10.1001/archpsyc.65.11.1324.
49. Berg SK, Pedersen PU, Zwisler AD, Winkel P, Gluud C, Pedersen BD, Svendsen JH. Comprehensive cardiac rehabilitation improves outcome for patients with implantable cardioverter defibrillator. Findings from the COPE-ICD randomised clinical trial. [Comparative study randomized controlled trial research support, Non-U.S. Gov't]. Eur J Cardiovasc Nurs. 2015;14(1):34–44. doi:10.1177/1474515114521920.
50. Fitchet A, Doherty PJ, Bundy C, et al. Comprehensive cardiac rehabilitation programme for implantable cardioverter-defibrillator patients: a randomised controlled trial. Heart. 2003;89:155–60.
51. Beattie J. Implantable cardioverter defibrillators in patients who are nearing the end of life. London: British Heart Foundation; 2007.
52. Gillon R. Medical ethics: four principles plus attention to scope. [Review]. Br Med J. 1994;309(6948):184–8.
53. Wright GA, Klein GJ, Gula LJ. Ethical and legal perspective of implantable cardioverter defibrillator deactivation or implantable cardioverter defibrillator generator replacement in the elderly. [Review]. Curr Opin Cardiol. 2013;28(1):43–9. doi:10.1097/HCO.0b013e32835b0b3b.
54. Lowery D, Carpenter CR. Cardiac patients at end of life in the emergency department. In: Goodlin SJ, Rich MW, editors. End-of-life care in cardiovascular disease. London: Springer; 2014. p. 91–105.
55. Mark DB, Anstrom KJ, Sun JL, Clapp-Channing NE, Tsiatis AA, Davidson-Ray LD, Bardy GH. Sudden Cardiac Death in Heart Failure Trial (SCD-HeFT) Investigators: Quality of life with defibrillator therapy or amiodarone in heart failure. N Engl J Med. 2008;359: 999–1008.
56. Dunbar SB, Langberg JJ, Reilly CM, Viswanathan B, McCarty F, Culler SD, O'Brien MC, Weintraub WS. Effect of a psychoeducational intervention on depression, anxiety, and health resource use in implantable cardioverter defibrillator patients. [Randomized controlled trial research support, N.I.H., Extramural]. Pacing Clin Electrophysiol. 2009;32(10):1259–71. doi:10.1111/j.1540-8159.2009.02495.x.

57. Crespo EM, Kim J, Selzman KA. The use of implantable cardioverter defibrillators for the prevention of sudden cardiac death: a review of the evidence and implications. Am J Med Sci. 2005;329:238–46.
58. Dougherty CM, Thompson EA, Kudenchuk PJ. Development and testing of an intervention to improve outcomes for partners following receipt of an implantable cardioverter defibrillator in the patient. [Randomized controlled trial research support, N.I.H., Extramural]. ANS Adv Nurs Sci. 2012;35(4):359–77. doi:10.1097/ANS.0b013e318271d2e8.
59. Miller PJ, Wikoff R. Spouses' psychosocial problems, resources, and marital functioning post-myocardial infarction. [Research support, non-U.S. Gov't]. Prog Cardiovasc Nurs. 1989;4(2):71–6.
60. Coyne JC, Rohrbaugh MJ, Shoham V, Sonnega JS, Nicklas JM, Cranford JA. Prognostic importance of marital quality for survival of congestive heart failure. [Comparative study research support, U.S. Gov't, P.H.S.]. Am J Cardiol. 2001;88(5):526–9.
61. Cleland JG, Ghosh J, Freemantle N, Kaye GC, Nasir M, Clark AL, Coletta AP. Clinical trials update and cumulative meta-analyses from the American College of Cardiology: WATCH, SCD-HeFT, DINAMIT, CASINO, INSPIRE, STRATUS-US, RIO-Lipids and cardiac resynchronisation therapy in heart failure. [Review]. Eur J Heart Fail. 2004;6(4):501–8. doi:10.1016/j.ejheart.2004.04.014.
62. Carlson LE, Bultz BD, Speca M, St Pierre M. Partners of cancer patients: Part II. Current psychosocial interventions and suggestions for improvement. J Psychosoc Oncol. 2000;18(3):33–43.
63. Kuhl EA, Sears SF, Conti JB. Using computers to improve the psychosocial care of implantable cardioverter defibrillator recipients. Pacing Clin Electrophysiol. 2006;29:1426–33.

Chapter 11
eHealth and mHealth to Manage Distress in Patients with an Implantable Cardioverter-Defibrillator

Gianluca Castelnuovo, Giada Pietrabissa, Gian Mauro Manzoni, Francesco Borgia, Gian Andrea Bertone, Mariella Montano, Ferruccio Nibbio, Anna Maria Titon, Luca Alessandro Gondoni, and Riccardo Proietti

Abstract One of the main benefits of the eHealth and mHealth approach is that it overcomes those limitations associated with the traditional, restricted and highly expensive in-patient treatment of many chronic pathologies, by reducing complications from a clinical, organizational and economic prospective. Mobile communication devices, therefore, may be an effective way to ensure long-term maintenance and improvement of health outcomes among patients with an implantable cardioverter-defibrillator (ICD). Employment of eHealth and mHealth usually increases participation, compliance, and engagement toward treatment and helps clinicians by motivating patients in remote settings to withstand medical treatments and to cope

G. Castelnuovo (✉) • G. Pietrabissa
Psychology Research Laboratory, Ospedale San Giuseppe, IRCCS Istituto Auxologico Italiano, Oggebbio (VCO), Italy

Department of Psychology, Università Cattolica del Sacro Cuore, Milan, Italy
e-mail: gianluca.castelnuovo@unicatt.it

G.M. Manzoni
Psychology Research Laboratory, Ospedale San Giuseppe, IRCCS Istituto Auxologico Italiano, Oggebbio (VCO), Italy

Faculty of Psychology, eCampus University, Novedrate, Como, Italy

F. Borgia
Department of Psychology, Università Cattolica del Sacro Cuore, Milan, Italy

G.A. Bertone • F. Nibbio • A.M. Titon • L.A. Gondoni
Division of Cardiological Rehabilitation, Ospedale San Giuseppe, IRCCS Istituto Auxologico Italiano, Oggebbio (VCO), Italy

M. Montano
Department of Cardiology, Ospedale Castelli, Verbania, Italy

R. Proietti
Department of Cardiology, Ospedale Luigi Sacco, Milan, Italy

Cardiac Center, Morriston Hospital, University of Swansea, Swansea, UK

© Springer International Publishing AG 2017

R. Proietti et al. (eds.), *Psychological, Emotional, Social and Cognitive Aspects of Implantable Cardiac Devices*, DOI 10.1007/978-3-319-55721-2_11

with chronic conditions, also in a stepped-care approach. Clinical experiences and best practices regarding mHealth based strategies used to tele-monitor patients with an ICD are reported/highlighted in this chapter which discusses methodological, clinical and technological issues. At the end of the chapter future trends of eHealth–mHealth applications for ICDs are discussed.

Keywords Implantable Cardioverter-Defibrillator • Distress • Stepped-care approach • eHealth • mHealth

New Opportunities Provided by eHealth and mHealth in Clinical Fields

eHealth recently emerged as a promising field for the implementation of better and more efficient healthcare delivery through the use of web-enabled services [1]. mHealth, instead, is the practice of medicine and public health specifically supported by mobile communication devices, such as mobile phones, tablets, computers, and PDAs, and the use of social media such as Facebook and Twitter, for health services and clinical data collection [2–10]. Mobile devices and smartphones can capture, analyze, store, and transmit health-related information from various sources including biosensors and other biomedical acquisition systems [11].

One of the main benefits of the mHealth approach is that it overcomes those limitations associated with the traditional, restricted and highly expensive in-patient treatment of many chronic pathologies, by reducing complications from a clinical, organizational and economic prospective [5, 12–15]. Mobile communication devices, therefore, may be an effective way to ensure long-term maintenance and improvement of health outcomes among patients with an implantable cardioverter-defibrillator (ICD) [16], since adherence to treatment recommendations, and observance of physical activity advice still appears challenging for recipients.

The employment of eHealth and mHealth usually increases participation, compliance, and engagement toward treatment [17, 18]. In fact the mHealth approach could be of help to clinicians by motivating patients in remote settings to withstand medical treatments and to cope with chronic conditions [19–21].

mHealth could, consequently, play a key role in the Chronic Care Model [22–24] which is based on the collaboration between a well-coordinated team of clinicians-providers and an activated-engaged patient, by permitting to track and share information regarding a patient's health status [25]. Through the use of mHealth it is possible to monitor a patient's progress by using a mobile platform or device that permits to access important information in real time [26, 27]. It might, therefore, possess the requirements necessary to be integrated and considered as a relevant part of the stepped-care model, as already suggested in the pioneering book *Stepped Care and e-Health Practical Applications to Behavioral Disorders* [25], where authors O'Donohue and Draper ([28], pp. 5–6) proposed a practical solution for managing chronic conditions. Starting from the previous work of Von Korff and

Tiemens [29], an advanced model of stepped care which integrates mHealth is proposed by O'Donnell ([25], p. 265): "The stepped care model is based on the acknowledgement that (1) different patients require different levels of care; (2) the most appropriate level of care is based on closely monitoring outcomes; and (3) moving from lower to more intensive levels of care based on patient response can increase the effectiveness of care while lowering overall costs". Stepped care is "potentially much more consistent with the ethical imperative of choosing the least intrusive intervention for one's patient" [30]. Taking into account this approach, research has to focus not only on the development of new clinical protocols or therapies, but on the validation of the efficacy, reliability and sustainability of this new technology-based model of healthcare [30–34].

eHealth and mHealth for ICD

Traditionally an ICD could be defined as "a battery-powered, fully implantable device that monitors heart rhythm and has the capacity to deliver an electrical shock to restore normal sinus rhythm when potentially life threatening ventricular arrhythmias are detected. An ICD system consists of the device and one or more leads which are implanted into the patient's body. The original devices simply offered defibrillation shocks. With improvements in sensing, the latest devices offer graded therapeutic responses to a sensed ventricular arrhythmia" (p. 7) [35].

The ICD is a highly technological device and its application can be improved by using additional technological solutions and opportunities such as mHealth-based monitoring and data management.

In fact tele-monitoring systems for ICDs are promising tools for reducing workload as well as improving the quality and reducing the costs of health services [36], and thus optimize patients' long-term adherence to treatment [37].

Since becoming the standard of care for prevention of sudden cardiac death, the number of patients with an implantable device has growing steadily and, typically, patients with an ICD need follow-ups every 3–6 months through traditional in-hospital visits.

However, biomedical data is periodically registered automatically by the device, and then send to the physician by use of a transmitter (*remote follow-up*).

In the era of communication technology, new options are available for remote patient follow-ups and monitoring of device integrity (i.e., battery status, lead impedance), programming issues (i.e., disabling of ventricular fibrillation therapy, insufficient safety margins for sensing or capture), or medical data (i.e., arrhythmias, indication of lung fluid accumulation) through periodic (Boston Latitude—LAT, Medtronic Carelink—MCL, St. Jude Merlin—SJM) or daily transmissions (Biotronik Home Monitoring—BHM) [38] of any pre-defined alerts to the physician [39].

Despite evidence of the effectiveness of mHealth-based strategies in tele-monitoring patients with an ICD has been reported in several studies [40–45], "in daily practice, remote monitoring has been implemented in uncoordinated and rather fragmented ways, calling for a more strategic approach" (p. 1) [39].

Specifically, Bohm et al. [46] highlighted that tele-medicine alerts on fluid status among recipients do not significantly improve patients' outcomes, but increase adherence to treatment protocols [46]. However, further research is needed, and the actual applicability of ICD tele-monitoring in daily routine has to be carefully investigated in order to enhance the benefits of mHealth and implement more effective treatment procedures. Siebermair et al. [37] noted, among the potential problems occurring during the implementation of a tele-monitoring system, a high rate of not-transmitted data, however this was due more to the patient's loss of interest and motivation than to technical problems [37]. Evaluating and improving patients' ability to self-care and readiness to adhere to both traditional and mHealth protocols plays, therefore, an important role in ensuring the reliability of these systems.

Notably, from a technological point of view, the Lumax and IEGM Online HD Evaluation study demonstrated that remote Intracardiac Electrograms (IEGM), are essential for assessing implantable ICD functions, and are "reasonably accurate in a remote monitoring system that transmits shorter IEGM than the full-length programmer IEGM for the sake of frequent, fully automatic data transmission" (p. 584) [47].

An important result was also obtained with the IN-TIME clinical trial, which involved 36 clinical centres and hospitals in Australia, Europe, and Israel, and came to the conclusion that "automatic, daily, implant-based, multiparameter tele-monitoring can significantly improve clinical outcomes for patients with heart failure. Such tele-monitoring is feasible and should be used in clinical practice" (p. 583) [48]. Tim Geach [49] deepened the IN_TIME study's results by noting that the new generations of ICDs are equipt to contain tele-monitoring options and functions such as recording technical and physiological information and automatically sending them to a clinical team via a mobile telephone link, coming to the conclusion that patients receiving ICD tele-monitoring have better outcomes in comparison with unmonitored control patients [49]. The author summarized that "the team believes that direct device tele-monitoring might enable clinicians to detect arrhythmias earlier, identify suboptimal device function, or initiate patient interviews that reveal worsening heart failure, which can subsequently be treated, which could explain the improved outcome in patients who received a tele-monitoring device" (p. 557) [49].

An important reduction in the length of hospitalizations for cardiovascular patients has been achieved in the CONNECT trial [50, 51], which showed that a wireless remote monitoring with automatic clinician alerts can reduce the time from a clinical event to a clinical decision after cardiovascular accidents of different gravity, in comparison with patients receiving a standard in-office treatment protocol.

The EuroEco (European Health Economic Trial on Home Monitoring in ICD Patients) study, based on 17 centres located in six different EU countries, confirmed the evidence that all the stakeholders receiving ICD monitoring might obtain benefits: "physicians and hospitals (the 'providers') may optimize performance by reducing the number of in-hospital visits, while specialist nurses and/or technicians can filter alerts from the remote system, hence possibly saving physician time. For patients, the technology provides a more continuous follow-up (FU) and saves time for visits to outpatient clinics that often do not result in specific actions" (p. 159)

[52]. Remote clinical results based on technology are non-inferior to classical in-office follow-up visits [40–45]. Particularly, "daily remote monitoring results in earlier detection of device and patient-related problems which translate into earlier clinical decision-making, less inappropriate shocks and improved device longevity" (p. 159) [52]. Notably, within the EuroEco study a rigorous and complete cost analysis of these technology based actions of care was carried out. In fact, "although remote monitoring technology of cardiac implantable devices entered the clinical field 10 years ago, EuroEco is the first trial estimating the cost for providers in setting up an organization based on such technology. Prior trials have shown that such FU is non-inferior clinically from a major events perspective, and even has clinical advantages like earlier actionability on clinical- or device-related findings, fewer and shorter hospitalizations, fewer inappropriate shocks, longer battery longevity, and even lower mortality … Taken together with data on the existing reimbursement situation (defining provider income) and on the costs from a payer perspective, EuroEco also allowed to estimate the impact on the net income of physicians and hospitals. The financial impact is an important determinant for physicians and hospitals when considering adoption of a remote monitoring-based FU. The findings in the overall EuroEco population showed no change in provider cost of HM based vs. classical FU, nor on their net income" (p. 164) [52]. Moreover, no worsening health-related quality-of-life outcomes, as measured by the Short Form Health Survey (SF-36) have been detected in the EuroEco study when comparing the technology-based monitoring approach with the traditional one [52].

Using the *HM (Home Monitoring) Acceptance and Satisfaction Questionnaire (HoMASQ)*, Ricci et al. [53] found that patients with an ICD periodically followed up by remote monitoring reported a high level of acceptance and satisfaction of this new technological approach [53]. Regarding the critical issue of patient-provider relationships, Ricci et al. [53] propose a model where "patients with (pacemaker or) ICD are followed up at scheduled in-hospital visits during which technical device performance and patient clinical status are checked. During the visit, the patient is informed about device functioning and clinical status and reassured by his/her nurse and physician when no abnormalities are detected. Such a personal contact is psychologically important for the patient. Whenever HM is started, the number or the frequency of personal contact with healthcare providers may be reduced, due to remote control. Therefore, the patient needs to receive clear, detailed, and convincing explanations on how HM works, in order to trust the system and to have a good compliance to remote monitoring. Our study showed that 97% of patients claimed to be satisfied with both initial training and successive contact with healthcare providers. Contact mostly occurred by phone with the dedicated nurses who definitely proved to play a critical role in keeping the human relationship with the patients" (p. 677) [53].

Moreover, the authors went on to state the following: "We could speculate that going on with the follow-up, patients may get more familiar with their transmitter and in turn its influence on daily life may even decrease. Ninety-two percent of patients claimed to receive a sense of security by their transmitter. Interestingly, this high rate was obtained despite the nurse and the physicians stressing during the initial training that the HM is not an emergency management system but simply a diagnostic tool" (p. 678) [53]. The sense of security and familiarity perceived by patients with an ICD about the HM approach has been further stressed by Cavaco [54], who noted that "One of the problems with face-to-face follow-up is that it is not continuous, but occurs at fixed times. This means that a problem that arises with a device the day after a consultation may not be detected until the next consultation, which could be six months later" (p. 965) [54]. Among the benefits of the mHealth approach, especially for the elderly and underserved populations, Cavaco underlines its potential in reducing the need to travel to hospitals, thus avoiding dangerous delays of clinical consultations and professional feedbacks.

Best Practices in eHealth-mHealth Applications for ICD

An interesting application of remote monitoring of patients with an ICD has been developed by Dario et al. [39], who implemented a multi-center, multi-vendor, controlled, observational, prospective study by enrolling 2101 patients to test the applicability of an innovative protocol characterized by six steps: "1. PMs and ICD periodically relay remote programmed transmissions (RPTs), and daily or weekly transmit serious recorded events to a home gateway; 2. The gateway automatically sends data to the vendor's Web server; 3. The nurse checks RPTs' data daily during regular working time, accessing them through the different vendors' Web-portals; 4. In case of an alert, the nurse receives a notification via email, fax, or short message service, and, still during regular working time, reviews data; 5. In case of a serious event, the nurse submits data to the physician. The physician evaluates data, and decides if the patient needs a specialist visit, in-clinic device follow-up, therapy modification, or other actions; and 6. When appropriate, the nurse contacts the patient to offer recommendations and care instructions" (p. 2) [39] Nurses and physicians played a key role in in this process and therefore received a specific training in cardiac electrophysiology, electro-stimulation and above all technology-based remote monitoring. Dario completed his contribution stating that this approach is "feasible, reliable, safe, and clinically useful" (p. 9) [39].

Similarly to the previous one, the EVOLVO study [55, 56] also aimed at comparing the remote management of ICD patients with standard-care. Research outcomes demonstrated that remote monitoring reduces inappropriate visits resulting from false alerts even if the alerting algorithms, created to promptly detect clinical worsening, may create unnecessary preemptive hospitalizations in patients who are not yet in crisis but only in a deteriorating state. Moreover, the EVOLVO study demonstrated that remote monitoring can limit emergency department/urgent in office visits. "Compared with standard follow-up through in-office visits and audible ICD alerts, remote monitoring results in increased efficiency for healthcare providers and improved quality of care for patients" (p. 2991), [55].

Trends in eHealth-mHealth Applications for ICD

According to Olderbung's recent contribution in the Handbook of Psychocardiology [57], the contemporary advances in new digital technologies have changed the communication and social interaction scenarios, deeply modifying the lifestyle change programs and the health care protocols. "By remembering preferences for content and mode of delivery, an algorithm-driven approach combined with new technologies that "crowd-source" feedback and "data" from thousands of participants in real time allows the delivery of program content to be adapted to multiple circumstances, contexts, and situations while remaining unique to individual users. Hence, while traditionally delivered health education and health promotion programs can be tailored for small numbers of individuals, new technologies can deliver highly personalized, standardized, and tailored messages to whole populations" (p. 1087) [57].

The expansion of eHealth applications and technology-based treatments for patients with an ICD is an interesting trend in the cardiovascular field and it is destined to grow over time. Web-based platforms are already available in order to provide patients with the possibility to track their cardiac functioning: for an updated list of websites developed by medical device companies please consider p. 990 of [58]. Educational websites for ICD Patients and their families are available at http://circ.ahajournals.org/ and http://campodayin.org/ (pp. 992–993, [58]).

References

1. Eysenbach G. What is e-health? J Med Internet Res. 2001;3:E20. doi:10.2196/jmir.3.2.e20.
2. Castelnuovo G, Manzoni GM, Pietrabissa G, Corti S, Giusti EM, Molinari E, Simpson S. Obesity and outpatient rehabilitation using mobile technologies: the potential mHealth approach. Front Psychol. 2014;5:559. doi:10.3389/fpsyg.2014.00559.
3. Castelnuovo G, Mauri G, Simpson S, Colantonio A, Goss S. New technologies for the management and rehabilitation of chronic diseases and conditions. Biomed Res Int. 2015;2015:180436. doi:10.1155/2015/180436.
4. Castelnuovo G, Pietrabissa G, Manzoni GM, Corti S, Ceccarini M, Borrello M, Giusti EM, Novelli M, Cattivelli R, Middleton NA, Simpson SG, Molinari E. Chronic care management of globesity: promoting healthier lifestyles in traditional and mHealth based settings. Front Psychol. 2015;6:1557. doi:10.3389/fpsyg.2015.01557.
5. Castelnuovo G, Zoppis I, Santoro E, Ceccarini M, Pietrabissa G, Manzoni GM, Corti S, Borrello M, Giusti EM, Cattivelli R, Melesi A, Mauri G, Molinari E, Sicurello F. Managing chronic pathologies with a stepped mHealth-based approach in clinical psychology and medicine. Front Psychol. 2015;6:407. doi:10.3389/fpsyg.2015.00407.
6. Cipresso P, Serino S, Villani D, Repetto C, Selitti L, Albani G, Mauro A, Gaggioli A, Riva G. Is your phone so smart to affect your states? An exploratory study based on psychophysiological measures. Neurocomputing. 2012;84:23–30. doi:10.1016/j.neucom.2011.12.027.
7. Eysenbach G. Can tweets predict citations? Metrics of social impact based on twitter and correlation with traditional metrics of scientific impact. J Med Internet Res. 2011;13:e123. doi:10.2196/jmir.2012.
8. Fiordelli M, Diviani N, Schulz PJ. Mapping mHealth research: a decade of evolution. J Med Internet Res. 2013;15:e95. doi:10.2196/jmir.2430.

9. Riper H, Andersson G, Christensen H, Cuijpers P, Lange A, Eysenbach G. Theme issue on e-mental health: a growing field in internet research. J Med Internet Res. 2010;12:e74. doi:10.2196/jmir.1713.
10. Whittaker R. Issues in mHealth: findings from key informant interviews. J Med Internet Res. 2012;14:e129. doi:10.2196/jmir.1989.
11. Adibi S. Introduction. In: Adibi S, editor. mHealth multidisciplinary verticals. New York: CRC, Taylor & Francis Group; 2015. p. 1–10.
12. Khaylis A, Yiaslas T, Bergstrom J, Gore-Felton C. A review of efficacious technology-based weight-loss interventions: five key components. Telemed J E Health. 2010;16:931–8. doi:10.1089/tmj.2010.0065.
13. Manzoni GM, Castelnuovo G, Molinari E. Weight loss with a low-carbohydrate, Mediterranean, or low-fat diet. N Engl J Med. 2008;359:2170. author reply 2171-2172
14. Manzoni GM, Pagnini F, Corti S, Molinari E, Castelnuovo G. Internet-based behavioral interventions for obesity: an updated systematic review. Clin Pract Epidemiol Ment Health. 2011;7:19–28. doi:10.2174/1745017901107010019.
15. Rao G, Burke LE, Spring BJ, Ewing LJ, Turk M, Lichtenstein AH, Cornier MA, Spence JD, Coons M. New and emerging weight management strategies for busy ambulatory settings: a scientific statement from the American Heart Association endorsed by the Society of Behavioral Medicine. Circulation. 2011;124:1182–203. doi:10.1161/CIR.0b013e31822b9543.
16. Kuhl EA, Sears SF, Conti JB. Internet-based behavioral change and psychosocial care for patients with cardiovascular disease: A review of cardiac disease-specific applications, Heart & Lung. J Acute Critical Care. 2006;35(6):374–382. DOI: http://dx.doi.org/10.1016/j.hrtlng.2006.02.004.
17. Graffigna G, Barello S, Riva G. Technologies for patient engagement. Health Aff (Millwood). 2013;32:1172. doi:10.1377/hlthaff.2013.0279.
18. Graffigna G, Barello S, Wiederhold BK, Bosio AC, Riva G. Positive technology as a driver for health engagement. Stud Health Technol Inform. 2013;191:9–17.
19. Castelnuovo G. Empirically supported treatments in psychotherapy: towards an evidence-based or evidence-biased psychology in clinical settings? Front Psychol. 2010;1:27. doi:10.3389/fpsyg.2010.00027.
20. Nguyen T, Lau DC. The obesity epidemic and its impact on hypertension. Can J Cardiol. 2012;28:326–33. doi:10.1016/j.cjca.2012.01.001.
21. Pietrabissa G, Manzoni GM, Corti S, Vegliante N, Molinari E, Castelnuovo G. Addressing motivation in globesity treatment: a new challenge for clinical psychology. Front Psychol. 2012;3:317. doi:10.3389/fpsyg.2012.00317.
22. Glasgow RE, Orleans CT, Wagner EH. Does the chronic care model serve also as a template for improving prevention? Milbank Q 2001;79:579–612, iv-v.
23. Wagner EH, Austin BT, Davis C, Hindmarsh M, Schaefer J, Bonomi A. Improving chronic illness care: translating evidence into action. Health Aff (Millwood). 2001;20:64–78.
24. Wagner EH, Glasgow RE, Davis C, Bonomi AE, Provost L, Mcculloch D, Carver P, Sixta C. Quality improvement in chronic illness care: a collaborative approach. Jt Comm J Qual Improv. 2001;27:63–80.
25. O'Donnell RR. Stepped care and E-health in behavioral managed care. In: O'Donohue WT, Draper C, editors. Stepped care and e-health: practical applications to behavioral disorders. New York: Springer; 2011. p. 263–82.
26. Javitt J. Case study: using mHealth to manage diabetes. mHealth News [Online]. 2014. http://www.mhealthnews.com/print/24916. [Accessed]
27. Moss Richins S. Emerging technologies in healthcare. New York: CRC, Taylor & Francis Group; 2015.
28. O'Donohue WT, Draper C, editors. Stepped care and e-health: practical applications to behavioral disorders. New York: Springer; 2011.
29. Von Korff M, Tiemans B. Individualized stepped care of chronic illness. West J Med. 2000;172:133–7.

30. O'Donohue WT, Draper C. The case for evidence-based stepped care as part of a reformed delivery system. In: O'Donohue WT, Draper C, editors. Stepped care and e-health: practical applications to behavioral disorders. New York: Springer; 2011. p. 1–16.
31. Mercer V. Chronic disease managemen. In: O'Donohue WT, Draper C, editors. Stepped care and E-health: practical applications to behavioral disorders. New York: Springer; 2011. p. 151–79.
32. Neumeyer-Gromen A, Lampert T, Stark K, Kallischnigg G. Disease management programs for depression: a systematic review and meta-analysis of randomized controlled trials. Med Care. 2004;42:1211–21.
33. Ofman JJ, Badamgarav E, Henning JM, Knight K, Gano AD Jr, Levan RK, Gur-Arie S, Richards MS, Hasselblad V, Weingarten SR. Does disease management improve clinical and economic outcomes in patients with chronic diseases? A systematic review. Am J Med. 2004;117:182–92.
34. Weingarten SR, Henning JM, Badamgarav E, Knight K, Hasselblad V, Gano A Jr, Ofman JJ. Interventions used in disease management programmes for patients with chronic illness-which ones work? Meta-analysis of published reports. Br Med J. 2002;325:925.
35. Buxton M, Caine N, Chase D, Connelly D, Grace A, Jackson C, Parkes J, Sharples L. A review of the evidence on the effects and costs of implantable cardioverter defibrillator therapy in different patient groups, and modelling of cost-effectiveness and cost-utility for these groups in a UK context. Health Technol Assess. 2006;10:iii–iv, ix–xi, 1–164.
36. Guedon-Moreau L, Finat L, Boule S, Wissocque L, Marquie C, Brigadeau F, Kouakam C, Mondesert B, Kacet S, Klug D, Lacroix D. Validation of an organizational management model of remote implantable cardioverter-defibrillator monitoring alerts. Circ Cardiovasc Qual Outcomes. 2015;8:403–12. doi:10.1161/CIRCOUTCOMES.114.001433.
37. Siebermair J, Clauss S, Martens E, Schuessler F, Oversohl N, Haserueck N, Estner HL, Kaab S, Wakili R. Remote monitoring of implantable cardioverter-defibrillators. Problems and implications using a telemonitoring system. Herz. 2015;40(Suppl 2):110–8. doi:10.1007/s00059-014-4080-7.
38. De Ruvo E, Sciarra L, Martino AM, Rebecchi M, Iulianella RV, Sebastiani F, Fagagnini A, Borrelli A, Scara A, Grieco D, Tota C, Stirpe F, Calo L. A prospective comparison of remote monitoring systems in implantable cardiac defibrillators: potential effects of frequency of transmissions. J Interv Card Electrophysiol. 2015; doi:10.1007/s10840-015-0067-4.
39. Dario C, Delise P, Gubian L, Saccavini C, Brandolino G, Mancin S. Large controlled observational study on remote monitoring of pacemakers and implantable cardiac defibrillators: a clinical, economic, and organizational evaluation. Interact J Med Res. 2016;5:e4. doi:10.2196/ijmr.4270.
40. Al-Khatib SM, Piccini JP, Knight D, Stewart M, Clapp-Channing N, Sanders GD. Remote monitoring of implantable cardioverter defibrillators versus quarterly device interrogations in clinic: results from a randomized pilot clinical trial. J Cardiovasc Electrophysiol. 2010;21:545–50. doi:10.1111/j.1540-8167.2009.01659.x.
41. Guedon-Moreau L, Lacroix D, Sadoul N, Clementy J, Kouakam C, Hermida JS, Aliot E, Boursier M, Bizeau O, Kacet S. A randomized study of remote follow-up of implantable cardioverter defibrillators: safety and efficacy report of the ECOST trial. Eur Heart J. 2013;34:605–14. doi:10.1093/eurheartj/ehs425.
42. Mabo P, Victor F, Bazin P, Ahres S, Babuty D, Da Costa A, Binet D, Daubert JC. A randomized trial of long-term remote monitoring of pacemaker recipients (the COMPAS trial). Eur Heart J. 2012;33:1105–11. doi:10.1093/eurheartj/ehr419.
43. Ricci RP, Morichelli L, Santini M. Remote control of implanted devices through home monitoring technology improves detection and clinical management of atrial fibrillation. Europace. 2009;11:54–61. doi:10.1093/europace/eun303.
44. Spencker S, Coban N, Koch L, Schirdewan A, Muller D. Potential role of home monitoring to reduce inappropriate shocks in implantable cardioverter-defibrillator patients due to lead failure. Europace. 2009;11:483–8. doi:10.1093/europace/eun350.
45. Varma N, Epstein AE, Irimpen A, Schweikert R, Love C. Efficacy and safety of automatic remote monitoring for implantable cardioverter-defibrillator follow-up: the Lumos-T Safely

Reduces Routine Office Device Follow-up (TRUST) trial. Circulation. 2010;122:325–32. doi:10.1161/CIRCULATIONAHA.110.937409.
46. Bohm M, Drexler H, Oswald H, Rybak K, Bosch R, Butter C, Klein G, Gerritse B, Monteiro J, Israel C, Bimmel D, Kaab S, Huegl B, Brachmann J. Fluid status telemedicine alerts for heart failure: a randomized controlled trial. Eur Heart J. 2016; doi:10.1093/eurheartj/ehw099.
47. Nagele H, Lipoldova J, Oswald H, Klein G, Elvan A, Vester E, Bauer W, Bondke H, Reif S, Daub C, Menzel F, Schrader J, Zach G. Home monitoring of implantable cardioverter-defibrillators: interpretation reliability of the second-generation "IEGM Online" system. Europace. 2015;17:584–90. doi:10.1093/europace/euu349.
48. Hindricks G, Taborsky M, Glikson M, Heinrich U, Schumacher B, Katz A, Brachmann J, Lewalter T, Goette A, Block M, Kautzner J, Sack S, Husser D, Piorkowski C, Sogaard P. Implant-based multiparameter telemonitoring of patients with heart failure (IN-TIME): a randomised controlled trial. Lancet. 2014;384:583–90. doi:10.1016/S0140-6736(14)61176-4.
49. Geach T. Device therapy: just IN-TIME for ICD telemonitoring. Nat Rev Cardiol. 2014;11:557. doi:10.1038/nrcardio.2014.130.
50. Crossley G, Boyle A, Vitense H, Sherfesee L, Mead RH. Trial design of the clinical evaluation of remote notification to reduce time to clinical decision: the Clinical evaluation of remote NotificatioN to rEduCe Time to clinical decision (CONNECT) study. Am Heart J. 2008;156:840–6. doi:10.1016/j.ahj.2008.06.028.
51. Crossley GH, Boyle A, Vitense H, Chang Y, Mead RH. The CONNECT (Clinical Evaluation of Remote Notification to Reduce Time to Clinical Decision) trial: the value of wireless remote monitoring with automatic clinician alerts. J Am Coll Cardiol. 2011;57:1181–9. doi:10.1016/j.jacc.2010.12.012.
52. Heidbuchel H, Hindricks G, Broadhurst P, Van Erven L, Fernandez-Lozano I, Rivero-Ayerza M, Malinowski K, Marek A, Romero Garrido RF, Loscher S, Beeton I, Garcia E, Cross S, Vijgen J, Koivisto UM, Peinado R, Smala A, Annemans L. EuroEco (European Health Economic Trial on Home Monitoring in ICD Patients): a provider perspective in five European countries on costs and net financial impact of follow-up with or without remote monitoring. Eur Heart J. 2015;36:158–69. doi:10.1093/eurheartj/ehu339.
53. Ricci RP, Morichelli L, Quarta L, Sassi A, Porfili A, Laudadio MT, Gargaro A, Santini M. Long-term patient acceptance of and satisfaction with implanted device remote monitoring. Europace. 2010;12:674–9. doi:10.1093/europace/euq046.
54. Cavaco D. Follow-up of implantable cardioverter-defibrillators: face-to-face or remote? Rev Port Cardiol. 2013;32:965–6. doi:10.1016/j.repc.2013.10.002.
55. Landolina M, Perego GB, Lunati M, Curnis A, Guenzati G, Vicentini A, Parati G, Borghi G, Zanaboni P, Valsecchi S, Marzegalli M. Remote monitoring reduces healthcare use and improves quality of care in heart failure patients with implantable defibrillators: the evolution of management strategies of heart failure patients with implantable defibrillators (EVOLVO) study. Circulation. 2012;125:2985–92. doi:10.1161/CIRCULATIONAHA.111.088971.
56. Marzegalli M, Landolina M, Lunati M, Perego GB, Pappone A, Guenzati G, Campana C, Frigerio M, Parati G, Curnis A, Colangelo I, Valsecchi S. Design of the evolution of management strategies of heart failure patients with implantable defibrillators (EVOLVO) study to assess the ability of remote monitoring to treat and triage patients more effectively. Trials. 2009;10:42. doi:10.1186/1745-6215-10-42.
57. Oldenburg B, Baptista S, Cocker F, O'Neil A. Changing lifestyle behaviors to improve the prevention and management of cardiovascular disease. In: Alvarenga ME, Byrne D, editors. Handbook of psychocardiology. Singapore: Springer; 2016. p. 1077–94.
58. Rosman L, Whited A, Ford JH, Nekkanti R, Cahill J, Sears SF. Adding psychological intervention to high-tech care for patients with implantable cardioverter defibrillators. In: Alvarenga ME, Byrne D, editors. Handbook of psychocardiology. Singapore: Springer; 2016. p. 1077–94.

Chapter 12
Quality of Life of Patients Over 80 Years Old with Implantable Cardioverter-Defibrillators

Ahmed AlTurki, Riccardo Proietti, and Francesco Borgia

Abstract Implantable cardioverter-defibrillators (ICD) are frequently used to prevent sudden cardiac death. ICDs are underutilized in the elderly population. Though randomized trials included few elderly patients over the age of 80, ICDs should not be withheld on the basis of age alone as the available evidence shows a mortality benefit in this population. Complication rates in the elderly are slightly higher in the early post-implantation period but late complications are significantly lower. Elderly patients more likely to have complications can be identified prior to implantation through use of a validated risk score. There is a paucity of evidence regarding quality of life after ICD implantation but current evidence suggests it is comparable to patients who did not receive a device. Younger patients were more likely to experience psychological distress though elderly patients who experienced complications also experienced distress. Psychological distress can be well managed with cognitive-behavioral therapy. There is no conclusive evidence to suggest worse psychological well-being after ICD shocks and further evidence is needed in this field.

Keywords Implantable cardioverter-defibrillator • Quality of life • Octagenerians

Introduction

Implantable cardioverter-defibrillators (ICD) have been progressively utilized to prevent sudden cardiac death due to malignant ventricular arrhythmias [1, 2]. Randomized controlled trials have shown their efficacy as primary prevention in

A. AlTurki, M.D. (✉)
McGill University Health Center, 1650 Cedar Avenue, Montreal, QC, Canada
e-mail: ahmedalturkimd@gmail.com

R. Proietti
Department of Cardiology, Ospedale Luigi Sacco, Milan, Italy

Cardiac Center, Morriston Hospital, University of Swansea, Swansea, UK

F. Borgia
Department of Psychology, Università Cattolica del Sacro Cuore, Milan, Italy

© Springer International Publishing AG 2017

R. Proietti et al. (eds.), *Psychological, Emotional, Social and Cognitive Aspects of Implantable Cardiac Devices*, DOI 10.1007/978-3-319-55721-2_12

patients with heart failure and reduced ejection fraction [3] and they remain one of the few successful strategies for secondary prevention in patients who experienced ventricular fibrillation or ventricular tachycardia [4]. However, randomized trials included few elderly patients over the age of 80 and some of the trials excluded patients over 80 [5, 6].

Access to an ICD remains an issue due to their high cost and the expertise required to implant them; older patients are less likely to receive an ICD. Hess et al. demonstrated in a large retrospective study that increasing age was associated with lower ICD use (odds ratio [OR] 0.89, 95% confidence interval [CI] 0.87–0.91 per 5-year increase in age, $p < 0.0001$) [7]. Data from real life registries also showed a low rate of ICD utilization in octogenarians. The US national ICD registry showed that 12% of patients who receive an ICD are over 80 years old. Similar rates could be found in an English registry and Ontario registry with rates of 5.3% and 8.0% respectively [8].

Given the cost and the ability to prevent sudden cardiac death and their impact on life, use of ICDs in the elderly remains a controversial decision that clinicians are faced with on a daily basis. We review the evidence for ICD implantation in the elderly for primary prevention, the complications associated with implantation as well as the impact of an ICD and ICD shocks on quality of life in the elderly.

Benefits of ICD in Elderly

Due to lack of enrolment in the randomized trials, uncertainty remained as to whether elderly patients derived survival benefit from an ICD for primary prevention of sudden cardiac death. Hess et al. in a meta-analysis of the five major randomized trials of ICD use found that a survival benefit exists in the elderly but that it is attenuated with age. However, this attenuation may have been explained by the small sample size of elderly patients, increased comorbidity or competing causes of death [9]. Compared to non-recipients, patients older than 75 had lower all-cause mortality (HR 0.54, 95% CI 0.37–0.78) [9]. In a retrospective study by Pellegrini et al., increased age was associated with higher total, cardiac, and non-cardiac mortality (all $P \leq 0.001$) [10]. Duray et al., in a retrospective study of 375 consecutive ICD patients showed a similar rate of appropriate shock and mortality in older compared to younger patients [11].

Chan et al., compared long-term mortality (mean follow up 34 months) of ICD recipients versus non-recipients in a prospective study of 965 patients with ischemic and non-ischemic cardiomyopathies, severe left ventricular dysfunction and no prior ventricular arrhythmias. ICD therapy decreased mortality by 31%, an effect that persisted across all age groups. Surprisingly, ICD implantation lead to a similar decrease in mortality in elderly patients despite higher annual mortality rates [12].

In a systematic review of randomized and observational studies, Earley et al., analyzed data from studies that included age subgroup analysis; there was no difference in mortality between patients younger and older than 65 years (Relative odds ratio 0.93, CI 0.73–1.20) [13]. Kong et al., in a meta-analysis of four RCTs (n = 579), demonstrated that in patients ≥75 years, primary prevention ICD therapy remains efficacious in reducing all-cause mortality (HR 0.73; 95% CI 0.51–0.974; p = 0.03). Furthermore, no difference could be found in ICD-related, operative, in-hospital, or long-term complications among older patients compared to younger patients. The authors comment however that it remains unclear if quality of life of the elderly is improved with an ICD—a point we shall address later on [14].

Healey et al., performed an individual patient analysis of three secondary prevention randomized controlled trials in which ICD use was compared to amiodarone. The ICD significantly reduced all-cause and arrhythmic death in patients younger than 75 years of age (all-cause death HR = 0.69, 95% CI: 0.56–0.85, P = 0.0001; arrhythmic death HR = 0.44, 95% CI 0.32–0.62; P = 0.0001), but not in patients above 75 years of age (all-cause death HR = 1.06, 95% CI 0.69–1.64; P = 0.79; arrhythmic death HR = 0.90, 95% CI 0.42–1.95; P = 0.79). The difference in all cause death is explained by the increased rate of non-cardiac death in the elderly group and the study was clearly underpowered to detect a difference in arrhythmia death in the elderly subgroup. Therefore, the authors conclude that while life-saving therapy should not be withheld on the basis of death, an assessment regarding the likelihood of non-cardiac death is needed and this should be factored into the decision to implant an ICD [15].

Risk scores for the prediction of mortality in ICD recipients have been developed in five separate studies including one by Goldenberg et al., which used data from the MADDIT-II randomized trial sub-study that has been validated twice [16]. All five studies using different cut-offs of 70, 75 or 80 showed that increasing age was a predictor of mortality in ICD recipients with the risk of death increasing with comorbidities such as AF, renal dysfunction, liver dysfunction, history of stroke, anemia and NYHA IV symptoms [8]. This information should be utilized when deciding which patients should receive an ICD.

At a time when health care costs are rising, cost effectiveness has become essential. Given the strong possibility that elderly patient are at a higher risk of nonarrhythmic death, the need to demonstrate cost-effectiveness is even more pressing. Sanders et al., developed a model using data from six randomized trials for primary prevention. The model showed that the use of an ICD was projected to add between 1.01 and 2.99 quality-adjusted life-years (QALY) and between 68,300 dollars and 101,500 US dollars in cost. A sensitivity analysis performed by the authors showed that the cost-effectiveness ratio would remain below 100,000 dollars per QALY only while ICD decreased mortality for seven or more years [17]. However, a meta-analysis of trials of secondary prevention showed that an ICD only extended life by around 5 months at a follow up period of 6 years which would increase the cost-effectiveness ratio significantly and this finding was also corroborated in another study [18]. These findings suggest that an ICD may not be cost-effective in the in elderly patients above 80 years old though further studies are needed to strengthen these findings and each patient's life expectancy would need to be taken into account.

Complications of ICD Implantation in the Elderly

The procedure of implanting an ICD is not without complications. This includes those occurring during the procedure and in the post-procedure period. ICD implantation has a 98% success rate; mortality is very low at 0.2–0.6%. The association of elderly age and perioperative complications after ICD implantation was assessed by Tsai et al. using data from 150,264 primary prevention patients who received ICDs from January 2006 to December 2008. Elderly patients over 80 had a complication rate of 4.5% compared to 2.8% in those younger than 65. There was no difference in the rate of complications in the subgroup of 80–84 years compared to 85 years and above [19]. In an individual data meta-analysis, Armaganijan et al., found an early complication rate of 5.1% in patients over 75 years of age compared to 3.4% in patients younger than75 years (P = 0.006) which was mainly due to an increased risk of pneumothorax (1.6% vs. 0.8%, P = 0.07). However, older patients had a lower risk of lead fracture (3.6% vs. 2.7%, P = 0.08) [20].

In contrast, Yung et al., in a prospective registry of 5399 ICD recipients in Ontario, Canada from February 2007 to September 2010, found no increase in perioperative complications with increasing age in the 45 days following implantation [21]. A meta-analysis of randomized control trials and a large observational study also demonstrated that age was not an independent predictor of perioperative complications [8]. Ozcan et al., examined all the cases of pacemaker implantation at a single institution. The complication rate was 39 (15.1%) out of 259 young patients and 24 (7.6%) out of 315 elderly patients which was statistically significant (P = 0.005). No clear explanation could be given for this higher rate of complication in younger patients [22].

Haines et al. developed a risk score consisting of ten variables that are easily obtainable that accurately identifies patients at high risk of complications [23]. The score was derived from the ICD registry with 268,701 ICD implants and showed a risk of any in-hospital complication increased from 0.6% among patients with a score of ≤5 to 8.4% among patients with ≥19 risk points. The score was also shown to correlate with in-hospital mortality [23]. This is a useful tool for discussing peri-implantation morbidity with patients and may assist in the decision-making process for ICD implantation.

Challenges of an Elderly Patient Living with an ICD

In heart failure patients, older patients have been show to give greater import to quality of life rather than length of life compared to younger patients [24]. Noyes et al., assessed the association between quality of life and age in ICD recipients using the data from the RCT MADDIT-II. The authors found no difference in quality of life between patients who received an ICD and those who did not. More significantly in this case, there was no difference QoL between patients older than 65 and those younger. No data was available for patients specifically above the age of 80 [25]. Though QoL is usually considered an important factor for ICD placement in the elderly, there is a dearth of evidence on this topic. Older patients with ICDs have decreased physical functioning, more co-morbid illness, and worse symptoms that negatively impact QoL, However, younger patients with ICDs tend to experience increased psychological distress, anxiety, and depression. In elderly patients who develop complications, psychological distress and depression are more likely to occur [26].

Looking at the current literature, a conclusion cannot be drawn regarding the effect of an ICD on quality of life due to the heterogeneity of the available studies. Tomzik et al., in a systematic review of five randomized and ten observational studies could not reach a conclusion. Nine studies found similar QoL in ICD patients and patients in the control groups, three studies found an improved QoL for ICD recipients, and three studies found a diminished QoL for ICD patients. Lower QoL was evident among ICD recipients who experienced several device discharges [27].

Barros et al., assessed the quality of life among PM recipients relating it to age and Gender in a descriptive, quantitative, cross-sectional, observational study of 107 patients. They found that as age increases, quality of life worsens in terms of functional capacity and discomfort; and the longer the pacemaker implantation timespan, the worse quality of life when it comes to vitality. It was unclear if these patients were pacemaker dependent or if the device was implanted for defibrillator purposes [28].

Due to a lack of large or randomized trials regarding QoL, it is difficult to reach a definitive conclusion. May et al., showed that after a period an initial period of worsening QoL that was mainly due to transient problems in the areas of emotional behavior, alertness, and social interaction, QoL returned to pre-implant levels by 12-month follow-up; 17% of patients felt their tiredness was due to their old age [29]. Using data from the CABG Patch trial in which patients after CABG were randomized to ICD versus no ICD, Namerow et al., found that QOL outcomes (mental and physical) for the ICD patients were significantly worse compared to patients with no ICD. However, non-shocked ICD patients had similar QoL to patients without an ICD; there was no association with age [30]. Herbst et al., compared the Qol of four different study arms: ICD only, ICD plus antiarrhythmic drug, antiarrhythmic drug alone and general cardiology patients. There was no significant difference on the 11 QOL scales between any of the groups even after factoring age differences [31].

Psychological Complications of ICD Shock in Elderly

An ICD shock is the most feared even in ICD recipients. Both appropriate and inappropriate ICD shocks have been shown to worsen mortality and even more so after an appropriate shock as that likely indicates worse underlying cardiac disease [32]. Regardless of it appropriateness, a shock can have a profound psychological effect on patients and the thought of shock and fear of recurrence produces anxiety and possibly depressive symptoms [26].

Credner et al., found that around 10% of their sample of 136 ICD patients experienced an ICD storm during the first 2 years following ICD implantation. The experience of an ICD storm may prompt catastrophic cognitions and feelings of helplessness; younger patients were more likely to experience these distressing symptoms [33]. In a randomized controlled study, cognitive—behavioral therapy was used to reduce psychological distress in patients with newly implanted ICD. At 9 months follow-up, active treatment patients reported less depression, less anxiety, and less general psychological distress than the no treatment group. This suggests that systematic psychological interventions for new ICD patients would likely improve psychological and QOL outcomes [34].

Manzoni et al., performed a systematic review to delineate the psychological and QoL effects of ICD shocks. No conclusion could be reached on this association due to the methodological heterogeneity of study methods being too varied thereby restricting any quantitative attempt to explain the mixed findings [35]. This further highlights the need for high quality research to address these issues.

Generator Replacement in an Elderly with an ICD

Should generators be replaced in very elderly patients? Guidelines to guide the decision are currently lacking and good evidence is also not available. Goodewardene et al., examined data from a retrospective analysis of a prospectively maintained database from a single tertiary unit that consisted of octogenarian patients with ICD implantation and elective unit replacement. After elective unit replacement, ventricular tachycardia occurred in very few patients with no episodes of ventricular fibrillation occurring. Another important finding was the lack of ICD therapy delivered to any patient who did not need ICD therapy prior to replacement. The authors suggest that a survival benefit from ICD EUR in this age stratum is not likely [36]. Rechecking the ejection fraction to see if patients remain eligible and considering explanting the device in patients with no previous ICD delivered therapies are reasonable strategies.

Conclusion

ICDs are life-saving devices. Although specific robust evidence for efficacy in patients over 80 is lacking, they should not be withheld due to age alone and patient selection is important. Complication rates in this age group is not excessive compared to younger patients and patients at higher risk of complications can be identified early. There is a paucity of evidence regarding quality of life of ICD recipients but this does not appear to be worse than patients on AADs and patients with symptoms may benefit from cognitive-behavioral therapy. There is no conclusive evidence to suggest worse psychological well-being after ICD shocks.

References

1. Cesario DA, Dec GW. Implantable cardioverter-defibrillator therapy in clinical practice. J Am Coll Cardiol. 2006;47(8):1507–17.
2. DiMarco JP. Implantable cardioverter-defibrillators. N Engl J Med. 2003;349(19):1836–47.
3. Ponikowski P, Voors AA, Anker SD, Bueno H, Cleland JG, Coats AJ, et al. 2016 ESC Guidelines for the diagnosis and treatment of acute and chronic heart failure: the Task Force for the diagnosis and treatment of acute and chronic heart failure of the European Society of Cardiology (ESC) developed with the special contribution of the Heart Failure Association (HFA) of the ESC. Eur Heart J. 2016;37(27):2129–200.
4. Kusumoto FM, Calkins H, Boehmer J, Buxton AE, Chung MK, Gold MR, et al. HRS/ACC/AHA expert consensus statement on the use of implantable cardioverter-defibrillator therapy in patients who are not included or not well represented in clinical trials. J Am Coll Cardiol. 2014;64(11):1143–77.
5. Kadish A, Dyer A, Daubert JP, Quigg R, Estes NA, Anderson KP, et al. Prophylactic defibrillator implantation in patients with nonischemic dilated cardiomyopathy. N Engl J Med. 2004;350(21):2151–8.
6. Higgins SL, Daubert JL, Akhtar M. Who are the MADIT patients? Multicenter automatic defibrillator implantation trial. Am J Cardiol. 1997;80(5B):42F–6F.
7. Hess PL, Grau-Sepulveda MV, Hernandez AF, Peterson ED, Bhatt DL, Schwamm LH, et al. Age differences in the use of implantable cardioverter-defibrillators among older patients hospitalized with heart failure. J Cardiovasc Electrophysiol. 2013;24(6):664–71.
8. Barra S, Providencia R, Paiva L, Heck P, Agarwal S. Implantable cardioverter-defibrillators in the elderly: rationale and specific age-related considerations. Europace. 2015;17(2):174–86.
9. Hess PL, Al-Khatib SM, Han JY, Edwards R, Bardy GH, Bigger JT, et al. Survival benefit of the primary prevention implantable cardioverter-defibrillator among older patients: does age matter? An analysis of pooled data from 5 clinical trials. Circ Cardiovasc Qual Outcomes. 2015;8(2):179–86.
10. Pellegrini CN, Lee K, Olgin JE, Turakhia MP, Tseng ZH, Lee R, et al. Impact of advanced age on survival in patients with implantable cardioverter defibrillators. Europace. 2008;10(11):1296–301.
11. Duray G, Richter S, Manegold J, Israel CW, Gronefeld G, Hohnloser SH. Efficacy and safety of ICD therapy in a population of elderly patients treated with optimal background medication. J Interv Card Electrophysiol. 2005;14(3):169–73.
12. Chan PS, Nallamothu BK, Spertus JA, Masoudi FA, Bartone C, Kereiakes DJ, et al. Impact of age and medical comorbidity on the effectiveness of implantable cardioverter-defibrillators for primary prevention. Circ Cardiovasc Qual Outcomes. 2009;2(1):16–24.
13. Earley A, Persson R, Garlitski AC, Balk EM, Uhlig K. Effectiveness of implantable cardioverter defibrillators for primary prevention of sudden cardiac death in subgroups a systematic review. Ann Intern Med. 2014;160(2):111–21.
14. Kong MH, Al-Khatib SM, Sanders GD, Hasselblad V, Peterson ED. Use of implantable cardioverter-defibrillators for primary prevention in older patients: a systematic literature review and meta-analysis. Cardiol J. 2011;18(5):503–14.
15. Healey JS, Hallstrom AP, Kuck KH, Nair G, Schron EP, Roberts RS, et al. Role of the implantable defibrillator among elderly patients with a history of life-threatening ventricular arrhythmias. Eur Heart J. 2007;28(14):1746–9.

16. Goldenberg I, Vyas AK, Hall WJ, Moss AJ, Wang H, He H, et al. Risk stratification for primary implantation of a cardioverter-defibrillator in patients with ischemic left ventricular dysfunction. J Am Coll Cardiol. 2008;51(3):288–96.
17. Sanders GD, Hlatky MA, Owens DK. Cost-effectiveness of implantable cardioverter-defibrillators. N Engl J Med. 2005;353(14):1471–80.
18. Connolly SJ, Hallstrom AP, Cappato R, Schron EB, Kuck KH, Zipes DP, et al. Meta-analysis of the implantable cardioverter defibrillator secondary prevention trials. AVID, CASH and CIDS studies. Antiarrhythmics vs Implantable Defibrillator study. Cardiac Arrest study Hamburg. Canadian Implantable Defibrillator study. Eur Heart J. 2000;21(24):2071–8.
19. Tsai V, Goldstein MK, Hsia HH, Wang Y, Curtis J, Heidenreich PA, et al. Influence of age on perioperative complications among patients undergoing implantable cardioverter-defibrillators for primary prevention in the United States. Circ Cardiovasc Qual Outcomes. 2011;4(5):549–56.
20. Armaganijan LV, Toff WD, Nielsen JC, Andersen HR, Connolly SJ, Ellenbogen KA, et al. Are elderly patients at increased risk of complications following pacemaker implantation? A meta-analysis of randomized trials. Pacing Clin Electrophysiol. 2012;35(2):131–4.
21. Yung D, Birnie D, Dorian P, Healey JS, Simpson CS, Crystal E, et al. Survival after implantable cardioverter-defibrillator implantation in the elderly. Circulation. 2013; 127(24):2383–92.
22. Ozcan KS, Osmonov D, Altay S, Donmez C, Yildirim E, Turkkan C, et al. Pacemaker implantation complication rates in elderly and young patients. Clin Interv Aging. 2013;8:1051–4.
23. Haines DE, Wang Y, Curtis J. Implantable cardioverter-defibrillator registry risk score models for acute procedural complications or death after implantable cardioverter-defibrillator implantation. Circulation. 2011;123(19):2069–76.
24. Lewis EF, Johnson PA, Johnson W, Collins C, Griffin L, Stevenson LW. Preferences for quality of life or survival expressed by patients with heart failure. J Heart Lung Transplant. 2001;20(9):1016–24.
25. Noyes K, Corona E, Zwanziger J, Hall WJ, Zhao H, Wang H, et al. Health-related quality of life consequences of implantable cardioverter defibrillators: results from MADIT II. Med Care. 2007;45(5):377–85.
26. Sears SF Jr, Conti JB. Quality of life and psychological functioning of ICD patients. Heart. 2002;87(5):488–93.
27. Tomzik J, Koltermann KC, Zabel M, Willich SN, Reinhold T. Quality of life in patients with an implantable cardioverter defibrillator: a systematic review. Front Cardiovasc Med. 2015;2:34.
28. Barros RT, Carvalho SM, Silva MA, Borges JB. Evaluation of patients' quality of life aspects after cardiac pacemaker implantation. Rev Bras Cir Cardiovasc. 2014;29(1):37–44.
29. May CD, Smith PR, Murdock CJ, Davis MJ. The impact of the implantable cardioverter defibrillator on quality-of-life. Pacing Clin Electrophysiol. 1995;18(7):1411–8.
30. Namerow PB, Firth BR, Heywood GM, Windle JR, Parides MK. Quality-of-life six months after CABG surgery in patients randomized to ICD versus no ICD therapy: findings from the CABG Patch Trial. Pacing Clin Electrophysiol. 1999;22(9):1305–13.
31. Herbst JH, Goodman M, Feldstein S, Reilly JM. Health-related quality-of-life assessment of patients with life-threatening ventricular arrhythmias. Pacing Clin Electrophysiol. 1999;22(6 Pt 1):915–26.
32. Proietti R, Labos C, Davis M, Thanassoulis G, Santangeli P, Russo V, et al. A systematic review and meta-analysis of the association between implantable cardioverter-defibrillator shocks and long-term mortality. Can J Cardiol. 2015;31(3):270–7.
33. Credner SC, Klingenheben T, Mauss O, Sticherling C, Hohnloser SH. Electrical storm in patients with transvenous implantable cardioverter-defibrillators: incidence, management and prognostic implications. J Am Coll Cardiol. 1998;32(7):1909–15.

34. Pauli P, Wiedemann G, Dengler W, Blaumann-Benninghoff G, Kuhlkamp V. Anxiety in patients with an automatic implantable cardioverter defibrillator: what differentiates them from panic patients? Psychosom Med. 1999;61(1):69–76.
35. Manzoni GM, Castelnuovo G, Compare A, Pagnini F, Essebag V, Proietti R. Psychological effects of implantable cardioverter defibrillator shocks. A review of study methods. Front Psychol. 2015;6:39.
36. Goonewardene M, Barra S, Heck P, Begley D, Fynn S, Virdee M, et al. Cardioverter-defibrillator implantation and generator replacement in the octogenarian. Europace. 2015;17(3):409–16.

Chapter 13
Importance of Counselling ICD Patients: The Role of Cardiac Physiologists

Parisha Khan

Abstract Implantable Cardiac Defibrillators (ICDs) have proven mortality benefits in those at risk of cardiac arrest due to Ventricular Fibrillation (VF) or Ventricular Tachycardia (VT). ICDs present challenges not only in the technical management of the device but also on the psychosocial impact it has on a patient. ICD counselling prior to implantation and in some instances during follow up, can allow a patient to address the concerns they may have and attempt to minimise any possible negative psychosocial impact. ICD counselling should be provided by appropriately experienced healthcare professionals, in some UK centres this service is provided by cardiac physiologists and specialist arrhythmia nurses. The chapter specifically focuses on the role of a cardiac physiologist which is reflective of practise within our centre (St Georges' Hospital, London, UK). ICD counselling prior to implantation is a way of protecting a patients' autonomy and allows informed consent by empowering the patient with appropriate detail as well as giving them the opportunity to discuss the positive and negative aspects of the device. ICD counselling presents many different patient related challenges. This chapter aim is to explore these and offer advice on how to overcome them based on experiences within our centre.

Keywords Implantable cardiac defibrillators (ICDs) • Ventricular fibrillation (VF) Ventricular tachycardia (VT) • Cardiac physiologists • Primary prevention • Secondary prevention • Cardiac resynchronization thearpy (CRT) • Channelopathies Anti-tachycardia pacing • Phantom shocks

P. Khan
Department of Cardiology, Kings College Hospital, Denmark Hill, London SE5 9RS, UK
e-mail: parisha.khan@nhs.net

© Springer International Publishing AG 2017

R. Proietti et al. (eds.), *Psychological, Emotional, Social and Cognitive Aspects of Implantable Cardiac Devices*, DOI 10.1007/978-3-319-55721-2_13

Introduction

The clinical benefits of Implantable Cardiac Defibrillators (ICDs) for those at risk of cardiac arrest from Ventricular Fibrillation (VF) or Ventricular Tachycardia (VT) have been well established through many randomised trials and registries. As a result, the number of patients receiving these devices is growing exponentially throughout Europe [1]. Advancement in ICD technology has been aimed at improving the patient's experience either through aesthetics by attempting to make devices more cosmetically pleasing to a patient or through sophisticated algorithms that provide lifesaving therapy without treating the patient inappropriately. Healthcare professionals are trained to understand and manage the complexities of an ICD as a medical device but often the psychosocial impact on a patient is over looked. The perceived psychosocial impact is not merely based on subjective experience but has been investigated in several studies where the outcomes have reinforced the benefits of ICD counselling. An example of one such study is by Sears et al. [2] who examined the psychosocial impact of ICDs and documented psychological morbidity in adult ICD patients with anxiety ranging from 13 to 46% and depression from 24 to 46% of patients. This is could be interpreted as surprising given the known benefits of ICD therapy however, it is often the negative or perceived 'downside' to having an ICD which could account for much of the anxiety that patients often exhibit and which may not have been discussed openly prior to implant.

Aims of Counselling

The success of an ICD implant should not only be measured by procedural success in the short term but in the long term, how well a patient adjusts and accepts having the device. The concept of acceptance is demonstrated in a study by Sears et al. [3] who looked at the quality of life outcomes for patients with ICDs. The study concluded that acceptance of the device and the impact it a has on lifestyle could positively influence the quality of life, with those who have high positive health expectations and high optimism reporting better mental health and social functioning at follow-up. One of the biggest challenges that an ICD patient faces is returning to what is perceived to be 'normal' life. In order to do so, a patient not only has to overcome the stress of being at risk of an abnormal arrhythmia but also coming to terms with a device that has the potential to deliver a shock if necessary. Lack of a detailed discussion could have implications on how informed a patient's consent is for an ICD procedure. The following will look at types of concerns and anxieties that a patient may have and how healthcare professionals, such as cardiac physiologists are in a unique to position to act as an advisor and maintain a patients' autonomy through education. Much of the opinions that are put forward in this chapter are based on the experience from follow-ups of ICD patients within our centre.

The challenge of educating a patient prior to implant is to provide information that is neither falsely optimistic nor alarming. Topics such as driving bans, inappropriate therapy, and deactivation in later life or limitations to work need to be sensitively addressed in order to allow the patient time to adjust to the implications of having the device. The conversation required in order to address patient concerns and work towards acceptance is often time consuming. Increased workflow through most hospital catheter labs in addition to greater clinical and administrative demands on healthcare professionals can sometimes impact the education a patient receives before undergoing an ICD procedure.

Who Are Cardiac Physiologists?

So, who is responsible for having this important discussion? In order to allow the patient enough time to process any given information, the discussion should ideally take place well before procedural consent is given. In the UK, some hospitals have a system of pre-procedural ICD counseling which is undertaken by either Specialized Cardiac Physiologists or Specialist Arrhythmia Nurses. This system is practiced in the majority of UK hospitals where cardiac physiologists or specialist nurses play a key role in the patient's clinical care once the device has been implanted. In fact, programming of the devices and follow up troubleshooting are performed by cardiac physiologists or specialist arrhythmia nurses in the majority of UK centers.

At St Georges Hospital in London, there is a dedicated device clinic run by highly specialized cardiac physiologists; however this may not reflect the practice of all hospitals. The following is an explanation of how a cardiac physiologist attains the appropriate specialization in order to fulfill this role. The pathway involves a cardiac physiologist attaining a degree in clinical physiology with a specialization in cardiology. Post graduate specialization is encouraged in echocardiography, electrophysiology or devices. Having gained sufficient experience in a particular area, a cardiac physiologist will gain certification in their chosen specialization area through a professional body exam. The British Heart Rhythm Society has put in place a standard which outlines how many device procedures and follow ups should be maintained per year in order to be deemed competent. Cardiac Physiologists therefore not only provide practical expertise but are also in a position to have a significant clinical impact on a patient. This puts them in the unique position of being able to build a relationship that is more open and informal than that between a patient and physician. A familiarity is built up over time through regular device checks and therefore patients often feel that a cardiac physiologist represents an important link to the hospital even though they may no longer be followed up by a cardiologist. In turn, cardiac physiologists are exposed to the genuine emotions and fears that patients often face and gain experience in dealing with them in a professional way. In order to give credence to a cardiac physiologists' role as an advisor, our centre provides counseling skills workshops. These are run by trained counselors who can offer advice on how ICD counseling should be approached in a professional way and how to deal with difficult patient scenarios. It is this experience that a cardiac physiologist can draw upon in a conversation about ICD implantation which is not only clinically informative but can lay the foundation towards acceptance.

Primary Prevention and Secondary Prevention Patients

The approach to the discussion should be based on the individual and the reason for referral. Although there are certain topics that should always be covered, it is important to realize that the reason for implantation can influence what concerns a patient may have. Primary prevention patients may have different expectations of the device compared to secondary prevention patients. Primary prevention patients often struggle to understand why the device is necessary in the first place particularly because they have no experience to draw upon in terms of surviving a dangerous arrhythmia. To the primary prevention patient, the device could represent an added complication rather than protection particularly the notion that it is capable of delivering a shock. It is with these patients that the most work needs to be done in order to help them accept the device. In this situation, it is important to make the patient understand what benefit having the device has to offer, however this should not be used as an opportunity to alarm. Although there is no definitive estimate of how many primary prevention patients will go on to develop ventricular arrhythmias, there is also a real possibility that these patients may never receive therapy while they have the device. The patients are then within their right to question if they need the device at all, this should be addressed in an objective manner by reassuring the patient this could be the case but implant of the device represents a small additional risk to them.

The different etiologies that primary prevention patients display can present various challenges in terms of counseling. Landmark trials have shown that heart failure patients are offered a significant reduction in mortality with an ICD and those with the wide QRS complexes due to bundle branch morphologies, further benefit from resynchronization therapy [4]. As a result, recent updates to national guidelines in the UK have recommended a larger proportion of population received a CRT-D (cardiac resynchronization therapy with defibrillator therapy) [5]. Heart failure patients may have the conception that the device could improve or ‘reverse’ their heart failure and this issue needs to be broached very carefully when providing counseling. False hope should never be given and heart failure patients should be made to understand that the device is not a ‘cure’ for their condition, rather once the device is implanted there is a process of optimization in order to provide the maximum benefit to the patient. The optimization is driven by how that patient responds to the therapy and although heart failure patients should be on optimal medical therapy at the time of implant, further changes may be required along with programming optimization.

Those primary prevention patients implanted due to channelopathies such as Long QT and Brugada or any other inherited cardiac conditions have the additional stress of having to deal with a condition which puts them at a higher risk of having dangerous ventricular arrhythmias. In some instances, a sudden death has occurred in the family which brings emotion turmoil that often does can't be processed before the family screening begins. Younger patients in particular may have more difficulty accepting the need for the device because the ICD could serve as a reminder that something is 'wrong' with them, the parallel could be drawn in this situation of an ICD being akin to having a breast removed when someone is suffering from breast cancer—there is a constant reminder of the condition. This may lead to elements of denial and resentment, which can impact the counseling in two ways—either the patient will not be receptive to counseling and therefore will not want to listen to the information being provided to them or they will use the session as a way to work through their anxiety. The challenge that this presents to the cardiac physiologist providing the counseling is to avoid getting emotionally involved, this objectivity must be maintained. Often in these situations a single counseling session is not enough to allow the patient sufficient time to work towards acceptance and counseling may even be required after the device has been implanted. In addition to ICD counseling, genetic counseling is also offered to patients with inherited cardiac conditions which helps them understand the condition and the impact it has on family members. This provides an important foundation which subsequently ICD counseling can build on when explaining the role of the device.

For those that are considered secondary prevention patients, the implantation of an ICD may be easier to accept. Presenting the ICD as a device that offers protection in the event of a dangerous arrhythmia can be comforting to a patient who has survived in part because they received defibrillation therapy. This, however, does not mean that a secondary prevention patient is always happy to accept the device. As with primary prevention patients, there may be an element of resentment and a feeling that the ICD serves as a reminder of what may be wrong. In our centre, we have also experienced patients who consider the ICD as having a profoundly restrictive impact on lifestyle and therefore don't see the benefits. Some patients also feel that the cause of the cardiac arrest should be reversible and therefore do not understand the need for the device. In these instances, again, the benefit of the device should be emphasized in an objective manner; although it may be very easy to fall into the trap of using methods to make the patient almost feel guilty that they are not agreeing to have the device. It is important to remember that the patient has autonomy over the final decision and therefore the position of the cardiac physiologist should be neutral, representing the mediator between a physician who places importance on the clinical benefit and a patient who could be driven by psychosocial anxieties.

Practicalities of ICD Counseling

The counseling session should ideally take place before procedural consent but in reality, this time may not be afforded to the patient particularly if the decision to implant is taken while they are in the hospital. The tone of the discussion may be affected by the circumstances under which the discussion takes place, with a difference between an outpatient and in-patient setting. If a patient is electively referred for an ICD, it is likely that he has had the time to speak to his appointed cardiologist regarding the need for the device and has already began the process towards acceptance. In some centers within the UK, patients are not only electively referred for the procedure but in addition for elective ICD counseling. Once the patient arrives for counseling, they are able to have the discussion in a private environment with minimal time constraint, giving them the opportunity to work through the concerns they may have with a healthcare professional.

Patients who are already in the hospital present different challenges. The environment in which the patients finds themselves in is often not conducive to an objective approach towards the discussion, in some instances where patients are already anxious about being in the hospital, this could further compound the fear and anxieties they may have about having an ICD implanted. Patients may not have had the necessary time in order to process their clinical diagnosis and may not experience continuity with regards to which physicians they talk to. There are steps taken to try and maintain some kind of privacy when counseling patients on a ward however this is not always practical and in addition there are small aspects that can have a negative impact on the discussion. Simple things like the patient not being in their own clothes can add to the perception of being in an unfamiliar environment. The job of the healthcare professional is then to almost try and create equality between the patients and themselves in order to achieve a sense of ease. The aim is to make the patient believe they are not just talking to someone in uniform but a person that represents their interests.

Importance of Capacity

In order to make the patient feel as if they are the centre of the conversation, it is important to start by assessing how much the patient knows about the device and reasons for implant. An opening line of 'how much have you been told about the ICD or how do you feel about the ICD' gives the patient an opportunity to set out their concerns from the beginning. It also gives the healthcare professional a chance to judge at what level the discussion should take place. The patients' cognitive ability is important it influences how the information is received. Factors to consider are learning difficulties, cognitive impairment secondary to medical condition and maturity. A patients' ability to determine what happens to their own body is fundamental to their wellbeing. A healthcare professional has a moral obligation to show respect for patients and their autonomous choices. When a patient becomes unable to make these choices then concern for the patient's welfare becomes the responsibility of the healthcare professional. Appropriate assessment of cognitive ability should be made before a patient is referred for an ICD, in England and Wales, decision making in this area is covered by the Mental Capacity Act [6]. According to the act, if there are concerns over capacity then there should be a documentation in the medical records along with any details from appropriate assessments. If there is no documentation, a cardiac physiologist can use the ICD counseling session to try and assess capacity. The key points to note when talking to the patient are, can the patient understand and retain the information given to them regarding the ICD? Patients who fully understand have a much greater degree of acceptance and therefore those who do not have the capacity are already at a disadvantage. The role of a cardiac physiologist or any healthcare professional counseling a patient for an ICD is not just to prepare them but also to make a judgment on whether a patient has the suitable capacity to have the device implanted. The ability of the patient to handle the psychosocial aspects of having an ICD is often overlooked in favor of the clinical need which can later lead to a struggle in making the patient take responsibility and ownership of the device. To further expand this idea, it is true that the patient's care is overseen by a clinic with regular checks however in order to reduce the anxiety associated with having an ICD the patient should have the capacity to understand its capabilities and when it is appropriate to seek advice. In this instance the cardiac physiologist can act as an impartial representative between the patient and the physician in order to ensure that the correct medical and ethical decision is taken.

Involvement of families or those close to the patient in counseling sessions has advantages and disadvantages. For those patients that are considered to have capacity, having family members can offer a balance to the conversation and the patient may feel more at ease with close family present. For those patients who lack capacity it is often necessary to involve those who are close to the patient or those designated as power of attorney. The disadvantage of involving family members arises when a conflict of interest exists between the patient's personal relationships. In this situation, a cardiac physiologist has to decide who is the best person to direct the counseling to without becoming involved in personal politics. It is advisable to make the discussion as concise as possible so to avoid influencing either side.

The Importance of Lifestyle

During the counseling session it is important to discuss the impact of the ICD on lifestyle. Patients are often concerned that the ICD will limit what they can do and is seen as an obstacle in returning to normal life. Patients should be reassured that although there may be certain limitations in the short term, for example, restricted arm movement and driving bans, a patient can return to normal life. Where there are restrictions, these should be explained so they are understood rather than considered an imposition. In the UK, the Driver and Vehicle Licensing Authority (DVLA) issues guidelines on the recommended driving ban for patients who receive ICD therapy. Primary prevention patients are subject to a 1 month ban, whereas secondary prevention patients are given a 6 month driving ban. There is a further 6 month driving ban if the patient received appropriate shock therapy [7]. Patients whose livelihood depends on driving may resist the device, even though they are clinically more at risk if they do not have it. The social and economic impact of not driving for whatever length of prescribed time is sometimes overlooked. During counseling, it is not only necessary to inform the patient about the ban, there should be an attempt to make the patient understand why this is necessary as a form of protection for the patient.

The Impact of Shocks

The most important topic to discuss is the devices ability to deliver a shock and the small risk of inappropriate shocks. Approximately one third of patients who receive an ICD may experience a shock during the first year [8]. Both meta-analysis and individual trials have indicated that shock is at least, temporarily associated with decrements in quality of life [9]. Although strategic programming and ATP reduces the incidence of shocks to 9% vs. 17% in primary prevention patients over the first year [10] there is still a significant psychological impact on the patient. Versteeg et al. [11], published a brief report showing ICD shock experience was the strongest determinant of post-traumatic stress disorder at 3 months post-implant. It is therefore evident that one of the most important steps in helping patients accept the device, is for them to accept that they may experience a shock and educate them on how to cope with this. The focus is often placed on how a shock will stop a dangerous arrhythmia but not how a patient may feel afterwards as well as the risk of inappropriate shocks. In ICD recipients, depressive symptoms may be caused by the perceived lack of control over necessary defibrillation discharges [2]. Although pre-implant counseling may not completely remove anxiety should a patient receive a shock it lays a foundation for ongoing future counseling.

A recently recognized phenomenon that occurs in some ICD patients which consists in a manifestation of an emotional response is known as a 'phantom shock'. This phenomenon occurs when the patient perceives that the device has discharged with describable sensations, however the device memory indicates that no shock was delivered. Swygman et al. [12], investigated this phenomenon further with a study population of 445 patients. Of these 445 patients, 30 reported phantom shocks. The study tried to determine if there were any demographic predictors such as age, gender, ejection fraction, number of shocks or inappropriate verses appropriate shocks that would suggest that specific groups were more susceptible to this phenomenon, however there were none. It was noted, however that phantom shocks were more likely to occur within the first 6 months after an ICD implant and as late as 52 months post. Although this phenomenon is rare, it does show how necessary it is to have a support network available for patients even after implant.

Deactivation

As patients live longer with the support of the device the question of deactivation arises. Patients should be afforded the opportunity to discuss their wishes in relation to deactivation of the shock function. If attempted prolongation of their life by the device is no longer appropriate for them, deactivation of the shock function may spare them (and those close to them) the distress and indignity of ICD shocks. Although this could be considered a topic that would add to a patient's anxiety, it has become more pertinent and is an example of a way to protect patient's autonomy. Patients do not always realize that they are entitled to instruct others on their wishes concerning the ICD in the context of palliative care. When a decision about deactivation of an ICD is being considered it is especially important that patients and those close to them have a clear understanding of what is being considered, for what reason and the expected effects of deactivation [13]. The responsibility of healthcare professionals involved with the patients' care is to act upon the patients' wishes at the appropriate time but also to ensure that these wishes are documented clearly. In the event that patients have not stated their preference for deactivation, there can often be a conflict between relatives and healthcare professionals. It is common for people to be alarmed by the false belief that deactivation will lead to immediate death, so sensitive, clear and unambiguous explanation is crucial in this situation, as it is in all aspects of end-of-life care. Any decision should be documented clearly by the physician, patient or the patients' representative. These types of joint decisions are more easily taken if the patient is in hospital; those that are in the community sometimes find themselves unable to access the relevant healthcare professionals. There is also the additional complication of not being able to complete the correct documentation that verifies the decision for deactivation in a community setting. In this situation it may be advisable to have the family doctor act as the patient's lead physician, however appropriate documentation should be sent to the centre where ICD follow-up occurs. There are other decisions which the physician is responsible for making regarding deactivation. To clarify this further, ICD patients suffer a wide range of illnesses and often those that are terminal are non-cardiac. The physician responsible for these patients is not specialized in dealing with ICDs therefore it is often more appropriate for a cardiologist to make this decision. Discussion about deactivation should be treated with care and presented to patients as a choice that they have the ability to make rather than an inevitable fact that comes with having an ICD.

Recalls and Advisories

Devices have become more sophisticated in recent times; however, they are still subject to recalls and sudden failures. This topic is difficult to discuss with patients during counselling as it can trigger patients' fears and anxiety making it even more difficult for them to accept the device. Depending on how well the counselling session has gone, the healthcare professional may choose not to discuss this topic if the patient is particularly anxious, withholding this information is never wise or it puts the patient in the situation of not being able to make an informed decision. Another relevant topic concerns the use of a magnet. Magnets are given to patients in the event the device delivers inappropriate shocks but a judgement has to be made on the patients' ability to use the magnet appropriately. This judgement can be based on the pre-procedural counselling. Although a patient may appear to have the suitable cognitive ability to understand the need for the device, they may not be able to make an appropriate decision on when and how to use the magnet. The discussion about inappropriate shocks should also include an introduction to the use of a magnet without necessarily going into great detail. Instructions on the use of a magnet can be given after implant, once the patient is over the initial trauma of the procedure. In our centre, the policy is to give all primary prevention patients magnets at the post day check if they are considered capable of making decisions concerning the use of the magnet.

Post Implant Support

Although the aim of the counselling session is to provide as much relevant information as possible in order to allow the patient to give informed consent, there is also the issue of giving too much information. A judgment has to be made on how much information a patient can retain without feeling overwhelmed. In these circumstances it may be more beneficial to have more than one session so that the patient has the time to process what has been said in each sitting, this approach reinforces the notion that ongoing counselling and support is essential. So far, we have focused on how to prepare the patient for the ICD before the procedure takes place but as we have previously discussed, a support network is essential after the device has been implanted. There are patients who are counselled appropriately and have an uncomplicated implant and seemingly have a good acceptance of their device, but the situation may arise where a problem occurs further down the line that can have a significant psychological impact. This is not limited to inappropriate shocks, procedural complications due to wounds or displaced leads can require further counselling. The patient has to adjust mentally and physically to having the device. There is a period when the patient can naturally be uncomfortable but there are situations in which a patients' anxiety manifests itself as a 'physical' rejection of the device. This concept has not been investigated scientifically, however it is based on experiences we have had with patients within our clinic. Patients can repeatedly come back to clinic because they are convinced that the device is causing them discomfort and pain even though there is no evidence of infection or abnormalities. Reassurance may not always be enough and it can become a longstanding issue. From the experience at our centre, we find that if these types of patients are presented with the possibility of undergoing another procedure in order to resolve the 'problem', they can be reluctant which may be indicative of a more psychological issue than a physical one. In these instances there has to be an ongoing form of counselling which may have to come from a professional counsellor as the issues may go beyond the expertise of a cardiac physiologist. When there are real infections, wound or lead problems which result in repeated procedures this can have an impact on the patients' confidence and therefore continued support is necessary.

Patient Support

In our centre, the need for ongoing counselling and patient support was ascertained which lead to the creation of an ICD support group in 1997. Reblin and Uchino [14] looked at findings from selected publications investigating links between social support and physical health. They concluded that social support from others can be protective of health which is why patient support groups are so important. The main aims of the ICD support group in our centre are as follows.

- To provide a forum for all ICD patients, their partners and families to discuss their concerns and problems.
- To help patients with ICDs to regain their confidence and morale when experiencing problems or during times of trouble.
- To provide literature and information on all topics that are relevant to ICD patients.
- To provide information about driving, insurance, holidays, interference and any other areas where ICD patients may experience problems in day-to-day life.
- To provide emergency and technical information to other healthcare workers such as A & E departments, ITU's and ambulance crews in order to promote better understanding of patients with implanted ICDs.

The group holds regular meetings where they have the opportunity to meet each other, there are also educational talks led by various healthcare professionals, ultimately the group allows patients to take ownership of their devices by gaining more information about their condition and how the device works.

Conclusion

Throughout this chapter, we have discussed the important role that a cardiac physiologist plays in counselling an ICD patient not only before but also after an implant. The focus of any discussion about an ICD should be on the patient and therefore it should be presented in such a way so it is within the patient's capability to understand it. When possible, technical language should be avoided and those providing the counselling should show that they are 'actively' listening to the patient i.e. demonstrate they have listened to and understood the patients concern. The aim of counselling should not be to either persuade or dissuade but to present the facts in a way that allows the patient to make an informed decision which then can be translated into informed consent.

Acknowledgment I would like to acknowledge Sue Jones, Pacing and ICD Manager at St Georges' Hospital, London, UK whose experience and guidance I drew upon when writing this chapter. Sue Jones was responsible for setting up the ICD counselling pathway that is used within our hospital as well as the ICD support group for patients that is an integral support for ICD patients.

References

1. Nicor. National audit of cardiac rhythm management devices 2013–2014. 2013. http://www.ucl.ac.uk/nicor/audits/cardiacrhythm/reports. Accessed 15 Aug 2015.
2. Sears SF, Todaro JF, Lewis TS, Sorile W, Conti JB. Examining the psychosocial impact of implantable cardioverter defibrillators: a literature review. Clin Cardiol. 1999;22:481–9.
3. Sears SF, Serber ER, Lewis TS, Walker RL, Conners N, Lee JT, Curtis AB, Conti JB. Do positive health expectations and optimisation relate to quality of life outcomes for patients with an implantable cardioverter defibrillator? J Cardiopulm Rehabil. 2004;24:324–31.
4. Cleland JG, Daubert JC, Erdmann E, Freemantle N, Gras D, Kappenberger L, Tavazzi L, Cardiac Resynchronisation-Heart Failure (CARE-HF) Study Investigators. The effect of cardiac resynchronization on morbidity and mortality in heart failure. N Engl J Med. 2005;352(15):1539–49.
5. NICE. Implantable cardioverter defibrillators and cardiac resynchronisation therapy for arrhythmia and heart failure (review of TA95 and TA120). 2014. http://www.nice.org/guidance. Accessed 20 Aug 2015.
6. Mental Capacity Act. 2005. http://www.legislation.gov.uk/ukpga/2005/9/contents. Accessed 26 Apr 2016.
7. DVLA. Atrial and ventricular defibrillators and driving. 2015. http://www.gov.uk/health-conditions-and-driving. Accessed 20 Apr 2016.
8. Connolly SJ, Dorian P, Roberts RS, Gent M, Boul WS, Fairi ES, Thorpe K, Champagne J, Talajic M, Coutu B, Gorefeld GC, Hohnloser SH, Optimal Pharamalogical Therapy in Cardioverter Defibrillator Patients (OPTIC) Investigators. Comparison of beta-blockers, amiodarone plus beta-blockers or sotalol for prevention of shocks from implantable cardioverter defibrillators; the OPTIC Study: a randomised trial. JAMA. 2006;295:165–71.
9. Francis J, Johnson B, Niehaus M. Quality of life in patients with implantable cardioverter defibrillators. Indian Pacing Electrophysiol J. 2006;6:173–81.
10. Sears SF, Matchett M, Conti J. Effective management of ICD patient psychosocial issues and patient critical event. J Cardiovasc Electrophysiol. 2009;20:297–307.
11. Versteeg H, Theuns DAMJ, Erdman RAM, Jordaens L, Pedersen SS. Post traumatic stress in implantable cardioverter defibrillator patients: the role of pre implantation distress and shocks. Int J Cardiol. 2011;3:438–9.
12. Swygman C, Link M, Cliff D. Incidence of phantom shocks in patients with implantable cardioverter defibrillators (abstract). Pacing Clin Electrophysiol. 1998;21:810.
13. Resuscitation Council (UK). British Cardiovascular Society and National Council for Palliative Care. Deactivation of implantable cardioverter defibrillators towards the end of life. 2015. https://www.resus.org.uk/search/?q=%27ICDs%27. Accessed 26 Apr 2016.
14. Reblin M, Uchino B. Social and emotional support and its implication for health. Curr Opin Psychiatry. 2008;21(2):201–5. doi:10.1097/YCO.0b013e3282f3ad89.

Chapter 14
The Patient's Informal Caregiver

Mitzi M. Saunders

Abstract The majority of care for patients with implantable cardioverter defibrillators (ICDs) and left ventricular assist devices (LVADs) takes place beyond hospital or clinic walls. Most patients share this unique experience in a committed relationship with another person. This person, often the patient's spouse, cares for the patient by supporting their physical and emotional healing. However this often comes with a price. This chapter reveals how the role of the informal caregiver can take a toll on a person's physical, emotional and spiritual health. Health care providers (HCPs) must take notice and act in ways that support these people in order for optimal patient outcomes to occur. This chapter focuses on the informal caregivers (ICs) responses in the provision of care for patients with ICDs and LVADs and offers recommendations to support them. Distinctions will be made as there are some differences in informal caregiving based on the type of device the patient has i.e., ICD or LVAD.

Keywords Implantable cardioverter defibrillator • Left ventricular assist device • Informal caregiving • Informal caregiver • Spousal caregiver • Partner • Family caregiver • Caregiver activities • Caregiver health • Health care providers • Sexual counseling • Caregiver outcomes • Caregiver research

The majority of care for patients with implantable cardioverter defibrillators (ICDs) and left ventricular assist devices (LVADs) takes place beyond hospital or clinic walls. Most patients share this unique experience in a committed relationship with another person. This person, often the patient's spouse, cares for the patient by supporting their physical and emotional healing. However this often comes with a price. This chapter reveals how the role of the informal caregiver can take a toll on a person's physical, emotional and spiritual health. Health care providers (HCPs) must take notice and act in ways that support these people in order for optimal patient outcomes to occur. This chapter focuses on the informal caregivers (ICs)

M.M. Saunders, R.N., Ph.D., A.C.N.S.-B.C.
University of Detroit Mercy, Detroit, MI 48221, USA
e-mail: saundemm@udmercy.edu

© Springer International Publishing AG 2017

R. Proietti et al. (eds.), *Psychological, Emotional, Social and Cognitive Aspects of Implantable Cardiac Devices*, DOI 10.1007/978-3-319-55721-2_14

responses in the provision of care for patients with ICDs and LVADs and offers recommendations to support them. Distinctions will be made as there are some differences in informal caregiving based on the type of device the patient has i.e., ICD or LVAD.

Who is the Informal Caregiver?

- Spouse/Partner
- Adult child
- Relative
- Friend
- Neighbor

A lack of research on ICs of patients with ICDs is evident and even sparser for ICs of patients with LVADs. Why does this matter? Since 1990, with the first documented study on this type of informal caregiving [1], there have been consistent reports that the role is challenging, demanding [2] and has an impact on patient and IC outcomes. Unfortunately, in most instances, ICs take on the caregiver role with very little guidance [3]. Thus, it is time to act on what we do know and devote more resources and time to assisting the ICs through research that examines the best strategies to support them.

Specifically, this chapter will uncover the following:

- Who are they (ICs) and what do they do for patients with ICDs and LVADs?
- How do they respond to this type of caregiving?
- What are the recommendations, guidelines and resources to help the IC?

Who Are They and What Do They Do?

Having a general understanding of informal caregiving in the U. S. provides a foundation for understanding ICs for patients with ICDs and LVADs. In the general population, the typical IC is a middle-aged adult child caring for an older relative but this person can also be a spouse/partner, relative, friend or neighbor [4]. Sometimes, informal caregiving goes beyond assistance with household chores and getting patients to doctor's appointments to include medical and nursing related tasks such as administration of medication, wound care, checking weight, blood sugar and blood pressure or managing special diets such as tube feeding [4]. With the development of measures that allow patients with chronic illnesses to live longer, the complexity of home care has grown. The problem however, is that the IC continues to do more but in the process is receiving very little training and support for these "expected" and "necessary" care activities [4]. There is no necessary test or assessment of the IC to even make sure they are competent at what they are doing. Thus, stress, burden, fatigue, anxiety, depression and missed time at work are well known consequences associated with informal caregiving [4]. But, there are positive aspects as well. Some ICs enjoy helping the patient and grow closer to them in doing so. They also learn new skills and feel they are making things better for the patient by permitting the patient to remain at home [4].

More specifically, ICs of patients with ICDs and LVADs are mostly spouses/partners of patients who range in age from the mid-50s to the upper 60s in most reports. Similar to the general IC population, most are Caucasian and female. At least 1/3–1/2 of ICs are also employed and have at minimum a high school education. Overall, this person watches over the patient, participates to a large extent in their daily care and assists the patient in decision-making [5]. The following is a list of the many care activities performed by the ICs of patients with ICDs and LVADs reported to date:

Pre-device

- Assist the patient in the decision to get the device [5]

Post-device

- Assist with physical needs like getting the urinal and providing pillows for positioning [3]
- Watch the patient (vigilance) [3, 6]
- Limit the patient's physical activity to support recovery and prevent shocks [7]
- Provide lots of encouragement [6]
- Drive the patient to appointments [6]
- Be present [6]
- Help with the exercise regimen [6]
- Shift of one's roles at home by doing more work such as cooking, shopping, finances, etc. [3, 6]
- Provide emotional support and protection from stressful situations [3]
- Help with treatments [3] and medications [6]
- Manage symptoms [6]

Many of the care activities listed above also apply to informal caregiving of patients with LVADs. But, there are others based on the specific needs associated with an LVAD device. The following list includes the additional care activities performed by ICs for patients with LVADs that grow in complexity:

- Assist with all basic cares such as dressing and bathing [8, 9]
- Assist with the bedtime routine and help the patient find a comfortable sleeping position [8]
- Monitor the patient's blood pressure, medications and weight [8, 9]
- Perform sterile dressing changes, handle battery issues and the docking system [8, 9]

- Monitor LVAD function and alarms [8]
- Have back up batteries charged and materials gathered for dressing changes [8]
- Prepare for emergency situations [8]

Transiantly, the greatest demands on the ICs of patients with ICDs occur in the first 3 months after implantation when the patient is most vulnerable and fragile [3]. This time frame also equates to more physician appointments [3]. By 12 months post-device, patients with ICDs tend to be more independent and by one report, closer to their baseline or pre-cardiac event state [10]. The 12 month mark has been found to coincide with a greater overall adjustment to the routine by the family [10] and a return to normality or acceptance of the new norm [7].

ICs of patients with LVADs seem to adapt over time to care routines as well [8] but report feeling overwhelmed [11]. For some ICs, it was getting the necessary equipment in place i.e., stethoscope, blood pressure cuffs and scales for weighing the patient that helped ICs adjust more quickly to the role [8].

How Do They Respond to This Type of Caregiving?

This section will highlight how ICs respond to caregiving for patients with ICDs and LVADS. This information was accumutated from studies of the ICs of these patient types through self-reports and open-ended interviews. Negative responses are reported first and diverse. Positive responses follow.

Negative Responses

Symptoms Experienced by Informal Caregivers

The demands placed on the IC may be greater than those experienced by the patient. Studies show that ICs when compared to patients with ICDs in the same time frame post-implantation have higher levels of anxiety [3, 12, 13], depression, greater felt demands on family functioning [12], less free time, assumption of more household chores [14], higher degrees of post-traumatic stress syndrome [11] and possibly experience more stress than patients when advisories or malfunctions of devices occur [5].

Higher levels of anxiety have persisted in ICs for up to 1 month post-implantation of the patient's device [3]. In one study, ICs were assessed on day 1 of the ICD procedure and again at a 6 month follow-up [13]. At both intervals, ICs had significantly higher levels of anxiety and depression than the patients with ICDs they were caring for [13]. Gender differences in ICs did not have an effect on symptoms [13] while having a Type D personality, smoking, low levels of education, being on psychotropic medications and device placement due to secondary prevention did [13]. At the 6 month follow-up, there was a decrease in levels of depression and anxiety in ICs [13] that suggests some level of coping occurs over time.

Feeling fatigued and "run-down" has also been reported among ICs and found to persist beyond the 12 months post-implantation [3]. Feelings of social isolation [6, 15], not having time away from the patient [6] and finding it hard to care for one's own needs have been identified [6]. Yet, one study found that ICs scores on quality of life survey were no different than scores in the general population matched in age and sex [16]. Thus, more research and use of qualitative measures are needed to fully capture and understand this unique caregiving experience.

To date, there is no evidence that suggests any correlations between IC outcomes and the frequency of shocks experienced by patients with ICDs. ICs are known to purposefully protect patients from stress for fear of triggering a shock [6]. It has also been suggested that this "overprotectiveness" of the patient might hamper patient progress over time, ideally patients should gradually be assuming more of their own care as they heal [10].

Among the few studies reporting on symptoms of ICs of patients with LVADs, there is one report that compared levels of anxiety and depression with ICs of patients with ICDs [17]. ICs of patients with LVADS had significantly higher levels in both [17]. This may correlate with the higher levels of complexity involved in the care of patients with LVADs. Patients with LVADs are generally sicker and in poorer physical health [8]. Markers for post-traumatic distress syndrome have also been significantly higher in IC spouses than patients' scores as have the values depicting levels of depression and anxiety [11].

Concerns of Informal Caregivers

A major concern of ICs of patients with ICDs is not being informed and not getting answers to their questions when needed. Specifically, they blame the HCPs [6, 14]. ICs want to be informed on what to do when things go wrong and on strategies that help prevent problems such as shocks to the patient [6]. They do not like when HCPs use "professional jargon," seem "uninterested" or "too busy" and neglect to tell them what the future might hold [14]. When things happen, ICs resort to calling 9:1:1 [6], a potentially unnecessary and costly service that can been averted by better informing the IC. It is also suggested that HCPs do not know enough about the experience of ICD patients to teach about it [14]. When ICs feel informed, they feel better [6].

Another major concern of ICs is the lack of attention to their needs. ICs have medical problems too and take medications [3]. Some ICs of ICD patients perceive declines in their own physical health since the patient's device was placed [3]. ICs of patients with LVADs feel their own health ranks second to the patients. In one study, the IC of a patient with an LVAD acknowledged the following when she knew the researcher was planning to ask her about her health: "Just before you [the researcher] knocked on the door, he [the patient with an LVAD] said you [the researcher] was going to be asking me about it [my own health] and I looked up the doctor's telephone number to make the call. I am going to do it. I have a plan now" ([9], p. 87). In another study, ICs had more outpatient visits to doctors for their own health issues in the first year of caring for patients with ICDs than before [3]. Caregiver health may be at risk.

The ICs of patients with LVADs, have significantly higher concerns about the patients having a stroke and being in pain than the patients themselves [11]. ICs of patients with LVADs seem to worry in general of the possibilities of infection and device malfunction [18]. This again, emphasizes that ICs are at risk of experiencing health issues because of the caregiver role and consequently need to be supported.

Adjustments in Sexual Activity and Other Areas

Because the majority of ICs of patients with ICDs and LVADs are spouses/partners of patients, adjustments to sexual activity is as important for them to understand as it is for the patient. IC spouses/partners express worry and fear about having sex and believe it might cause a shock [19]. Spouses worry what the shock experience might be like during sex [19]. Seeing the patient's scar from the ICD when the patient's shirt is off is difficult for some and a represents a constant reminder of the situation [19]. Others have expressed the importance of engaging in other intimate acts such as hugging and cuddling as they might be less apt to promote a shock [19]. Some ICs choose relaxation techniques before sexual activity such as having a glass of wine [19]. One IC spouse of a patient with an LVAD indicated how she and the patient find themselves watching the flow and rate of the LVAD while having sex and being afraid of too much exertion [11]. Overall, they blame HCPs for being reluctant to discuss this topic with them [19].

Other adjustments by ICs include staying at home more, doing more household chores and spending a great deal of time caring for the patient [14]. Overall, time might be the greatest adjustment [6]. Major adjustments to spending have occurred when patients can no longer work [20] and finances need to be readjusted [6]. One family reported having to sell their mobile home [14].

Positive Responses

ICs of patients with ICDs and LVADs also have positive responses to this experience. While fewer, they may be meaningful enough to negate or offset the negative responses. These responses are:

- Better communication with the patient [3, 14]
- More honest and loving relationship with the patient [11, 14]
- Being grateful of having a second chance [8, 11]
- Supporting each other [3]
- Security in feeling the device is supporting the patient [10]
- Becoming more lighthearted [3] and optimistic [11]
- Enjoying just today [6]

When Involved in a Support Group

- Ability to help others in similar situations [15]
- Helping the next generation [15]

Contrary to reports by ICs of patients with ICDs, ICs of patients with LVADs have felt supported by HCPs both educationally and psychologically in their transition from hospital to home. As stated by one IC of a patient with an LVAD: "I have very good support from the transplant team. The nurses answered a million questions. The training was excellent." ([20], p. 198). Some believe they could not have coped without that support [11].

What Are the Recommendations, Guidelines and Resources to Help the IC?

Recommendations from Informal Caregivers

In this section we will discuss the strategies used by the ICs, who are the ones most intimately involved by the experience. The following is a list of their recommendations. It is subdivided in areas of greatest potential to support one's physical, emotional or spiritual health. Many however, could fit in two or more categories simultaneously. The importance of spiritual health is that the very act of comforting and caring for the patient is an act of merciful giving of oneself to help another. Many may also experience spiritual distress in their attempts to find meaning in the situation.

Physical Health

- Practice healthy behaviors like eating well, exercising [6] and giving up smoking [14]

Emotional Health

- Having a support system or others to talk to who are experiencing the same situation [14, 21]
- Join a support group [15]
- Get out of the house [14, 21]
- Keep a positive attitude [6]
- Get back to work and enjoy hobbies like riding a bike [6, 14] or shopping [11]
- Get/hire the help needed [6, 8]

- Use time management skills [6]
- Slow down the pace [6]
- Spend time with family [6]
- Share feelings with others and the patient ([6, 20, 21])
- Take one day at a time [6]
- Be patient [6, 21]
- Establish a routine [6, 20]
- Use relaxation techniques [6, 21]
- Make end-of-life care plans [6]
- Screen phone calls [6]
- Control the environment [6]
- Engage with HCPs [20, 22]
- Make needed lifestyle changes [8, 11]
- Be confident you can do it [11]
- Learn manufacturer information [6, 15]
- Have sex [11]

Spiritual Health

- Find meaning in the experience [6]
- Be committed to the informal caregiver role [20]
- Pray [14]

While the list is extensive and involves dealing with both practical and more difficult adjustments which this type of informal caregiving implies, we must appreciate the changes and growth that ICs undergo and encourage their efforts in the process.

Guidelines

HCPs

Firstly, HCPs need to take special notice of the ICs. Involving the IC in patient care is very important [23, 24]. In their role as caretakers they could be suffering physically, mentally and spiritually. The concerns and needs of the ICs should be addressed from the moment that the device is proposed to the patient [2]. It is suggested that by including the IC, both the patient's and IC's experience is better and as a result this may even permit to lower the costs of care for patients [23].

While the literature identifies negative responses to this type of caregiving experience, very little evidence supports positive solutions. However, we gleaned from ICs of patients with LVADs that when they did feel supported by HCPs, they were able to cope better [11]. We also know that ICs have questions that need answers. One pilot study considering a small sample showed how having nurses available by telephone, made a difference in IC responses in the first 3 months following implantation of the ICD [23]. This study fostered a larger randomized control study that is currently being investigated. The idea here is to extend the reach of nurses to patients and their ICs beyond the hospital experience where the majority of care occurs [23]. However it should not begin and end with nurses. All HCPs need to be involved in the care of the ICs so that not even one IC who needs help is neglected. This strategy that all HCPs need to offer supportive interventions is the best way to provide a safety net so that not one IC feels alone in his role. If we garner anything from the telephone call approach [23], it is the need to reach out, listen, ask questions and give helpful responses in a way that ICs can understand.

Until more research is done to guide interventions, we suggest the following strategies for HCPs.

- Evaluate the ICs needs along with the patients [24] including sexual concerns [25]
- Listen and give lots of information readily [15]
- Offer strategies on how they (IC) can help [6] and not be overprotective [21]
- Be honest of the realities of the situation [15]

Sexual Counseling

In most cases, the IC is the patient's spouse/partner. It is important therefore to elaborate specific guidelines related to sex. It is also advisable that HCPs use a "just ask," proactive approach in talking about sex that is on-going and should occurs across all health care settings of various HCPs [25]. Any strategies to help the patient in this area should likewise be extended to their spouse/partner [25]. IC spouses/partners of patients with LVADs need to know the importance of checking battery function, monitoring the device as well as modifying positions during sexual activities [25]. Patients and their IC spouses/partners should be encouraged to continue to have sex unless there are specific contraindications [25] and to explore ways to minimize stress on the patient's heart function [19]. Finally, IC spouses/partners should be informed that they will not be shocked if the patient is shocked during sex [21].

End-of-Life Care

The literature suggests that ICs have a poor and incomplete knowledge when it comes to end-of-life (EOL) care planning for these types of patients [14]. Besides the need to initiate discussions about EOL care with patients and ICs, there are specific aspects that must be addressed. The goal of EOL care is a peaceful death, sometimes the patient might die of other non-cardiac causes, the need to inform ICs of eventual plans to deactivate the device is mandatory [14]. Frank discussions about shocking the body at the time of death and thus permitting a peaceful dying experience must take place.

Web-Based Resources for the Informal Caregiver

There are web-based resources for ICs of patient with heart related conditions. The American Heart Association (AHA) web-site provides information that can assist the IC in learning what an ICD is and its use in arrhythmias [28, 29]. This site includes a picture of an ICD implanted in a patient. Another AHA web-site includes the eight R's of caregiving that can help the caregiver to cope with their role. The eights R's are rights, responsibility, reality check, refresh, rejuvenate, replenish, reach-out and resources [30]. Additionally, there is information on caring for one-self both physically and emotionally with tips for success as well as specific contact information for accessing a support group [28, 29]. ICs of patients with ICDs have found that being in support groups and talking to others going through the same experience is beneficial [15].

More Research

While it is evident that the role is challenging for ICs, we know very little about selecting the right interventions to adequately support ICs. It is very important to invest time into research studies that evaluate interventions for ICs on outcomes that impact both the IC and the patient [17]. Studies should also consider investigating differences in ICs for race/ethnicity, gender, level of education as well as being employed or not so no IC group is underrepresented in research. For example, in one study on the effects of employment on IC outcomes when caring for home bound patients with heart failure, employed ICs had higher well-being than those not employed [26]. It is important too that these studies assess both quality and cost-related type outcomes such as worsening IC health that might lead to higher usage of health care services by the IC. HCPs should likewise encourage ICs participation in studies that may actually benefit them. The use of 24/7 on call services for problems ICs encounter might be a great area to investigate. If HCPs can argue the benefits of such interventions, then insurance agencies might be more apt to cover the additional time afforded in caring for the IC. Under the current Medicare guidelines, custodial related cares such as helping patients with activities with daily living is not a covered service because these activities can be done by someone without medical training [27]. However, these ICs are performing more complex cares and there is no current payment system that subsidizes any of these cares or HCPs time in caring for the IC. More research is needed to validate interventions that support the IC to promote changes in policy.

Conclusion

Whether by choice or not, the IC provides the emotional and physical support needed by patients with ICDs and LVADs. Many ICs experience negative responses in their role that could easily be averted if HCPs were more supportive of to the IC's needs. HCPs must explore every aspect of the IC's experience. This type of assessment should be on-going for the needs of the IC and patient change over time. Providing adequate education and monitoring for negative responses will surely necessitate increased care strategies. ICs must be assisted in order to be effective in caring for the patient. More research is needed so that HCPs can select the best interventions to adequately support the IC. Most importantly, the role of the IC must be recognized and HCPs must be willing to help.

References

1. Pycha C, Calabrese JR, Gulledge AD, Maloney JD. Patient and spouse acceptance and adaptation to implantable cardioverter defibrillators. Cleve Clin J Med. 1990;57:441–4.
2. Dunbar SB, Dougherty CM, Carroll DL, McDaniel G, Schron E. Educational and psychological interventions to improve outcomes for recipients of implantable cardioverter defibrillators and their families. Circulation. 2016;216:2146–72. doi:10.1161/CIR.0b013e31825d59fd.
3. Dougherty CM, Thompson EA. Intimate partner physical and mental health after sudden cardiac arrest and receipt of an implantable cardioverter defibrillator. Res Nurs Health. 2009;32:432–42.
4. Reinhard SC, Levine C, Samis S. Home alone: family caregiving providing complex chronic care. AARP Public Policy Institute. 2012. http://www.aarp.org/content/dam/aarp/research/public_policy_institute/health/home-alone-family-caregivers-providing-complex-chronic-care-rev-AARP-ppi-health.pdf. Accessed 27 Apr 2016.
5. Ottenberg AL, Mueller LA, Mueller PS. Perspectives of patients with cardiovascular implantable electronic devices who received advisory warnings. Heart Lung. 2013;42:59–64.
6. Dougherty CM, Pyper GP, Benoliel JQ. Domains of concern of intimate partners of sudden cardiac arrest survivors after ICD implantation. J Cardiovasc Nurs. 2004;19(1):21–31.
7. Palacios-Cena D, Losa-Iglesias ME, Alvarez-Lopez C, Cachon-Perez M, Reyes RAR, Salvadores-Fuentes P, Fernandex-de-las-Penas C. Patients, intimate partners and family experiences of implantable cardioverter defibrillators: qualitative systematic review. J Adv Nurs. 2011;67(12):2537–50. doi:10.1111/j.1365-2648.2011.05694.x.
8. Kitko LA, Hupcey JE, Gilchrist JH, Boehmer JP. Caring for a spouse with end-stage heart failure through implantation of a left ventricular assist device as destination therapy. Heart Lung. 2013;42:195–201.
9. Saunders MM. Perspectives of family caregivers receiving home nursing support. Home Healthc Nurse. 2012;30(2):82–90.
10. Kamphuis H, Verhoeven N, de Leeuw R, Derksen R, Hauer R, Winnubst J. ICD: a qualitative study of patient experiences the first year after implantation. J Clin Nurs. 2004;13:1008–16.
11. Bunzel B, Roethy W, Znoj H, Laederach-Hofmann K. Psychological consequences of life-saving cardiac surgery in patients and partners: measurement of emotional stress by the impact of event scale. Stress Health. 2008;24(5):351–63. doi:10.1002/smi.1194.
12. Dougherty CM, Fairbanks AM, Eaton LH, Morrison ML, Kim MS, Thompson EA. Comparison of patient and partner quality of life and health outcomes in the first year after and implantable cardioverter defibrillator (ICD). J Behav Med. 2016;39(1):94–106.
13. Pedersen SS, Van Den Berg M, Erdman R, Van Son J, Jordaens L, Theuns D. Increased anxiety in partners of patients with a cardioverter-defibrillator: the role of indication for ICD therapy, shocks, and personality. PACE. 2009;32:184–92.
14. Imes CC, Dougherty CM, Pyper G, Sullivan MD. Descriptive study of partners' experiences of living with severe heart failure. Heart Lung. 2010;40:208–16.
15. Williams AM, Young J, Nikoletti S, McRae S. Reasons for attending and not attending a support group for recipients of implantable cardioverter defibrillators and their carers. Int J Nurs Pract. 2004;10:127–33.

16. Jenkins LS, Powell JL, Schron EB, McBurnie MA, Bosworth-Farrell S, Moore R, Exner DV. Partner quality of life in the antiarrhythmics versus implantable defibrillators trial. J Cardiovasc Nurs. 2007;22(6):472–9.
17. Brouwers C, Caliskan K, de Jonge N, Theuns D, Constantinescu A, Young QR, Cannon C, Denollet J, Pedersen SS. A comparison of the health status and psychological distress of partners of patients with a left ventricular assist device versus an implantable cardioverter defibrillator: a preliminary study. Heart Lung. 2015;44:27–32.
18. Dew MA, Kormos RL, Winowich S, Stanford EA, Carozza L, Borovetz H, Griffith B. Human factors issues in ventricular assist device recipients and their family caregivers. ASAIO J. 2000;46(3):367–73.
19. Steinke EE, Gill-Hoppie K, Valdez D, Wooster M. Sexual concerns and educational needs after an implantable cardioverter defibrillator. Heart Lung. 2005;34(5):299–308. doi:10.1016/j.hrtlng.2005.03.002.
20. Baker K, Flattery M, Salyer J, Haugh KH, Maltby M. Caregiving for patients requiring left ventricular assistance device support. Heart Lung. 2010;39(3):196–200.
21. Hazelton AG, Sears SF, Kirian K, Matchett M, Shea J. Coping with my partner's ICD and cardiac disease. Circulation. 2009;120:e73–6. doi:10.1161/CIRCULATIONAHA.109.877613.
22. Casida J. The lived experience of spouses of patients with a left ventricular assist device before heart transplantation. Am J Crit Care. 2005;14(2):145–51.
23. Dougherty CM, Thompson EA, Kudenchuk PJ. Development and testing of an intervention to improve outcomes for partners following receipt of an implantable cardioverter defibrillator in the patient. Adv Nurs Sci. 2012;35(4):359–77.
24. Van Den Broek KC, Habibovic M, Pedersen SS. Emotional distress in partners of patients with an implantable cardioverter defibrillator: a systematic review and recommendations for future research. Pacing Clin Electrophysiol. 2010;33:1442–50.
25. Steinke EE, Jaarsma T. Sexual counseling and cardiovascular disease: practical approaches. Asian J Androl. 2016;17:32–9.
26. Saunders MM. Working and caregiving: a comparison of employed and unemployed caregivers of older heart failure patients. Home Healthc Nurse. 2010;24(1):16–22.
27. Center for Medicare and Medicaid Services. Your medicare benefits. 2016. https://www.medicare.gov/Pubs/pdf/10116.pdf. Accessed 29 Apr 2016.
28. American Heart Association. How should I care for myself as a caregiver? 2015. http://www.heart.org/idc/groups/heart-public/@wcm/@hcm/documents/downloadable/ucm_300662.pdf. Accessed 27 Apr 2016.
29. American Heart Association. What is an arrhythmia? 2015. http://www.heart.org/idc/groups/heart-public/@wcm/@hcm/documents/downloadable/ucm_300290.pdf. Accessed 27 Apr 2016.
30. American Heart Association. 2016. http://www.heart.org/HEARTORG/Caregiver/Caregiver_UCM_001103_SubHomePage.jsp. Accessed 27 Apr 2016.

Chapter 15
Ethical Aspects of Withdrawing Cardiac Device Therapy at End of Life

Vilma Torres and William R. Lewis

Abstract Cardiac device therapies are associated with improved survival in patients at risk for sudden cardiac death due to ventricular arrhythmias. The number of implants for both primary and secondary prevention continues to rise both in the United States and European countries. As the population ages and technology advances, patients with implantable devices continue to live longer. When terminal illness becomes apparent, patient's goals may change to comfort care and painful shocks from ICDs become unwanted and inappropriate. This chapter discusses the challenges that patients and medical caregivers face as these patients deal with terminal illnesses. It also discusses the latest information available in the medical literature related to ethics and patient's and physician's attitudes. Ethics will aid the clinician's management of the goals of care related to potentially complex end-of-life issues. With some pre-planning a potentially stressful situation can become more manageable for all those involved.

Keywords End-of-life • Deactivation • ICD withdrawal • Terminally ill and ICD • Withdrawing cardiac device • Withholding CIED's

Cardiovascular Implantable Electronic Devices (CIEDs) have been associated with reduced mortality in patients with structural heart disease [1–4]. Cardiac resynchronization therapy (CRT) devices have recently been shown to improve congestive heart failure symptoms as well as survival [5]. As indications for device therapy continue to expand, the population of patients with these devices continues to grow [6]. Despite the tremendous advances in technology, all patients will reach the end of their lives, due to their underlying heart condition, such as end stage congestive heart failure but additionally diseases such as severe lung disease, neurological disorders such as Parkinson's disease, dementia, fatal infections as well as terminal cancers will also lead to their death. Unplanned events can also occur such as

V. Torres, M.D. (✉) • W.R. Lewis, M.D.
Department of Medicine, MetroHealth Campus of Case Western Reserve University, 2500 MetroHealth Drive, Cleveland, OH 44109, USA
e-mail: vtorres@metrohealth.org; wlewis@metrohealth.org

© Springer International Publishing AG 2017

R. Proietti et al. (eds.), *Psychological, Emotional, Social and Cognitive Aspects of Implantable Cardiac Devices*, DOI 10.1007/978-3-319-55721-2_15

automobile accidents or other forms of trauma leading to similar terminal scenarios. Due to the nature of physiological changes such as electrolyte imbalance, hypoxia or pH changes that can occur with many of these illnesses there is a higher probability that supraventricular or ventricular arrhythmias are triggered especially during an acute decompensation. The defibrillator functions as programmed and thus, appropriate as well as inappropriate therapies, including shocks, are delivered to the patient. In patients suffering from terminal illness, these shocks are painful and may be intolerable and inconsistent with treatment goals [7]. Because of the potentially higher number of shocks what had been a tolerable experience because it was life-saving, is no longer appropriate.

In the last weeks of their lives, 20% of ICD patients receive shocks which are painful and known to decrease quality of life [7]. This greatly contributes to the distress of patients and their families. In patients with terminal illnesses, minimizing discomfort and maintaining quality of life should be a priority for everyone involved in their care.

The goals of this chapter are:

- To educate clinicians regarding the legal, ethical, religious principles and rights and responsibilities of health care providers associated with withdrawal of life-sustaining therapies, specifically CIED deactivation or removal, in patients who have made this decision.
- Discuss published data regarding variations in current clinical practices, knowledge, perception and provider preferences.
- Develop a framework or strategies to guide the health care providers involved in assisting patient and families when a request is made to withdraw CIED therapy.
- Encourage a team/multidisciplinary approach to care for these patients and their families.

Although the main focus of this discussion is on patients nearing the end of life, it will also address patients who have made a decision for device deactivation at other times of their lives.

The issue of managing patients nearing end of life was initially addressed in the 2008 ACC/AHA/HRS Guidelines for device therapy of Cardiac Rhythm Abnormalities [8]. As the number of ICD implants continued to rise and the number of instances where therapy withdrawal becomes appropriate, the interest and number of publications in this area has risen. Two excellent consensus statements have been written outlining the principles and suggested best practices of Cardiovascular Implantable Electronic Devices (CIEDs) management in patients nearing end of life. These provide a very balanced and detailed discussion to guide health care providers in the management of what can be a very stressful time for all those involved, including but not limited to health care providers, patients, their families as well as industry professionals.

The United States Expert Consensus was developed by the Heart Rhythm Society (HRS) in collaboration with and endorsed by American College of Cardiology

(ACC), American Geriatric Society (AGS), American Academy Of Hospice and Palliative Medicine (AAHPM), American Heart Association,(AHA), European Heart Rhythm Association (EHRA) and Hospice and Palliative Nurses Association (HPNA) and published in 2010 [9]. The European Heart Rhythm Association published similar guidelines several months later [10]. It highlights the differences arising from the diversity of national laws in Europe. There are countries where the deactivation of anti-bradycardia pacing function in a pacemaker dependent patient is prohibited by law. It is therefore important to be aware of the laws that apply to the country of practice.

Legal, Ethical and Religious Issues in Withdrawing Cardiac Device Therapy

This discussion begins with a clinical scenario that will help illustrate some of the salient points:

A 65 year old retired college professor is admitted to the hospital with altered mental status. She had a permanent pacemaker implanted for complete heart block (CHB) 5 years prior to the current illness. She resulted being pacemaker dependent at every office pacemaker evaluation. She is now critically ill with sepsis, a newly diagnosed stroke and as part of the clinical evaluation was found to have metastatic ovarian cancer. She has an older spouse and 3 children. She has no advance directive (AD). Her oncologist contacts her cardiologist who implanted the pacemaker to consult regarding the patient's request to have her pacemaker turned off as she feels it is keeping her alive against her wishes. Her cardiologist is hesitant to deactivate the pacemaker given his own personal values as well as the fact that opinions are divided among her family members.

Question #1. Does She Have the Capacity to Make Such a Request Given the Acuity of Her Illness? How Is That Determination Made?

The following discussion on basic legal principles will shed some light into this question.

Legal Principles

Request for deactivation of a CIED, can originate with the patient, a family member or a health care provider who feels it should be considered based on their knowledge of the CIED's function. Some of these requests are made based on knowledge or the lack thereof. It is known that many patients and family members have not thought about or are not aware of the consequences of CIED device shocks associated with illnesses near the end of life [11]. Others have misconceptions of being kept artificially alive by CIED's [11].

Before any deactivation or removal is performed or non-replacement of a device is elected, the patient or surrogate must give consent. *Informed consent* is paramount and is at the very core of these discussions. As very clearly explained by Zellner et al. "Informed consent derives from the ethical principle of respect for persons; autonomy is maximized when patients understand the nature of their diagnoses and treatment options and participate in decisions about their care [12]. Informed consent is the most important legal doctrine in the clinician patient relationship. Clinicians are ethically and legally obligated to ensure that patients are informed and allowed to participate in decision making regarding their diagnoses and treatment options" [13, 14].

The elements of informed consent include information, patient voluntariness, and patient decision-making capacity. *Decision-making capacity* is a clinical term and refers to a patient's ability to make informed health care-related decisions. Clinicians determine decision-making capacity by whether a patient is able to:

1. Make and communicate choices.
2. Understand relevant information.
3. Appreciate the clinical situation and its consequences.
4. Manipulate information rationally.
5. Make a decision that is consistent with the patient's values and goals [14–16].

Because of these requirements, proof of decision making capacity can vary according to the complexity of the decision that has to be made; e.g., the graver the consequences of the decision, the greater the proof of decision-making capacity the clinician should require. Clinicians should not presume incapacity in patients who make clinical decisions contrary to the clinicians' recommendations [13, 14]. In contrast, *competence* is a legal term and is determined by courts [16]. In most situations it is acceptable to act on the physician's determination of capacity without formal legal declaration of incompetence" [14]. According to the July 2010 Heart Rhythm Society consensus document, a psychiatry consult is not necessary to determine capacity [9]. The physician determines that a patient is gravely ill and therefore not able to make an informed decision. Some of these capacity decisions can change as clinical conditions improve or deteriorate.

Most patients who have lost decision-making capacity due to illness have not been declared incompetent by the courts [9, 13]. With the loss of capacity, the decision making will fall to a surrogate. "For patients who lack decision-making capacity and those declared incompetent by a court, clinicians must rely on *surrogates* to make decisions. If the patient has an advance directive (AD) that identifies a surrogate, legally as well as ethically the patient's choice of surrogate must be respected [13].

In the absence of an AD, clinicians must identify the legally recognized appropriate surrogate. The ideal surrogate is one who best understands the patient's health care-related goals and preferences. In the United States, most states specify by law a hierarchy of surrogate decision-makers (e.g., spouse, followed by adult child, etc.). Clinicians should be aware of the definition of legal surrogate in their locality [17]. When making decisions, a surrogate should adhere to the instructions in the patient's AD (if one exists) and base decisions on the patient's (not the surrogate's) values and preferences if known (i.e., the "substituted judgment" standard) [18].

A corollary to informed consent is *informed refusal*. A patient has the right to refuse any treatment, even if the treatment prolongs life and death would follow a decision not to use it. A patient also has the right to refuse a previously consented treatment if the treatment no longer meets the patient's health care goals, specifically if those goals have changed (e.g., from prolonging life to minimizing discomforts), or if the perceived burdens of the ongoing treatment now outweigh the perceived benefits of that treatment (e.g., quality of life) [19–21]. Honoring these decisions is an integral part of patient-centered care. As described in the AMA Statement on end-of-life care, "[patients are entitled] to trustworthy assurances that preferences for withholding or withdrawing treatment will be honored" [13].

It may not be appreciated by clinicians that "If a clinician initiates or continues a treatment that a patient (or his/her surrogate) has refused, then ethically and legally the clinician is committing *battery*, regardless of the clinician's intent" [14, 15, 22, 23].

After a long discussion with his pastor (religious support), the spouse decides to abide by his wife's wishes and he asks the cardiologist to deactivate his wife's pacemaker. He gives him a written document stating so.

As per the newer 2010 HRS consensus statement, written consent by the patient or surrogate is not required for CIED deactivation [9]. The conversations and rationale for the actions to be undertaken however should be clearly documented by the health care practitioner in the patient's medical record.

Question #2. Is It Legal for the Health Care Provider to Deactivate the Pacemaker According to the Patient and Surrogate Wishes?

The legal precedents and ethical principles are clear on this issue. The patient has the right to refuse and request the withdrawal of CIED therapies regardless of whether he or she is terminally ill or not, and regardless of whether the therapies prolong life and hence death would follow as a consequence of a decision not to use them [13, 14].

Question #3. The Cardiologist Feels Deactivating the Pacemaker in This Pacemaker Dependent Patient Is Akin to "Pulling the Plug" and He Does Not Want to Be Part of Physician Assisted Suicide or Euthanasia. Is Deactivation in This Setting Physician Assisted Suicide (PAS) or Euthanasia?

This issue is very well presented by Zellner et al. [12] in their response to an article in Circulation under the Controversies in Arrhythmia and Electrophysiology by Kay and Bittner and also addressed in the 2010 HRS consensus statement: [9] "Clinicians may be concerned that withdrawing life-sustaining treatments such as CIED therapies amounts to assisted suicide or euthanasia. However, two factors differentiate withdrawal of an unwanted therapy from assisted suicide and euthanasia: the intent of the clinician, and the cause of death." First, in withdrawing an unwanted therapy, the clinician's intent is not to hasten the patient's death, but rather, to remove a treatment that is perceived by the patient as a burden [9, 12]. In contrast, in assisted suicide, the patient intentionally terminates his/her own life using a lethal method provided or prescribed by a clinician. In euthanasia, the physician intentionally terminates the patient's life (e.g. lethal injection). Second, in assisted suicide and euthanasia, the cause of death is the intervention provided, prescribed, or administered by the clinician. In contrast, when a patient dies after a treatment is refused or withdrawn, the cause of death is the underlying disease [12]. United States Supreme Court decisions have made a clear distinction between withholding or withdrawing life-sustaining treatments, and assisted suicide or euthanasia" [24]. The Court ruled that all patients have a constitutional right to refuse treatment, but no one has a constitutional right to assisted suicide or euthanasia. In another case, the Court ruled that "clinicians can legally (and should, from an ethical perspective) provide patients with whatever treatments are needed to alleviate suffering (such as morphine) even if the treatments might hasten death. Criminality is determined by the clinician's intent" [9, 25]. This is a very passionate subject with an extensive body of philosophical literature addressing these issues. For those who want to research this further they can refer to the work of Sulmasy [26].

On a personal level many physicians have not totally come to terms with the philosophical aspects of this issue. This is especially true with regards to the legal aspects of deactivating a pacemaker in a pacemaker dependent patient. A number of surveys have been published in the medical literature expressing the attitudes of physicians of various specialties and subspecialties towards this issue. Over the past decade the comfort level in making these decisions has increased and the associated anxiety has decreased [27, 28].

Question #4. Is the Health Care Provider Obligated to Carry Out the Patient's Wishes?

If a healthcare provider is not able to perform the requested deactivation function, he or she has the right to refuse, but the patient cannot be abandoned and the patient should be referred to a provider who feels comfortable carrying out the wishes of the patient. These wishes are supported by the laws of the United States as discussed above. Even if a patient is not terminally ill, device deactivation can be justified based on the perceived balance of the benefits vs. burdens of such device therapy [12].

Question #5. Is This Clinical Scenario Preventable?

In unexpected situations where undesired ICD shocks are delivered, emergency deactivation can occur. However, situations of surrogates struggling with making a determination or carrying out the wishes of the patient can be prevented by doctor-patient interactions before an illness becomes serious. As stated by Lewis et al. [29], "the time has come to teach and understand" even though two excellent guideline consensus papers on the management of CIED in patients nearing end-of-life exist, there are still a significant number of patients that are dying with their devices active and who are experiencing significant discomfort [7, 29, 30]. The fact that many patients are dying with their ICD devices in an active mode is confirmed by Kramer and colleagues in a recent Circulation publication reporting new data on hospice utilization following cardioverter defibrillator implantation in the older patient population. This is based on data obtained from the National Cardiovascular Data Registry (NCDR) and the Medicare Hospice Data Base and is discussed in more detail below [31].

These CIED end-of-life issues and challenges can be potentially preventable in many cases by evaluating patients and dialoging with them well in advance. These discussions are likely to take place in the primary care doctor's office. As already discussed, there are an increasing number of primary prevention devices that are being implanted [6]. Most of the care that these uncomplicated patients receive is being performed by their primary care providers such as internists, family practitioners or nurse practitioners. These providers may not be knowledgeable as to how CIEDs function nor the technique for withdrawing therapy at the end of life. The issues associated with cardiac device withdrawal are usually not addressed at the CME conferences that they attend [32]. The bulk of this literature has appeared in either the electrophysiology or palliative care literature. In order for these efforts to be successful there has to be a team approach and a greater educational effort directed at all medical specialties, as they all will be coming into contact with a device patient at one point or another. There has to be a network where health care providers are able to consult with each other regardless of their specialty, that enables them to face issues associated with cardiac device withdrawal.

Another potential barrier that has made the teaching and the planning for end-of-life care including withdrawal of device therapy more difficult has been the increased mobility of the patient due to either health insurance plan coverage changes or socio-economic mobility. For example, families moving from one county to another or to different states in search of a better life. A dialogue started by one particular group of medical healthcare providers in terms of teaching and end-of-life planning may not be reinforced or carried out at all in a different facility.

Data on Current Knowledge, Clinical Practices and Perceptions

Patient Knowledge, Perception and Attitudes Towards ICD Withdrawal at End-of-Life

Most of the studies regarding this issue have been done in the form of interviews or surveys and involved a small number of patients. A small study of 54 patients from the United Kingdom by Rafael et al. [33] demonstrated that most patients were not aware that the ICD could be deactivated. Approximately 84% of the patients wanted to be involved in the deactivation decision of end-of-life issues. Forty percent of patients surveyed felt that this discussion should be held prior to ICD implantation while 16% felt it should be done while the patient was terminally ill and 5% felt it should be done in the last days of life. In another survey study from Prague, 109 patients completed 13 survey questions [34]. About 45% of patients stated that they had never considered ICD deactivation during near end-of-life situations. The topic had only been discussed with 7.3% of patients and 40% of patients wanted more information about ICD deactivation. However 41% of patients who had ICDs for secondary prevention and 22% of patients for primary prevention refused additional information or further discussion on the topic [34].

In a larger study from Sweden, published in PACE in 2014, Stromberg et al. surveyed 3067 patients [35]. The broad aim of the study was to correlate knowledge in relation to end-of-life issues and decisions. The instrument had three domains including experiences, attitudes and knowledge. The experience domain included ten items about patients' actual discussion experiences such as "I have discussed what a battery replacement involves with my ICD doctor or nurse". The answers were scored in a simple yes or no; can't understand, agree or don't agree format. The attitude domain included 18 items about "patient's attitudes toward potential future events." Example: "I want to have the battery in my ICD replaced even if I am seriously ill suffering from another disease". Or "I want to have the defibrillator shocks in my ICD even if dying of cancer or another serious disease". In the knowledge domain, they were presented with 11 statements concerning end-of-life issues as well as their knowledge of practical functions of the ICD. Only 3% of respondents scored correctly on all of the 11 knowledge questions. Approximately 29% of participants had insufficient knowledge. The authors conclude that insufficient knowledge was associated with indecisiveness in making decisions about ICD deactivation in end-of-life situations and in making decisions about replacing a defibrillator even if seriously ill or dying from a terminal illness [35].

In a more homogeneous study group from the Thoraxcenter Erasmus Medical Center Database in Rotterdam, Netherlands a total of 294 patients completed the survey out of the intended 440 [11]. They were divided into three groups based on the length of ICD therapy from recent implantations to implantation of more than 10 years. Sixty-eight percent of the patients were aware that it was possible to turn the ICD off and 95% of the patients believed that it was important to inform the patient about this possibility. Additionally, 84% of the patients indicated a choice for or against ICD deactivation. The authors concluded that the wish for a "worthy death" at the end-of-life was an independent predictor of a favorable attitude. During the studies the author noted that there was a trend for anxiety and suggested that physicians should take into account patient's anxiety levels when discussing the issue of deactivation [11].

The results of these studies highlight the lack of consensus among patients with implantable devices on the issues of device deactivation at the end of life. However, a large number of patients seem receptive to the idea of better understanding and having open discussions regarding the subject, therefore there is fertile ground for these discussions take place prior to the initial defibrillation implantation. The same can be said for the completion and filing out of an advanced directive (AD). A study from the Mayo Clinic in 2012 showed that about one third of patients in their studies had an advanced directive but only two patients specifically mentioned the ICD in the AD [36]. The conclusion from this paper is that patients should be encouraged to have an advanced directive, which should be updated if done prior to ICD implantation and they should be very clear their desire of deactivation of the ICD or the pacemaker in order to avoid any ethical dilemmas. Clinicians tend to prefer treatment specific statements as opposed to general statements regarding life-sustaining treatments. Is important to emphasize that the thrust of this discussion is not to promote device deactivation or withdrawal of device therapy as a goal of care but to support the patient's decision to have control over his medical treatment and to do it in such a way that allows patients and their families to have an honorable and peaceful death.

Patient opinions regarding who has the responsibility for discussing device deactivation or advanced directives with them were also varied and lacked consensus. In a study from the University of Pennsylvania, Kirkpatrick et al. reported that 35% of responders said the electrophysiologist should discuss the AD; 45% said it should be the general cardiologist and 14% said the primary care physician [37]. Ideally, the physician who has the greatest rapport with the patient should be the one approaching the issue early in the implantation process with support from the cardiologist or electrophysiologist if necessary. Even though a primary care provider may not be able to go into an in depth discussion of the technical aspects or logistics of cardiac device deactivation, they can approach the subject of the goals of care towards the end of life in the same manner that a Do Not Resuscitate (DNR) order is obtained. Even though there is a DNR order in place, a number of these CIED patients do not have their devices deactivated prior to death. The reasons are multi-factorial and can include a simple oversight of the existence of an ICD by the care team. Surprisingly, a significant number of ICD patients that qualify for hospice care do not even have DNR orders towards the end-of-life [31]. The reality is, that most of these discussions do not occur at the time of implant and goals of care change over time. Thus, these discussions require updates to assure that therapies are consistent with treatment goals in the near and long term. Continued educational efforts at every level are paramount and we cannot make assumptions that CIED patients know or have retained information on basic ICD functioning. As discussed earlier [35] lack of device function knowledge could be associated with inability to make some critical end-of-life decisions.

To date, there has been no demonstrated ownership of this issue by any particular specialty. This educational process can take place through cooperation with other specialties, physicians can reach out to each other and consult each other permitting the patient to access to the most accurate information.

There are pamphlets with educational information from medical specialty societies such as the Heart Rhythm Society addressing this issue for patients and their care givers [38]. They discuss the purpose of cardiac devices and options that are available to deactivate an ICD or pacemaker. These pamphlets can be given to patients at the time of their device discharge teaching as part of their discharge packet. It goes without saying that there has to be an introductory discussion otherwise the booklet becomes another "dust catcher" or "trash" as it is the fate of many educational brochures. It should also be available in the device clinics to educate patients and caregivers at all times during their device evaluations. New patients to the device clinic from other geographic areas who have not had any education on this subject should also be exposed. This educational tool can serve as a link for approaching what can be a difficult subject for some medical providers, patients and families. Table 15.1 adapted from the 2010 HRS consensus statement contains useful ideas that we feel can be incorporated in a teaching/planning strategy [9].

Table 15.1 Communicating with patients and families about goals of care relating to CIEDs

1.	Determine what patients/families know about their illness
2.	Determine what patients/families know about the role the device plays in their health both now and in the future
3.	Determine what additional information patients/families want to know about their illness
4.	Correct or clarify any misunderstandings about the current illness and possible outcomes, including the role of the device
5.	Determine the patient/family's overall goals of care and desired outcomes
6.	Using the stated goals as a guide, work to tailor treatments, and in this case, management of the cardiac device in conformity to these goals

Adapted from HRS Expert Consensus Statement [9]

Clinicians' Knowledge, Perception and Attitudes Towards ICD Withdrawal at End-of-Life

There is limited data evaluating the perception, opinions or perspectives of healthcare providers with regards to withdrawal or withholding of device therapy or dealing with these issues at end-of-life. What can be said in reviewing the literature is that some of these opinions and perspectives have changed significantly over the last decade. Farber et al. in 2006 surveyed 1000 internist and internal medicine subspecialists about their views on withholding or withdrawing life-sustaining treatment [28]. Only 41% of those surveyed responded. The survey included 32 hypothetical cases where 51% of responders were willing to withhold or withdraw treatment in all of the 32 hypothetical scenarios. Respondents were less likely to withhold or withdraw treatments in patients who were not terminally ill. The authors noted that 49% of respondents would be unwilling to withhold or withdraw treatment in at least one scenario. This is in contrast to the results of a study from the Mayo Clinic from 2010 where 658 medical and legal professionals were surveyed, (that survey also included patients) [39]. In this study there was almost complete consensus among legal professionals, medical professionals and patients that if a terminally ill patient requested that his or her ICD be turned off that they would agree. The opinions began to differ when it came to turning off a pacemaker in a pacemaker dependent patient. In this case, 81% of legal professionals compared to 58% of medical professionals agreed with turning off the pacemaker in a pacemaker dependent patient. Medical professionals were more likely to perceive turning off an ICD as being legal compared to turning off a pacemaker (85 vs. 41% $P < 0.001$) [39].

Even though there have been significant educational and philosophical discussions over the years regarding this issue in the medical literature, healthcare providers continue to struggle in coming to terms with some of these decisions. It is clearly easier for legal professionals to see pacemakers and defibrillators as similar and to accept readily withdrawal or withholding medical therapies even in non-critically ill patients. Obviously, they have a comfort level that most physicians will probably never achieve. This is highlighted in a recent online survey conducted by physicians from the University of Pennsylvania and New York University Langone Medical Center [27]. Email surveys were sent out to 1894 electrophysiology practitioners. Out of these 384 responses were collected. The sample included respondents from Europe, Asia, Australia, South America and Africa but the majority were from North America (78%). The electrophysiologists surveyed felt that deactivation of the ICD shocking function in agreement with patient wishes and a pre-existing DNR order would not be considered physician-assisted suicide (93.2%). Surprisingly, however, only 77.1% felt that it was not ethical/moral for doctors to deactivate ICD *against* patients' or family/surrogates' wishes. The international sample of responders considered ICD and pacemaker deactivation to be ethically distinct. Cardiac pacemakers were considered to be like dialysis therapy that keep these patients alive [27]. These views as mentioned above are different compared to legal professionals.

These views or opinions are influenced by a number of factors including prior experiences, social up-bringing, religion as well as other unknown variables. In a recent survey published in the Journal Religious Health, physician religiosity was associated with finding withdrawal more ethically problematic, but not finding it more psychologically difficult [40]. The authors concluded that most United States physicians find withdrawing life-sustaining therapies not only more psychologically difficult but more ethically problematic than withholding such treatment.

Framework or Strategies to Guide Providers in the Withdrawal of Device Therapies

As background to this section, the legal, ethical and religious principles surrounding withdrawal of cardiac device therapies have been discussed. The perceptions of patients as well as healthcare providers that are available in the medical literature were reviewed. It is now important to develop a framework for providers to engage patients in identifying goals of care and execute strategies for CIED therapy withdrawal if appropriate. Withdrawal of cardiac device therapy can be requested at any time by patients or caregivers. The most familiar scenario is that associated with the potential of frequent painful shocks toward the end-of-life especially in the setting of a terminal illness. Goldstein et al. reported that 20% of patients can receive painful shocks which can decrease the quality of life during the last days or weeks of their lives [7].

Other authors have reported that up to 31% of patients received shocks in the last 24 h of life [30]. In a MADIT-II trial Substudy, Sherazi et al. reported similar findings [41]. Lewis et al. confirmed this, but in addition they demonstrated that a strategy that minimizes pain and suffering at end-of-life can be implemented [29]. This was a retrospective study that reviewed the charts of 90 patients who died between 1994 and 2004. Sixty-three patients were included. Group 1 (20) were patients whose defibrillator was turned off through a comprehensive comfort care approach. Group 2 (43) included patients whose clinical course was so rapid that the defibrillator could not be turned off before their illness arose. As the pacing function was not withdrawn in either group, important information regarding pacing at the end-of-life was not addressed in this study. The patients in Group 1 had chronic illnesses that were identified from a medical history obtained during their visits to the clinic. Ideally, the goals of care would be to avoid painful or inappropriate shocks towards the end-of-life. In this study even with careful planning patients in Group 1 received shocks but significantly less than those in Group 2 [29]. The timing of a compassionate care strategy can be difficult because shock therapy needs to be available to patients up until death from the terminal illness is imminent. In Group 1, the actual time between the device being turned off and death was short at 49 +/−89 days [29]. Adopting a compassionate strategy as discussed above can potentially alleviate stressful end-of-life situations for healthcare providers, patients and their loved ones.

Ten years after the above paper was written, the demographics are much different. The number of primary prevention ICDs in elderly patients with chronic illness has increased dramatically, with over 50,000 devices being inserted annually in patients over the age of 65 [42]. The recent study by Kramer et al. is the only study to date to evaluate hospice care in ICD patients over 65 years of age [31]. Only patients that were matched to the Medicare database were included. Probabilistic matching to the Medicare data yielded the final analytic cohort of 194,969 patients. The results showed that 11.5% of patients were enrolled in hospice during the 5 year follow-up period. For those patients that were enrolled in hospice, the median time from ICD implantation to hospice enrollment was 1.3 years. A total of 36.8% of decedents received hospice services. The data presented above according to the authors "underscores the need for hospital hospice providers to prepare to care for dying ICD patients including establishing protocols for turning off such devices and avoiding shocks at end-of-life" [31]. This includes simple measures such as having a doughnut magnet that when applied over the defibrillator site can inhibit shocking therapies from the defibrillator as long as the magnet is in contact with the skin or thin clothing over the device. Once the magnet is removed ICD function can resume as was initially programmed (Fig. 15.1). This problem is further compounded by the fact that 5 years post implantation 51% of the older ICD patients were either dead or in a hospice and thus calls for a greater understanding of the broader palliative care needs of the older ICD patients and how to improve strategies to deliver that care. Even though the emphasis of this chapter is on withdrawing cardiac device

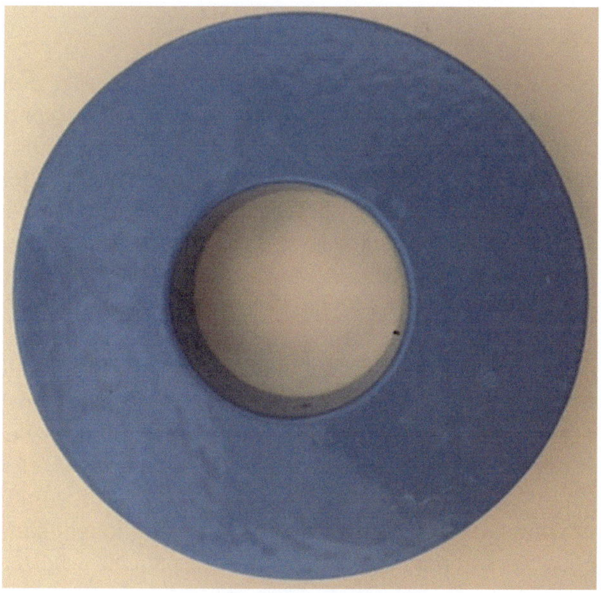

Fig. 15.1 A "doughnut" magnet used to disable therapies from an implantable defibrillator. This magnet is placed directly over the ICD to stop unwanted ICD shocks

therapy, in our opinion the hospice data presented above highlights the importance of appropriate patient selection for ICD therapy while refraining from offering it to very high risk patients, whose prognosis from other comorbid conditions tips the scale of the potential risk/benefit ratio [43].

The appropriate selection criteria for patients who will benefit the most from a primary prevention ICD has eluded electrophysiologists for years. This area is very fertile for future research especially when it comes to elderly patients with multiple comorbidities. In the data presented by Kramer and Associates, some of the factors that were most strongly associated with shorter time to hospice enrollment where older age, Class IV heart failure, and ejection fraction less than 20% [31]. If we had a better way of risk stratifying these patients who will be entering hospice soon after their device implantation perhaps these withdrawal issues could be minimized. As reviewed earlier it is easier for physicians to accept withholding device therapies than withdrawing and the decision could be made even easier with more guideline appropriate data [27, 37, 39]. With better patient selection, the problem of withholding therapies would not completely resolve but could potentially be decreased. In the current literature, there are a number of already published clinical variables that can help identify potentially high risk patients for death not preventable by an ICD. Perhaps an algorithm can be developed to help manage this clinical issue. Updating recommendations to the device therapy guidelines based on current or new data seems like a good place to start.

Conclusion

As discussed above the pain from an implantable cardioverter defibrillator ICD shock during the terminal phase of an illness or the anxiety of potentially receiving such a shock can be contrary to the goal of dying a peaceful death in comfort and dignity. When a patient with an ICD develops a new diagnosis of a terminal illness, the options of disabling defibrillator therapies should be included in the broader discussion of end-of-life care much like a do not resuscitate status is discussed. Over the years physicians have become more comfortable with obtaining a "code status" i.e. DNR status in patients who have chronic terminal illnesses. Discussions regarding deactivation of ICDs or turning off pacemakers could achieve the same level. Patients with these implantable devices should be encouraged to complete an advanced directive in which they should specify their decisions regarding the device. Educating patients about the many options available would aid patients in making these decisions. Early education and conversations at the time of referral for device implantation can make end of life transition more focused on comfort and not on frantically attempting to stop undesired shocks. Careful thought and consideration should be given when offering device therapies to patients who have competing risks and who will have minimal benefit from preventing an arrhythmic death. It is important to remember that according to current device therapy guidelines implantation in those whose potential survival is less than a year is considered a class III indication.

It is our hope that the information provided in this chapter will help to educate and support healthcare providers, in making these challenging and emotionally draining decisions.

References

1. The Antiarrhythmics Versus Implantable Defibrillators (AVID) Investigators. A comparison of antiarrhythmic-drug therapy with implantable defibrillators in patients resuscitated from near-fatal ventricular arrhythmias. N Engl J Med. 1997a;337:1576–83.
2. Bokhari F, Newman D, Greene M, Korley V, Mangat I, Dorian P. Long-term comparison of the implantable cardioverter defibrillator versus amiodarone: eleven-year follow-up of a subset of patients in the Canadian Implantable Defibrillator Study (CIDS). Circulation. 2004;110: 112–6.
3. Goldenberg I, Gillespie J, Moss AJ, Hall WJ, Klein H, McNitt S, Brown MW, Cygankiewicz I, Zareba W, Executive Committee of the Multicenter Automatic Defibrillator Implantation Trail II. Long-term benefit of primary prevention with an implantable cardioverter-defibrillator: an extended 8-year follow-up study of the Multicenter Automatic Defibrillator Implantation Trial II. Circulation. 2010;122:1265–71.
4. Wever EF, Hauer RN, van Capelle FL, Tijssen JG, Crijns HJ, Algra A, Wiesfeld AC, Bakker PF, Robles de Medina EO. Randomized study of implantable defibrillator as first-choice therapy versus conventional strategy in postinfarct sudden death survivors. Circulation. 1995;91:2195–203.
5. Bristow MR, Saxon LA, Boehmer J, Krueger S, Kass DA, de Marco T, Carson P, Dicarlo L, Demets D, White BG, Devries DW, Feldman AM, Comparison of Medical Therapy, Pacing, and Defibrillation in Heart Failure Investigators. Cardiac-resynchronization therapy with or without an implantable defibrillator in advanced chronic heart failure. N Engl J Med. 2004;350:2140–50.
6. Kurtz SM, Ochoa JA, Lau E, Shkolnikov Y, Pavri BB, Frisch D, Greenspon AJ. Implantation trends and patient profiles for pacemakers and implantable cardioverter defibrillators in the United States: 1993–2006. Pacing Clin Electrophysiol. 2010;33:705–11.
7. Goldstein NE, Lampert R, Bradley E, Lynn J, Krumholz HM. Management of implantable cardioverter defibrillators in end of life care. Ann Intern Med. 2004;141:835–8.
8. Epstein AE, Dimarco JP, Ellenbogen KA, Estes NA III, Freedman RA, Gettes LS, Gillinov AM, Gregoratos G, Hammill SC, Hayes DL, Hlatky MA, Newby LK, Page RL, Schoenfeld MH, Silka MJ, Stevenson LW, Sweeney MO, American College of Cardiology, American Heart Association Task Force on Practice Guidelines, American Association for Thoracic Surgery, Society of Thoracic Surgeons. ACC/AHA/HRS 2008 guidelines for device-based therapy of cardiac rhythm abnormalities. Heart Rhythm. 2008;5:e1–62.
9. Lampert R, Hayes DL, Annas GJ, Farley MA, Goldstein NE, Hamilton RM, Kay GN, Kramer DB, Mueller PS, Padeletti L, Pozuelo L, Schoenfeld MH, Vardas PE, Wiegand DL, Zellner R, American College of Cardiology, American Geriatrics Society, American Academy of Hospice and Palliative Medicine, American Heart Association, European Heart Rhythm Association, Hospice and Palliative Nurses Association. HRS Expert Consensus Statement on the management of cardiovascular implantable electronic devices (CIEDs) in patients nearing end of life or requesting withdrawal of therapy. Heart Rhythm. 2010;7:1008–26.
10. Padeletti L, Arnar DO, Boncinelli L, Brachman J, Camm JA, Daubert JC, Hassam SK, Deliens L, Glikson M, Hayes D, Israel C, Lampert R, Lobban T, Raatikainen P, Siegal G, Vardas P, Reviewers: Kirchhof P, Becker R, Cosio F, Loh P, Cobbe S, Grace A, Morgan J, European

Heart Rhythm Association and Heart Rhythm Society. EHRA Expert Consensus Statement on the management of cardiovascular implantable electronic devices in patients nearing end of life or requesting withdrawal of therapy. Europace. 2010;12:1480–9.

11. Pedersen SS, Chaitsing R, Szili-Torok T, Jordaens L, Theuns DA. Patients' perspective on deactivation of the implantable cardioverter-defibrillator near the end of life. Am J Cardiol. 2013;111:1443–7.
12. Zellner RA, Aulisio MP, Lewis WR. Should implantable cardioverter-defibrillators and permanent pacemakers in patients with terminal illness be deactivated? Deactivating permanent pacemaker in patients with terminalillness. Patient autonomy is paramount. Circ Arrhythm Electrophysiol. 2009;2:340–4; discussion 340.
13. American Medical Association, Council on Ethical and Judicial Affairs. AMA code of medical ethics: current opinions and annotations. Chicago, IL: AMA Press; 2010.
14. Snyder L, Leffler C. Ethics manual fifth edition. Ann Intern Med. 2005;142:560–82.
15. Annas GJ. The rights of patients, third edition: the authoritative ACLU guide to patient rights. Carbondale, IL: Southern Illinois University Press; 2004.
16. Ganzini L, Volicer L, Nelson WA, Fox E, Derse AR. Ten myths about decision-making capacity. J Am Med Dir Assoc. 2004;5:263–7.
17. Menikoff JA, Sachs GA, Siegler M. Beyond advance directives—health care surrogate laws. N Engl J Med. 1992;327:1165–9.
18. Cantor NL. Twenty-five years after Quinlan: a review of the jurisprudence of death and dying. J Law Med Ethics. 2001;29:182–96.
19. Annas GJ. "Culture of life" politics at the bedside—the case of Terri Schiavo. N Engl J Med. 2005;352:1710–5.
20. Hook CC, Mueller PS. The Terri Schiavo saga: the making of a tragedy and lessons learned. Mayo Clin Proc. 2005;80:1449–60.
21. Wiegand DL, Kalowes PG. Withdrawal of cardiac medications and devices. AACN Adv Crit Care. 2007;18:415–25.
22. New York Court of Appeals. Schloendorff v. Society of New York Hospital. *Northeastern Reporter*. New York: New York Court of Appeals; 1914.
23. United States Court of Appeals for the District of Columbia Circuit. Canterbury v. Spence. *F.2d*. Washington, DC: United States Court of Appeals for the District of Columbia Circuit; 1972.
24. Meisel A, Snyder L, Quill T, American College of Physicians–American Society of Internal Medicine End-of-Life Care Consensus Panel. Seven legal barriers to end-of-life care: myths, realities, and grains of truth. JAMA. 2000;284:2495–501.
25. Supreme Court of the United States. Washington v. Glucksberg. Washington, DC: Supreme Court of the United States; 1997b.
26. Sulmasy DP. Within you/without you: biotechnology, ontology, and ethics. J Gen Intern Med. 2008;23(Suppl 1):69–72.
27. Daeschler M, Verdino RJ, Caplan AL, Kirkpatrick JN. Defibrillator deactivation against a patient's wishes: perspectives of electrophysiology practitioners. Pacing Clin Electrophysiol. 2015;38:917–24.
28. Farber NJ, Simpson P, Salam T, Collier VU, Weiner J, Boyer EG. Physicians' decisions to withhold and withdraw life-sustaining treatment. Arch Intern Med. 2006;166:560–4.
29. Lewis WR, Luebke DL, Johnson NJ, Harrington MD, Costantini O, Aulisio MP. Withdrawing implantable defibrillator shock therapy in terminally ill patients. Am J Med. 2006;119:892–6.
30. Kinch Westerdahl A, Sjoblom J, Mattiasson AC, Rosenqvist M, Frykman V. Implantable cardioverter-defibrillator therapy before death: high risk for painful shocks at end of life. Circulation. 2014;129:422–9.
31. Kramer DB, Reynolds MR, Normand SL, Parzynski CS, Spertus JA, Mor V, Mitchell SL. Hospice use following implantable cardioverter-defibrillator implantation in older patients: results from the NCDR(R). Circulation. 2016;133(21):2030–7.
32. Sherazi S, Daubert JP, Block RC, Jeevanantham V, Abdel-Gadir K, Disalle MR, Haley JM, Shah AH. Physicians' preferences and attitudes about end-of-life care in patients with an implantable cardioverter-defibrillator. Mayo Clin Proc. 2008;83:1139–41.

33. Raphael CE, Koa-Wing M, Stain N, Wright I, Francis DP, Kanagaratnam P. Implantable cardioverter-defibrillator recipient attitudes towards device deactivation: how much do patients want to know? Pacing Clin Electrophysiol. 2011;34:1628–33.
34. Herman D, Stros P, Curila K, Kebza V, Osmancik P. Deactivation of implantable cardioverter-defibrillators: results of patient surveys. Europace. 2013;15:963–9.
35. Stromberg A, Fluur C, Miller J, Chung ML, Moser DK, Thylen I. ICD recipients' understanding of ethical issues, ICD function, and practical consequences of withdrawing the ICD in the end-of-life. Pacing Clin Electrophysiol. 2014;37:834–42.
36. Tajouri TH, Ottenberg AL, Hayes DL, Mueller PS. The use of advance directives among patients with implantable cardioverter defibrillators. Pacing Clin Electrophysiol. 2012;35: 567–73.
37. Kirkpatrick JN, Gottlieb M, Sehgal P, Patel R, Verdino RJ. Deactivation of implantable cardioverter defibrillators in terminal illness and end of life care. Am J Cardiol. 2012;109:91–4.
38. Heart Rhythm Society. End of life and heart rhythm devices [Online]. 2014. http://www.hrsonline.org/Patient-Resources/Patient-Information-Sheets. Accessed 21 Apr 2016.
39. Kapa S, Mueller PS, Hayes DL, Asirvatham SJ. Perspectives on withdrawing pacemaker and implantable cardioverter-defibrillator therapies at end of life: results of a survey of medical and legal professionals and patients. Mayo Clin Proc. 2010;85:981–90.
40. Chung GS, Yoon JD, Rasinski KA, Curlin FA. US physicians' opinions about distinctions between withdrawing and withholding life-sustaining treatment. J Relig Health. 2016;55(5): 1596–606.
41. Sherazi S, McNitt S, Aktas MK, Polonsky B, Shah AH, Moss AJ, Daubert JP, Zareba W. End-of-life care in patients with implantable cardioverter defibrillators: a MADIT-II substudy. Pacing Clin Electrophysiol. 2013;36:1273–9.
42. Epstein AE, Kay GN, Plumb VJ, McElderry HT, Doppalapudi H, Yamada T, Shafiroff J, Syed ZA, Shkurovich S, Investigators ACT. Implantable cardioverter-defibrillator prescription in the elderly. Heart Rhythm. 2009;6:1136–43.
43. Barsheshet A, Moss AJ, Huang DT, McNitt S, Zareba W, Goldenberg I. Applicability of a risk score for prediction of the long-term (8-year) benefit of the implantable cardioverter-defibrillator. J Am Coll Cardiol. 2012;59:2075–9.

Chapter 16
Natural Kinds, Similarity, and Individual Cases: Ontological Presuppositions and Ethical Implications

Paolo Valore

Abstract The ethical implications of medical research and clinical practice are addressed by (a) questioning the ontological presuppositions of such notions as *kinds* and *similarity*, both object-to-object and object-to-category; (b) applying this strategy to the particular case of medicine and biomedical science, with a focus on the notion of *kinds of patients*; and (c) suggesting a way for researchers and clinicians to take advantage of the ontological perspective, connecting creative approaches to responsible, ethical choices.

Keywords Ontology • Natural kinds • Kinds of patients • Conceptual relativity • Medical ethics

The rapidly changing technology in invasive cardiology, and in particular in cardiovascular intervention and cardiac devices implantation, encouraged a wide spectrum of reflections: epistemological, methodological, social and economical. In addition, an evaluation of the ethical implications of this practice seems more and more urgent and, together with the general codes for medical ethics and responsible conduct of research, the best analyses available so far, despite their high quality, are indeed sporadic [5, 6, 8, 15, 31]. Leaving aside important advice on issues such as informed consent, conflicts of interest and professional self-regulation, the typical approach has obviously been the recommendation of the welfare of the patients and this is surely always advisable since it is, incidentally, not only a minimum requirement of any medical ethics but also the very goal of the whole medical enterprise. Here I would like to suggest a slightly more technical approach to the ethical implications of cardiovascular practice and research: one conducted from the point of view of an ontological, *prima facie* unrelated question.

My starting point will be the standard and good practice in taking the correct stand when facing a new case, which fundamentally relies on the acknowledgment

P. Valore, Ph.D.
Department of Philosophy, University of Milan, Via Festa del Perdono 7, Milan 20122, Italy
e-mail: paolo.valore@unimi.it

© Springer International Publishing AG 2017
R. Proietti et al. (eds.), *Psychological, Emotional, Social and Cognitive Aspects of Implantable Cardiac Devices*, DOI 10.1007/978-3-319-55721-2_16

of the individual case as an exemplification of a typical kind of patient and/or clinical situation, questioning its philosophical implications. A typical example, among several possible ones, is the evaluation of the optimal assessment of long-term dual antiplatelet therapy following a percutaneous coronary intervention with an implantation of stent: we work with general cases built, basically, on the statistical frameworks resulting from the randomized controlled trials of the different models of medical devices appearing on the market. Overlooking the obvious and irrelevant differences, we focus on the similarities among individuals to build the general cases that will be the guide for our future practice (object-to-object similarity). Taking advantage of these general cases, we associate singular individuals with common kinds of patients, to which they are similar (object-to-category similarity). In general, any field of medical research and clinical practice presupposes a division of syndromes, organisms and events into *categories*, identified with *natural kinds* [4]. On closer inspection, the very concept of "disease" results from the selective act of grouping different events, selected from a composite background and gathered for the sake of our intervention, overlooking their obvious particular differences to focus on their similarity.

The complication with the previous picture is that, in contemporary formal ontology and in the analysis of theoretical knowledge embedded in human representation of categories, it is widely assumed that, while playing a crucial role in our capability in extending limited samples to general paradigms of "typical cases", the notions of "kind" and "similarity" are concepts worthy of further philosophical and scientific *clarification*, if not utterly puzzling.

I will firstly recap the problems with the notions of "similarity" and "kind" with reference to contemporary research in ontology and conceptual analysis. Secondly, I will suggest that these problems affect medical research and clinical practice as well, taking the notion of "kinds of patients" as a case study. Lastly, I will suggest a way to gain a better understanding of the question which would allow researchers in cardiology to take advantage of an ontological result, taking in consideration also the medical practice and its ethical implications.

The Hidden Dangers of Taxonomies Based on Similarities

The awareness that the very idea of "having something in common" might be logically elusive can be traced back to Kant [14], Husserl [35] and classical American Pragmatism [13], but such awareness has more recently gained renewed attention in the development of ontology as a formal discipline.

We know that, given a plurality of individuals, there are many ways of classifying them in classes according to their similarities, grouping them by color, size, distance from a given point, and so on. Let's consider the set of individuals $I = \{a, b, \ldots, n\}$ and the set of predicates $P = \{P_1, P_2, \ldots, P_n\}$ such that we can assign to any member of I any member of P or its negation (in the easiest case in which properties do not come in degrees). For instance, we can build the subset S_1 such that all elements of

S_1 are the elements of I for which the property expressed by the predicate P_1 holds, and the subset S_2 such that all elements of S_2 are the elements of I for which the property expressed by the predicate P_2 holds, and so on. Clearly, these subsets of I may or may not overlap, partially or completely. Consequently, we can define two or more individuals "similar" if they share the same property. Let's call this similarity among individuals "object-to-object similarity" or OTO similarity. In particular, we can define all the elements of S_i "similar according to the property P_i", since the property P_i holds for all of them. The last clarification displays that the very idea of OTO similarity requires the choice of a property that selects the intended way to generate the subset.

However, this strategy works in theory only. Complications arise when we consider that the individuals we need to classify do not come with a list of preferred properties for the sake of our conceptual work and that, at least theoretically, all the choices are of equal value. Everything is, in fact, "similar" to everything else in *some* respect [34]. We could try to ground OTO similarity on the sharing of properties, through a comparison such as "*a* is more similar to *b* than *c*" if *a* and *b* jointly belong to more sets than *a* and *c*. Properties can indeed be defined on such terms, but since sets are generated by the exhaustion of combinations, the number of sets to which any two elements jointly belong isn't determined by the features shown by those elements, i.e. their similarity, but rather by the total quantity of elements [26]. Any number of things are jointly members of any number of sets; therefore, given a domain of individuals, any coherent classificatory principle determines a set of things but this cannot be the OTO similarity we are looking for, in order to grasp (or generate) general kinds [2, 4, 7]. We should be able to identify *significant sets* and, for this purpose, we need a criterion to make the *right* choice.

There might be choices that we consider unwanted or unfitting, but, clearly, we need first to set our aims and the context, according to which we build our sense of what is appropriate or fitting—that is, we need a generating principle that we can trust in producing the correct, or suitable, grouping for our aims. The big problem being, at this point, that aims are chosen from an evaluative perspective, which spins data in a certain direction with reference to a preferred perspective among the many possible.

If on the one hand it seems puzzling to find a red thread that guides us among the different ways of grouping a variety of objects of a given domain in absence of an a priori strategy of intended relevant properties and a hierarchy of preferences, on the other hand we expect it to be easier to find the right association between a new case and one of the kinds once the correct grouping is given. Unfortunately, if we are not able to specify the strategy of the intended relevant properties and the hierarchy of preferences, the empirical data themselves do not help us do the job. The grouping, even when correct, does not come with a label specifying the reason why the individuals are gathered. In this case, we need to specify an object-to-category (OTC) similarity that allows us to choose among several properties of a given object in order to match it to the right category.

It should be clear that, when we take in consideration proprieties that come in degrees, and the greatest part of our properties do, the complications ramify exponentially and the interference among alternative ordering strategies requires further decisions in giving sense to the data under investigation. Therefore, the previous arguments apply here once again, multiplied in levels.

The philosophical worry about the notion of OTO similarity in generating categories and OTC similarity in associating an individual to the proper category seems reinforced by experimental psychology. With reference to saliency parameters, empirical results confirm that participants in experiments in categorization and similarity rating produce different patterns of classification guided by theoretical assumptions about the properties they handle, and shows that the configuration of features plays a crucial role in category classification [1, 27].

A first conclusion might be that we should be suspicious of the very idea of a *single* taxonomy of kinds or of a unique correct grouping of individuals established independently of any consideration about what should count as a *relevant* or *perspicuous* property [17]. "Relevant" and "perspicuous" are pragmatic and evaluative qualities. If we are suspicious of any pragmatic and evaluative injection in our science, we may conclude that the very notion of similarity and kind are to be dispensed with and even that "we can take it as a very special mark of the maturity of a branch of science that it no longer needs an irreducible notion of the similarity and kind" [26]. Nevertheless, this conclusion is far from being mandatory. If we are justified in mistrusting the necessity of any particular structure of ideal types based on similarity, it does not follow that our ontology can do without a scheme or hierarchical taxonomy. Some strategy for ordering in perspicuous kinds seems in need, even though this might take us to determine the ordering case by case, according to our theoretical concerns and evaluating the consequences of each choice, taking in consideration out field of interest and the ethical dimension of our aims. In this case, we speak in terms of "conceptual schemes" or "categorial frameworks" as the guiding background of our grouping options, which determine the acknowledgment of a certain structure of kinds instead of another [34].

How These Problems Affect Clinical Research and Practice

The notion of kind is involved in at least two concepts central to the healthcare disciplines: namely, "disease" and "kinds of patients". While the concept of "disease" seems more epistemologically characterized and the ontology of disease has been scrutinized from researchers working in philosophy of science in general and philosophy of medicine in particular [9, 12, 18, 28, 32, 33], the concept of "kinds of patients" seems more ontologically elusive and not yet adequately examined. The reason is that we may well debate if there is (if it literally *exists*) a thing called "disease" or if it is merely a fiction we build in order to give our various, different data a more functional manageability. We may well debate if there is a cultural, social and historical aspect to what counts as disease. However, there is surely no need to philosophically debate the trivial fact that clinicians do *not* treat kinds of patients but singular individual patients. Therefore, I prefer to focus on the notion of "kinds of patients" as the most challenging and disturbingly fragile version of natural kinds requested by medical research and clinical practice.

The idea of "kinds of patients" suggests that individuals behave in a similar way, given the same conditions, since they exhibit the same "nature" or "disposition" or "essence" [3, 4, 10, 16, 19, 20, 23], which we identify with an ideal entity that is our real object of study. In the research phase, such an idea is gained through an act of empirical abstraction, with a rather thin inductive base and a thick metaphysical assumption: we observe a (relatively small) amount of individuals in randomized controlled trials, looking for what the individuals share, with the aim of grasping the universal kind they exhibit (OTO similarity). In the practice phase, clinicians need to determine whether the individual cases exemplify one or another kind of patient that shall benefit from specified medical or surgical treatments and procedures (OTC similarity) [11].

These ideal kinds may be either *stipulated* (a) or *real* (b).

(a) If they are fictitious models stipulated in order to give sense to experimental data, they may work with the conjectural research or the theoretical assessment of trial outcomes but are out of place with reference to clinical practice. The latter interacts exclusively with actual individual patients and not abstract models and the ethical responsibility in this applicative phase is too high to ignore the elusiveness of our conceptual tools. A fictitious model clearly cannot do the job.

(b) Apparently, when medicine and biomedical science are concerned, we are interested in *real* kinds, rather than in kinds resulting from acts of grouping built artificially on the interests and decisions of human beings. Or, paradoxically, our particular interest in this case is the discovery of taxonomies and classifications that correspond to *real* kinds *in nature* and not our particular interests and decisions [4, 30]. Therefore, a simple reply to the previous concerns could be that some similarities are less relevant than others, from an *objective* point of view, without bringing any evaluation or particular preferences into it. We could select, for instance, only those factors that we know usually play a role in determining a medical condition and, once we have restricted the variations to this limited field of factors and, in case of multiple alternative classifications according to *those* factors, we might introduce a hierarchy of preference according to their likely relevance.

Now, there are at least two main levels of difficulties with this strategy. The first level is more general and concerns the fact-value distinction; the second level is more specific of medical research and clinical practice.

From the general point of view, there is a widespread agreement that the fact-value dichotomy cannot be simply assumed without qualification, since there are good reasons to suspect that a *strict distinction* between factual statements and evaluative statements is nothing short of a philosophical myth. Referring to the standard literature on the topic [22, 25], it is enough here to mention that requesting an objective, factual point of view with no mention of values and decisions as a way out from the previous troubles with OTO and OTC similarity imports difficulties that are as challenging as the ones we are thinking to solve, if not worse.

From a more specific point of view, requesting a selection of the only factors that objectively play a role in determining a medical condition conflicts with the evidence that we do not know in advance which factors do and which do not play a role. In order to comply with this request, we should be able to identify *significant sets*, such as "diabetic" and "aspirin-resistant", and not, for instance, "vegan"; but what if the vegan diet plays a role in the outcome of patients undergoing cardiac surgery? A real example from epidemiology is the category "homosexual" in HIV transmission: it is all but clear that individuals put in this category share some property relevant for the medical condition or the disease transmission, despite the fact that the empirical data suggested, at a certain point, a common *disposition* to get infected. As we saw earlier, empirical data themselves do not come with a specification of what should count as the relevant property for a certain group in order to account for their *disposition*. To follow the previous suggestion to focus exclusively on factors that we know usually play a role in determining a medical condition could even make us blind to some variables that we excluded a priori: a selection that trades the feasibility of the inquiry at the expenses of our unbiased freedom of research. An additional problem, with the second part of the suggestion concerning the hierarchy of preference according to the likely relevance of factors is that a hierarchy requires further criteria that needs to be disclosed. Even if we imagine reaching an agreement on such criteria, there is the additional problem that the likeliness of their relevance relies on previous results and on the way the previous research has been conducted, limiting again our ability to consider the data from an innovative point of view, that takes in consideration aspects that have been neglected [21].

We already know that fictitious models to make sense of empirical data based on our interests and decisions do not work for our applicative aims. A provisional conclusion is that looking for independent taxonomies and classifications without bringing evaluations or preferences into the field does not seem to work as well.

Being Aware of the Issue: A Call for a Responsible Creativity

Taking in consideration the aforementioned issues does not necessarily conflict with our practical strategy that needs to work with ideal models and kinds. Actually, there is no other way to do the job. In fact, I am not contesting a kinds-based approach to medical research and clinical practice, favoring a yet-to-clarify approach to the patient uniqueness. Here I am just suggesting that being aware of such complications may be useful in reminding us that *any* act of modeling is "biased", if you are willing to use such an expression, and that this limit is unavoidable. When I question the "natural" character of the categories used in both research and practice, I do not want to suggest that, since they are, at least partially, human creations, they are arbitrary and no one grouping is more correct than any other. If natural kinds are natural insofar as they lead to groups of natural objects that behave with a regularity independent of conscious human activity, their objectivity rests on the objectivity of natural laws [29]. What I am questioning is the fact that, while not completely dependent on human interests and decisions, they are taken to be completely independent. The mere fact that there are available alternatives, that is equally justified categorizations of the same data, raises doubts about their complete independency.

Moreover, that one grouping is more correct than some other can be justified only when it is possible to disclose the a priori set of criteria, preferences and choices that generate our ontological categorization of individual cases in general kinds.

When we speak of different alternatives in shaping the categorial frameworks of our taxonomy of kinds, each based on different assumptions of preferences and choices—ethical and evaluative decisions included—it seems we risk ending up in ontological relativism. How can we claim that the existence of "kinds of patients" depends on a conceptual scheme? Existence is itself independent from our categories and conceptualizations and so should be for the existence of kinds in medicine and biomedical science. However, this line of argument is misleading. The existence of kinds cannot be *wholly* dependent on conceptual schemes or categorial frameworks if we take this to mean that concepts and categorizations themselves generate kinds as things. This enigmatic act of institution is much more than any of our theories can do. The existence of kinds can be said to depend on conceptual schemes or categorial frameworks *in the following sense*: questions on existence or reality can only be asked relative to some background assumptions that cannot be found, as such, in our empirical data [34].

For this reason, I am characterizing these kinds as *quasi-natural*, since they are "natural" in the sense that they are not arbitrary and they are intimately connected with natural laws, but they are not "natural" if we intend "natural" as "opposed to kinds resulting from acts of grouping built on the interests and decisions of human beings".

Therefore, in pursuing our aims, while using *quasi-natural* kinds, we can keep an eye open to the always-available alternative ordering strategies. The risk, in fact, is to forget that taxonomies and classifications that we have been using for a long time sound "natural" and prevent us to explore new territories. In selecting relevant properties guiding our taxonomies in kinds, we should not look condescendingly at manifestation of ethical preference in assessing our aims, as it was the case with an old positivistic attitude towards science in general and medicine in particular. Even with reference to the most applicative field of one of the most empirical sciences, as it is the case of cardiac intervention, the best *objective* results can be gained when we face frankly the possibility that our preferential evaluative *subjective* perspective may be our best guide in organizing the data. It may indeed seem too hazardous to give space to creativity, but the risky face of the subjective qualification of such a perspective may just be neglecting or hiding the relevance of a factor that is inescapable anyway. The problem with implicit bias is that they are implicit. A more creative and responsible approach can be gained when these implications are not omitted or kept quiet, as if they were a birthmark that stains the purity of our science. It is desirable that in future research, alongside a disclosure of financial interests, studies and applications of cardiac surgery find the space to declare the *evaluative* perspective and the *ethical* interests that guided the ontological arrangement of singular cases in kinds, since there are so many different ways to organize objects in categories and so many different ways to justify the choices we made.

In a nutshell, natural kinds with a human face! [24].

References

1. Ahn W, Kim NS. The causal status effect in categorization: an overview. In: Medin DL, editor. The psychology of learning and motivation. San Diego, CA: Academic; 2000.
2. Beebee H, Sabbarton-Leary N, editors. The semantics and metaphysics of natural kinds. New York: Routledge; 2010a.
3. Beebee H, Sabbarton-Leary N, editors. Are psychiatric kinds real? Eur J Anal Philos. 2010b;6:11–27.
4. Bird A, Tobin E. Natural kinds. In: Zalta EN, editor. The Stanford encyclopedia of philosophy (Spring 2016 editon); 2016. http://plato.stanford.edu/archives/spr2016/entries/natural-kinds/.
5. Block M, Khitin L, Sade RM. Ethical process in human research published in thoracic surgery journals. Ann Thorac Surg. 2006;82:6–12.
6. Cameron AC, Laskey WK, Sheldon WC. Ethical issues for invasive cardiologists: society for cardiovascular angiography and interventions. Catheter Cardiovasc Interv. 2004;61:157–62.
7. Campbell JK, O'Rourke M, Slater MH, editors. Carving nature at its joints: natural kinds in metaphysics and science. Cambridge, MA: MIT; 2011.
8. D'Amico TA, McKneally MF, Sade RM. Ethics in cardiothoracic surgery: a survey of surgeons' views. Ann Thorac Surg. 2010;90:11–3.
9. Dragulinescu S. Diseases as natural kinds. Theor Med Bioeth. 2010;31:347–69.
10. Fine K. Essence and modality. In: Tomberlin JE, editor. Philosophical perspectives 8: logic and language. Atascadero, CA: Ridgeview; 1994. p. 1–16.
11. Hadorn DC. Kinds of patients. J Med Philos. 1997;22:567–87.
12. Hesslow G. Do we need a concept of disease? Theor Med Bioeth. 1993;14:1–14.
13. James W. In: James H, editor. Letters of William James. Boston: Atlantic Monthly; 1920.
14. Kant I. The critique of the power of judgment. In: Guyer P, Matthews E (editors and trans.). Oxford: Cambridge University Press; 2002.
15. Kavarana MN, Sade RM. Ethical issues in cardiac surgery. Futur Cardiol. 2012;8:451–65.
16. Kripke S. Naming and necessity. Cambridge, MA: Harvard University Press; 1980.
17. LaPorte J. Natural kinds and conceptual change. Cambridge: Cambridge University Press; 2004.
18. Lemoine M. Defining disease beyond conceptual analysis: an analysis of conceptual analysis in philosophy of medicine. Theor Med Bioeth. 2013;34:309–25.
19. Leslie SJ. Essence and natural kinds: when science meets preschooler intuition. Oxford Stud Epistemol. 2013;4:108–66.
20. Lowe J. A problem for a posteriori essentialism concerning natural kinds. Analysis. 2007;67:286–92.
21. Manzoni GM, Castelnuovo G, Compare A, Pagnini F, Essebag V, Proietti R. Psychological effects of implantable cardioverter defibrillator shocks. A review of study methods. Front Psychol. 2015;6:39. doi:10.3389/fpsyg.2015.00039.
22. Marchetti G, Marchetti S, editors. Facts and value: the ethics and metaphysics of normativity. London: Routledge; 2016.
23. Putnam H. The meaning of 'Meaning'. In: Putnam H, editor. Mind, language, and reality. Cambridge: Cambridge University Press; 1975. p. 215–71.
24. Putnam H. Realism with a human face. Cambridge, MA: Harvard University Press; 1992.
25. Putnam H. The collapse of the fact/value dichotomy and other essays. Cambridge, MA: Harvard University Press; 2004.
26. Quine WV. Natural kinds. In: Quine WV, editor. Ontological relativity and other essays. New York: Columbia University Press; 1969. p. 114–38.
27. Rehder B, Hastie R. Causal knowledge and categories: the effects of causal beliefs on categorization, induction, and similarity. J Exp Psychol Gen. 2001;130:323–60.
28. Reznek L. The nature of disease. New York: Routledge; 1987.
29. Riggs PJ, editor. Natural kinds, laws of nature and scientific methodology. Dordrecht: Springer; 1996.

30. Roy IC. The nature of natural kinds: natural kinds in biology and medicine. Berkeley, CA: University of California; 1998.
31. Sade RM, Williams T, Haney C, Perlman D, Stroud M. The ethics gap in surgery. Ann Thorac Surg. 2000;69:326–9.
32. Schwartz P. Decision and discovery in defining 'Disease'. In: Kincaid IH, McKitrick J, editors. Establishing medical reality. Essays in the metaphysics and epistemology of biomedical science. Amsterdam: Springer; 2007. p. 47–63.
33. Sulmasy DP. Diseases and natural kinds. Theor Med Bioeth. 2005;26:487–513.
34. Valore P. Fundamentals of ontological commitment. Berlin: De Gruyter; 2016.
35. Husserl, E. Logical Investigations. Volume 1 and 2. Translated by J. N. Findlay, with a new Preface by M. Dummett and edited with a new Introduction by D. Moran. New York: Routledge; 2001.

Chapter 17
Patient ICD Support Groups

Wendy Churchouse

Abstract Patients with implantable cardiovertor defibrillators (ICD) have to live with the fear of shock therapy and/or sudden death. These have to be balanced against the mortality benefit that the ICD provides. A persons' ability to cope and adjust positively to such a life changing circumstance is multifactorial. Support groups for patients with cardiac devices such as ICDs have progressed slowly. They have evolved from the concept of self-sought support and meeting of others who have experienced similar life events or ill health. They offer empathy, advice and comfort outside the patient's immediate family. Researchers have identified positive trends for their use. Cardiac charities often provide financial support for the introduction and cataloguing of the support groups which raises awareness of their availability and uptake.

Keywords Support • Coping • ICD • Patient

Support groups have evolved from the concept of self-sought support and meeting of others who have experienced similar life events or ill health. They provide an outlet for empathy, advice and comfort outside the patient's immediate family.

Patient support groups seem to have first developed in cancer care and slowly moved to other conditions such as post myocardial infarction and cardiac surgery. More recently support groups for patients with cardiac devices such as ICDs have been established. Early quantitative research by Badger and Morris [1], Dickerson et al. [2], Molchany and Peterson [3] and Williams et al. [4] identified some positive trends for their use. National cardiac charities such as the British Heart Foundation (BHF) [5] pioneered a more strategic approach and financial support for the introduction and cataloguing of support groups. This facilitated patients, relatives and health professionals (HPs) awareness of their availability and increased the uptake of this invaluable patient focused support network.

W. Churchouse, B.E.M., M.Sc., R.G.N., Dip. N., En(G)
Cardiac Centre, Morriston Hospital, Swansea, UK
e-mail: wendy.churchouse@wales.nhs.uk

© Springer International Publishing AG 2017

R. Proietti et al. (eds.), *Psychological, Emotional, Social and Cognitive Aspects of Implantable Cardiac Devices*, DOI 10.1007/978-3-319-55721-2_17

ICD support groups provide a haven of support for people who have either survived a cardiac arrest or because of their cardiac diagnosis are deemed at a significant risk of experiencing a life threatening arrhythmia [3]. It is without doubt that ICDs provide mortality benefit [6–8]. However patients with ICDs have to live with the thought or fear of shock therapy and/or sudden death [9]. A persons ability to cope and adjust positively to such a life changing circumstance is multifactorial and influenced by their personality type, pre-implant presence of anxiety and/or depression, social/family support and whether they experience shock therapy [9, 10].

Anxiety and depression affect a significant number of ICD patients ranging between 11–38% and 11–28% respectively [11, 12]. The prevalence of these reduces within the first year of implantation [13]. But sadly, around 10% still experience significant psychological trauma after 12 months [13] with approximately one in five patients living with an ICD having post traumatic stress disorder (PTSD).

One of the biggest challenges is managing post shock anxiety or PTSD, unlike other situations that can cause PTSD, is the re-occurrence of the trauma (shocks) cannot be eliminated so it is ever present for the patient which can complicate their recovery [9]. Therefore, an ICD support group can provide an opportunity for people to meet others who have experienced similar situations. This sharing of experiences and seeing others who have dealt with them normalises the situation and provides both practical and emotional support. This form of true empathy is something that most health professionals cannot provide.

For relatives or close friends of a patient with an ICD, they too have often witnessed a traumatic event such as their husband or wife collapsing and requiring resuscitation. They also have to cope with concerns about mortality, shock therapy, employment and family finances, and how to support their loved one resume a normal life etc. [14].

These factors are compounded by inadequate information being provided to both patients and relatives during the pre and post ICD implant phase [15]. Even in institutions where pre and post ICD implantation information is prioritised, patients and their relatives' ability to understand, synthesise and recollect information is reduced due to emotions and stress. This is exacerbated by shortened hospitalisation for secondary prevention (post cardiac arrest) ICD insertion and day-case care for primary prevention (prophylactic) ICD insertion. In addition, the introduction of remote ICD monitoring reduces the number of times patients and relatives attend ICD follow up clinic. This in turn decreases their opportunity to have face to face interaction and support from health professionals and the opportunity to ask questions and raise concerns related to coping with the device [15].

Because of these factors, the reviewed National Institute for Health and Care Excellence (NICE) ICD guidelines (2014) [16] emphasised the importance of pre and post ICD implant counselling consisting of a minimum information set of expected outcomes, living with the device and ICD deactivation in the context of palliative care. Therefore, providing information that is user-friendly and appropriate is an essential component of an ICD care pathway and a requirement of informed consent and best practice [16–18].

All of these factors contribute to the role of patient ICD support groups. Such groups are encouraged and deemed of benefit by the British Heart Rhythm Society (2015) [19]. An ICD support group connects people who have experienced similar life events or challenges but there is no universal format to develop an ICD support group as they tend to be organic. However there are often themes or factors that seem to be present in a successful viable group.

First, there are a small number of key individuals who act as leaders or driving forces. These leaders are often a combination of patients, their friends or relatives and occasionally a health care professional. This cluster of like-minded people have either had good experiences and want to help others or have had negative experiences and want to protect others from similar scenarios. Frequently, these individuals form a committee which takes on the responsibility for the organisation and running of the ICD support group.

The committee will formulate terms of reference or aims and objectives of the support group. This is often helpful so that all members of the committee and subsequent ICD support group members agree a common purpose and role.

Health professionals are not an essential part of an ICD support group. However, nurses, doctors, psychologists, cardiac physiologists, occupational therapists or physiotherapists are the types of professional genres that tend to be involved with a support group. Some health professionals sit on the support group committee and have a more proactive role. Other health professionals attend on an ad hoc basis providing education talks/updates. However, on both a personal and professional perspective, it has been useful attending the ICD support group, firstly to provide clarity when misconceptions are evident or being abounded. Secondly, there are times when the health professional needs to act as an adjudicator to ensure that every ones view/opinion/experience is valued and dealt with utmost sensitivity within the support group. For example, some patients who have received shock treatment from their ICD may need to talk about their experience. Conversely, others who have not had a shock and are fearful of them may find the account frightening. This leads to the importance of agreeing "ground rules" when the ICD support group is set up.

Another benefit for a health professional attending an ICD support group is the opportunity to listen to patients and relatives views and opinions about the service and care they have received. Many patients and relatives are more relaxed within a peer group setting. When they realise that others have similar views/experiences this in turn can make an individual feel more at ease to express both positive and negative outcomes.

The more established ICD support groups tend to offer a combination of components. These include an education session provided by a health professional, for example "how an ICD works" or "why drugs are important in the prevention of arrhythmias". Another component may be group and/or one to one discussions that are often based on the individuals' experiences. These are often described as patient stories and can be an invaluable mechanism of shared experiences and are cathartic for all concerned.

Whether part of the education component or not, the ICD support group provides an opportunity for patients and their relatives to ask questions. Ideally the questions or queries are answered by other group members or the patient themselves via discussion, problem solving or reflection. The ICD support group can be a medium to discuss/highlight sensitive or emotive aspects of living with an ICD such as sexual relationships or deactivation of the ICD in a patient who has a terminal illness or is frail and elderly. The latter is frequently overlooked by health professionals [20, 21].

The social element of the ICD support group for some individuals is particularly important. Following a traumatic event such as having a cardiac arrest or shock therapy, patients can adopt avoidance or isolating behaviour (emotion-focussed coping) [22] which is a negative coping strategy. The social element of the group often evolves around the making and serving of simple refreshments such as tea, coffee, biscuits and cakes. These rudimental elements of the ICD support group should not be overlooked as in all cultures so much is shared or off loaded when enjoying a beverage and talking to others. Some ICD support groups organise social events like meals out or cinema trips. For some people, being involved in the ICD support group can restore their personal worth and role. For example, if a person has become unemployed or ill health prevents them working they can contribute to the organisational aspects of the support group—chairperson or secretary of the support group.

The location for the meetings can be challenging. Some people prefer the meetings to be held on hospital premises which may reduce or eliminate the costs of room rental charges. Others prefer to meet in coffee shops or restaurants to help to de-medicalise the support group. Either option is successful.

The development of the intranet has revolutionised modes of communication. This in turn has had an impact on ICD support groups. Individuals attending the support groups frequently exchange mobile phone numbers and opt to use text messaging instead of telephoning to ask each other questions or gain support. For some texting can de-personalise the mode of communication and allow them to ask questions that they would not broach face to face or ask verbally. This concept of anonymity or loss of personal contact has also increased the use of on-line forums and chat rooms as a form of “virtual” ICD support groups. The use of Facebook ICD support groups is increasing in popularity. These “virtual” forms of ICD support groups are particularly popular with younger patients who have an ICD implant. Teenagers or young adults with an ICD often have issues related to not wanting to be “different” to their peers and concerns of physical appearance related to the device and wound scarring [23]. Such negative feelings are compounded by restrictions on recreation or sporting activities, future occupation/career restrictions [24]. All of which are exacerbated by unrecognised depression/anxiety [24].

ICD support groups are a relatively new phenomena in the care of patients living with an ICD. They provide a medium of support for both patients, their relatives or close friends. They provide the opportunity for individuals to “listen to others” and to be “listened to” [3]. This allows people to make sense of their situation within the context of others who have experienced similar events/challenges.

The ICD support group offers a sense of fellowship and the possibility of making new friendships based on a common theme (living with an ICD). The group concept is void of stereotyping, commitment, and status etc. as the only common bond is the presence of having or being linked directly or indirectly by the ICD. This concept appears to help some patients and their relatives by normalising their situation [22]. This process of normalization (proactive problem-focused coping) is an important aspect of acceptance [22].

A persons need to attend the ICD support group varies from individual to individual and may be based on their personality type, experience of living with the device, social/family support or the individuals ability to cope and make sense of the situation.

Anecdotally, there seems to be specific stages in the patients recovery when the ICD support group appears to be needed. These are either in the early post implant phase or after a new event such as receiving their first ICD shock. Conversely, for a small number of people they attend all meetings—year in year out. And of course, the "leaders" of the ICD support group/committee members are often involved for many years and are essential factors in the longevity of the support group.

From a health professional perspective, it is advantageous to support and engage with the ICD support group in order to provide on-going information and continuity from the acute hospital care to living with the ICD long term. In addition, there is an element of empathetic learning related to observing the patient and relatives "lived experience" with the ICD. This cannot be gained from conventional education or training.

An ICD support group seems to nurture expert patients who wish to give something back and help others [3]. This attribute is unquantifiable as is the benefit gained from ICD support groups [24]. The latter is surprising when there are numerous support groups throughout the United Kingdom and Ireland. Secondly, primary prevention ICD implant rates are increasing causing a growing population of patients living with ICDs. Sadly, any of these patients will experience psychological trauma and have difficulty living with the device [22, 23] and health professionals currently offer little to assess or address these issues. Therefore, it would seem that ICD support groups do and could offer a solution to some of these problems. Most health institutions are working in a climate of austerity with increasingly complex clinical workloads yet they have not investigated this "free" therapy/service (ICD support groups) which could potentially benefit so many patients and their relatives. There is very limited and dated research investigating or demonstrating the benefits of ICD support groups [24]. As evidence remains tentative there is a strong case to explore this subject area with a large representative study.

References

1. Badger JM, Morris PL. Observations of a support group for automatic implantable cardioverter-defibrillator recipients and their spouses. Heart Lung. 1989;18:238–43.
2. Dickerson SS, Posluszny M, Kennedy MC. Help seeking in a support group for recipients of implantable cardioverter defibrillators and their support persons. Heart Lung. 2000;29:87–96.
3. Molchany CA, Peterson KA. The psychosocial effects of support group intervention on AICD recipients and their significant others. Prog Cardiovasc Nurs. 1994;9:23–9.

4. Williams AM, Young J, Nikoletti S, McRae S. Reasons for attending and not attending a support group for recipients of implantable cardioverter defibrillators and their careers. Int J Nurs Pract. 2004;10(3):127–33.
5. British Heart Foundation. How to start up a BHF support group. http://www.bhf.com/how_to_start_a_heart_support_group. Accessed 30 Sept 2016.
6. Goldenberg I, Gillespie J, Moss AJ, Hall WJ, Klein H, McNitt S, Brown MW, Cygankiewicz I, Zareba W. Executive Committee of the Multi-center Automatic Defibrillator Implantation Trial II. Long-term benefit of primary prevention with an implantable cardioverter-defibrillator: an extended 8-year follow-up study of the Multicenter Automatic Defibrillator Implantation Trial II. Circulation. 2010;122:1265–71.
7. Smith T, Jordaens L, Theuns DA, vanDessel PF, Wilde AA, Hunink MG. The cost- effectiveness of primary prophylactic implantable defibrillator therapy in patients with ischaemic or non-ischaemic heart disease: a European analysis. Eur Heart J. 2013;34:211–9.
8. Goldenberg I, Kutyifa V, Klein HU, Cannom DS, Brown MW, Dan A, Daubert JP, Estes NA III, Foster E, Greenberg H, Kautzner J, Klempfner R, Kuniss M, Merkely B, Pfeffer MA, Quesada A, Viskin S, McNitt S, Polonsky B, Ghanem A, Solomon SD, Wilber D, Zareba W, Moss AJ. Survival with cardiac-resynchronization therapy in mild heart failure. N Engl J Med. 2014;370:1694–701.
9. Sears SF, Hauf JD, Kirian K, Hazelton G, Conti JB. Post traumatic stress and the implantable cardioverter defibrillator patient. What the electrophysiologist needs to know. Circ Arrhythm Electrophysiol. 2011;4:242–50.
10. Versteeg H, Theuns DAMJ, Erdman RAM, Jordaens L, Pedersen SS. Posttraumatic stress in implantable cardioverter defibrillator patients: the role of preimplantation distress and shocks. Int J Cardiol. 2011;3:438–9.
11. Sears SF, Todaro JF, Lewis TS, Sorile W, Conti JB. Examining the psychosocial impact of implantable cardioverter defibrillators: a literature review. Clin Cardiol. 1999;22:481–9.
12. Ladwig KH, Baumert J, Marten-Mittag B, Kolb C, Zrenner B, Schmitt C. Posttraumatic stress symptoms and predicted mortality in patients with implantable cardioverter defibrillators: results from the prospective living with an implanted Cardioverter-Defibrillator Study. Arch Gen Psychiatry. 2008;65:1324–30.
13. Kapa S, Rotondi-Trevisan D, Mariano Z, Aves T, Irvine J, Dorian P, Hayes DL. Psychopathology in patients with ICDs over time: results of a prospective study. Pace. 2010;33:198–208.
14. Dougherty CM. Psychological reactions and family adjustment in shock versus no shock groups after implantation of internal cardioverter defibrillator. Heart Lung. 1995;24:281–91.
15. Pederson S, Knudson C, Dilling K, Sandgaard NCF, Johanse JB. Living with an implantable cardioverter defibrillator: patients' preferences and needs for information provision and care options. Europace. 2016. doi:10.1093/europace/euw109. First published online: 5 June 2016. Accessed 1 Oct 2016.
16. National Institute for Health and Care Excellence (NICE). Implantable cardioverter defibrillator and cardiac resynchronisation therapy for arrhythmia and heart failure (review of TA95 and TA120). 2014. http://www.nice.org. Accessed 29 Sept 2016.
17. General Medical Council. Consent: patient and doctors making decision together. 2008. http://gmc-uk.org. Accessed 1 Oct 2016.
18. Patient Information Forum. Making the case for information. 2013. http://tinyurl.com/mm19ezm. Accessed 30 Sept 2016.
19. British Heart Rhythm Society. Clinical guidance Standards follow up of cardiac implantable electronic devices for cardiac rhythm management (appendix to standard for implantation and follow up of cardiac rhythm management devices in adults. p. 7 4.2 (c). http://bhrs.com.standards. Accessed 1 Oct 2016.
20. Churchouse W, Seaman S, Rees P, Cawsey-Williams J, Roberts K, Anderson M. Deactivation of ICDs in end-of-life care: A Welsh perspective. Br J Cardiac Nurs. 2012;7(7):333–7.
21. Resuscitation Council (UK), British Cardiovascular Society and National Council for Palliative Care. Deactivation of implantable cardioverter defibrillators towards the end of life. 2015. http://www.resus.org. Accessed 30 Sept 2016.

22. Hallas CN, JL B, White DG, Connelly DT. Pre-ICD illness beliefs affect post implant perceptions of control and patient quality of life. Pacing Clin Electrophysiol. 2010;33:256–65.
23. Sears SF, Burns JL, Handberd E, Sohle WM, Conti JB. Young at heart. Understanding the unique psychosocial adjustment of young implantable cardioverter defibrillator recipients. Pacing Clin Electrophysiol. 2001;24:1113–7.
24. Dunbar S, Dougherty CM, Sears SF, Caroll DL, Goldstein NE, Mark DB, McDaniel G, Pressler SJ, Schron E, Wang P, Zeigler VL. Educational and psychological interventions to improve outcomes for recipients of implantable cardioverter defibrillators and their families. Circulation. 2012;126(17):2146–72.

Chapter 18
Living with an Implantable Cardioverter Defibrillator: The Road to Resilience

Serena Santagostino, Giada Pietrabissa, Gianluca Castelnuovo, and Francesco Borgia

Abstract This chapter recounts the story of my brother Valerio, a carrier of Brugada syndrome, and his experience with the Implantable Cardioverter Defibrillator (ICD). My name is Serena, I am a 25 year old psychologist, and with the present contribution I would like to give the reader an idea of what it means to face, from both my personal point of view and, indirectly, though my brother's words, the diagnosis of a genetic disease that makes ICD implantation necessary to survive. Specifically, I would like to try to explain how the implantation of the device affects the individual's life, relationships, and even parenting; but also how a person can successfully learn to live with a defibrillator, seeing the ICD as an important resource.

Keywords Implantable Cardioverter Defribilator • Brugada syndrome • Clinical Case

Valerio's Experience

Valerio was 25 when on March 22, 2004 after an evening spent swimming for about 2 h (he was not training) at the pool with a friend, he stared feeling very tired. Despite this, they went out for dinner, and afterwards my brother stopped for a chat at his friend's house before returning home.

I was only 14, but I still vividly remember waking up at around 11:45 p.m. because of the heavy rain and then hearing the home phone ring. It was my brother's

S. Santagostino (✉) • F. Borgia
Department of Psychology, Università Cattolica del Sacro Cuore, Milan, Italy
e-mail: serena.santagostino@gmail.com

G. Pietrabissa • G. Castelnuovo
Department of Psychology, Università Cattolica del Sacro Cuore, Milan, Italy

Psychology Research Laboratory, Ospedale San Giuseppe, IRCCS Istituto Auxologico Italiano, Oggebbio (VCO), Italy

© Springer International Publishing AG 2017

R. Proietti et al. (eds.), *Psychological, Emotional, Social and Cognitive Aspects of Implantable Cardiac Devices*, DOI 10.1007/978-3-319-55721-2_18

friend telling my father to go quickly to his house because Valerio was unconscious, and that the ambulance was coming. My father rushed to the scene, while my mother and I remained at home, terrified and helpless.

Several people were gathered around my brother's car, and his friend, together with his parents, tried to revive him by rubbing his chest, but with no results. Valerio appeared lifeless, not breathing and with no heartbeats. My brother remembers feeling a strong sense of fatigue after waking up, which made even the slightest movement very hard for him; he didn't understand what was going on, despite discerning a huge concern on the staring faces of the people around him.

Rescuers asked our father if Valerio took drugs since he seemed to be going into overdose, but they were immediately proven wrong, thereafter they began assuming that the malaise was due to excessive swimming or too much water in his lungs.

In the meantime, my mother and I sat in the living room desperate, praying and waiting for news. We did not know what to think. I remember a strong sense of helplessness and anxiety until, after having cried uncontrollably for hours, I finally fell asleep.

In the emergency room, Valerio was first visited around 7 a.m., and blood tests showed that the value of CPK, which reported muscular effort, was too high. The cardiologist affirmed it was simply due to a pressure drop, but the trainee doctor insisted on hospitalization. After the change of shift, Valerio was visited by another cardiologist, who suspected an arrhythmia and, for the following 10 days, Valerio underwent several tests, including an EEG, a Tilt test, a cardiogram under stress, TACs, etc., none of which revealed that anything was wrong with him. Therefore, he was discharged from the hospital.

Despite feeling physically well, however, Valerio started to experience discomfort and dizziness, especially in association to noisy places, confusion, bright lights, and car travel, limited in his activities, he seriously began to look for an explanation, he went through a series of tests and doctor visits consulting several specialists, including ENT, neurologist, cardiologist, etc., since no medical explanation as found, professionals started to speculate that there were no physical causes for his discomfort, but that everything was in his mind.

Our parents were worried and confused; I was angry with the doctors, judging them incompetent. Also, in June, my brother's girlfriend who could not stand the pressure of the situation, interrupted their relationship, destabilizing him even more. In the same period, the presence of a small heart murmur was detected, and physicians agreed for the insertion of a stent, positioned by a probe and threaded from the groin through the femoral vein.

In July, Valerio had a second syncope while sitting in a pub with some friends. That night he had not exerted too much, he had only skated after work as he usually did. In the emergency room the doctors observed the presence of arrhythmias and prescribed an anti-arrhythmic. We were all tired and stressed, and needed to find the cause of the problem, we were hoping that the intervention would solve everything.

In August, Valerio went on vacation without any particular concerns and, in September he met Dr. C, an arrhythmologist, who finally identified the presence of Brugada syndrome from the reaction to Flecainide, the anti-arrhythmic drug that had been given to Valerio during the previous hospitalization. It is a genetic disease although not scientifically proven to be so. Since potentially dangerous. Dr. C. immediately suspended the use of Flecainide. However, since Valerio had two arrhythmias within 3 months (in addition to a fourth episode, that occurred while he was asleep, as we later discovered), further investigation was necessary in order to understand the symptoms' severity. My brother was, therefore, subjected to an electrophysiological study, which revealed that he was at high-risk of death for arrhythmia. Dr. C. explained that the most malignant arrhythmias are those that occur at rest, especially during sleep, without the person's awareness, and that they can be triggered by different factors, including a high fever. He, therefore, strongly advised the implantation of an ICD, in addition to drug therapy (precisely, Quinidine to stabilize the heartbeat and "reset" the memory of the heart).

At this point, Valerio had two options: to live with a defibrillator or to refuse both the surgery and the recommended drug therapy by signing a paper relieving the professionals from any responsibility in case of death. The discovery of suffering from Brugada syndrome and the idea of living with an ICD totally destabilized my brother. He, in fact, went from being considered a healthy "visionary" to being at risk of death because of his heart condition and thus requiring implantation of an ICD—"I always thought defibrillators were devices used to resuscitate seventy-year olds who smoked three packs of cigarettes a day or who had a malfunctioning heart" he stated "and not a treatment option for a 25 year old".

What dismayed Valerio the most was the realization that he would have to live with a foreign body in his chest forever—"it seemed to me" affirmed Valerio "that the choice was between an impaired but secure life or a healthy highly-at-risk existence".

In the following days, Valerio's emotional state worsened, also due to aesthetic concerns, since after the intervention he would have visible scars, and he would be able to see the shape of the defibrillator under his skin. He was not afraid of dying, but of remaining without oxygen for several minutes after an episode of arrhythmia, which would cause him brain-damage.

After obtaining all the information required, he carefully evaluated his options, and finally agreed to the ICD implantation, which took place on Sept. 21, 2004, the day of his 26th birthday.

The surgery lasted about 4 h, the procedure was not an easy one. Valerio was sedated with local anesthesia, which made the experience even more traumatic for him—"I was awake, and I saw everything (…) the surgeon had mirrored sunglasses, and there were no curtains (…) It was one of the worst experience of my life".

The surgery went well, but Valerio was asked to remain in bed for another 3 days. He was, then, monitored for about another month. Moreover, for 6 months, Valerio could not drive, or go back to work—"After the operation, I started to concentrate deeply on my body, and to write down everything I felt in a diary, (…) pain, dizziness" admitted Valerio "but when the doctor, after careful medical checks, could not detect anything, he then advanced the hypothesis of the presence of anxiety" (…) "I do not remember when, but I know for sure that at some point I realized there was nothing I could do to prevent this emotional state of anxiety, that is when I said to myself <*and so be it*!>".

Gradually, Valerio put his life back together: he got back with his girlfriend and progressively pursued a more dynamic and healthy lifestyle, while concluding his drug therapy. In late 2005, he bought a house and moved. In the same period, my parents asked for a genetic and molecular screening of the SCN5A gene, traditionally implicated in Brugada syndrome. No genetic mutation was found.

In November 2007, 3 years after implantation, another tense moment occurred: the defibrillator batteries discharged, my brother was alarmed by a peculiar repetitive sound made by the ICD. Valerio immediately contacted Dr. C., who explained that he needed a new operation in order to replace the old batteries. The batteries should, instead, have lasted 5 years—"I was in my bed when I hear a buzzer ringing" said Valerio "I did not understand what it was (…) I thought it might be the neighbors alarm, but soon I realized that the noise was coming from my chest, at regular intervals. I got worried and called the hospital, I was then told that it was necessary to replace the batteries."

The doctors reassured Valerio by explaining that the upcoming surgery was going to be easier and faster than the previous one, guaranteeing him that he would be able to return to work in a week. But my brother was still worried due to the uncertainly of the situation—"As you start to feel serene believing you have finally got your normal life back, all of a sudden you have to go back; same department, same faces, same procedures."

The second defibrillator installed was half the size of the first one, and lasted nearly 8 years—"An acceptable interval of time" stated Valerio.

Meanwhile, in 2008, my brother got married and, a year later, had a son.

The following years were very difficult for him for several reasons. Concerns related to his marriage and son led him to not sleep at night, and he also began to experience palpitations. At a race organized by his son's kindergarten class, Valerio had an "inappropriate shock" of the defibrillator, triggered by mistake as he ran with the child on his shoulder. Valerio described the ICD discharge as "an internal detonation that stuns you". When Valerio received the electric shock, in order to protect his son, he threw himself on the ground injuring his head and cracking two ribs. Fortunately, my parents, his wife, his mother and some neighbors were there. He was taken to the emergency room by ambulance, kept under observation and discharged the same evening, with a prescription to rest due to the broken ribs. During the days that followed, he was visited by Dr. L. who, after monitoring the ICD, observed that the shock was "inappropriate", due to an error of calibration, and affirmed that no arrhythmias had occurred during the race.

That episode scared all of us. It was like reliving the same experience, but with the difference that my brother was a father now.

A few months later, in 2014 Valerio and his wife got separated. Also, in 2015, Dr. C. and his team told Valerio that they were moving to another Hospital, he had to choose whether to follow them or not, Valerio decided to remain with them, in September 2015 he faced another ICD replacement, because of a new batteries discharge.

What It's Like Living with a Defibrillator

Being a carrier of Brugada syndrome causes irreversible changes to a person's life, since it seriously impairs the physical, psychological, emotional and social status of the individual. Recipients must learn to live with a visible, foreign and uncomfortable body in their chest, this is difficult to accept, especially at a young age, when death is perceived only at a distance. Negative emotions, such as fear, anxiety, worry, sadness, anger and helplessness, therefore, commonly arise among patients with an ICD. Despite permitting you to continue to carry out everyday activities, still it is not recommended to engage in competitive sports or heavy work; a person should also avoid exposure to the sun for too long or during hot hours. In hearing Valerio's words, his ambivalence about the ICD was clear to me: "The defibrillator makes you an adult, no matter how old are you. Of course, there are people who face worse events, such as losing a leg (…). The fact is, that the defibrillator causes great discomfort. It does not really cause pain but it does annoy you. At the same time, however, it allows you to keep doing things, to be involved in different activities. For example, if my friends go rafting, as it happened a few years ago, I can go, or I can go mountain climbing if I feel like it! However, it is not a natural thing. Something foreign is present in your body something that does not belong there, your body knows that and tries to knock it out (…)".

To date, my brother has experienced three different types of defibrillators. The first ICD, implanted in 2004, was extremely big and formed a visible lump on his chest, it looked like he had a pack of cigarettes in his pocket; Valerio also says that it was heavy and annoying. The wounds bothered him only when fresh, but once they healed, they did not create any additional discomfort other than on a psychological and aesthetic level. For this reason, Valerio initially used to hide it as much as possible by wearing large shirts with pockets. The following ICD models were lighter and less annoying, but Valerio still felt still uncomfortable about showing his bare chest, mostly he feared other peoples' reactions—"If you go to the beach or the pool you perceive, people looking at you (…) and even if you are physically well, you still feel awkward".

Despite these concerns, the device did not limit my brother's daily life, except for the pool and the beach, since they are respectively associated with the memory of the first syncope and the initial embarrassment in relation to other people.

Progressively, however, my brother gave less importance to the aesthetic issues related to the ICD, he started to get used to its presence, the changes it comported and learned to live with the device. Knowing that it was possible to have a normal life, without major limitations and problems, allowed him to be more accepting of the ICD and to see it as a resource, rather than a limitation—"After many years, the defibrillator is no longer a fixed idea (…) This year I went on vacation with my son, I went rafting with my friends (…) I consider it a minor cosmetic problem now, even if people stare at it, I don't really care … I'd be more ashamed to say to my son that I do not want go to the beach with him because I am ashamed of the ICD."

Another cause of demoralization for Valerio was that he was without a driver's license for a while, since additional medical certifications were required. Due to his risky health conditions, he then had to renew it annually for a few years and to date, medical checks are scheduled every 2 years. Still, every time the "healthy" fear that the license will not be renewed is present, and the consequent feeling of frustration arises. One more annoyance is that, at the airport, for example, the ICD cannot go through the metal detector and needs to be marked with a special badge, since the strong magnetic field may damage its functioning or cause an improper electrical discharge.

The greatest difficulty, for my brother is the need to periodically undergo surgical interventions in order to service the defibrillator, with the ever-present fear that something might go wrong; and another contraindication for him is the sound that the unloaded defibrillator makes, similar to a buzzer or an alarm clock that comes from the inside of your body at hourly intervals.

To date, Valerio has not yet had to face the replacement of the device, this operation is a bit more complex than a battery change, the fear of possible complications makes it very hard to undergo surgery and to cope with its consequences.

Over time, Valerio learned to handle the stress due to his condition, by trying not to worry about potential problems beforehand, and to address them step by step. This way of coping with the situations was essential to help him develop resilience—"Is the ICD something invasive? Yes, it is! Is it necessary? Yes, it is, and as soon as you realize it represents the only way you have for maintaining a normal life and avoid further concerns, you learn to accept it, I learned to compensate this difficulty with other things, such as being with my son or taking pictures."

Valerio did not receive any proper psychological support. He did not find it necessary—"Why should I look into the psyche? I do not need to create more problems to myself. I have good friends and a very supportive family; I also have a sunny personality. Today, I would to go to a psychologist more for curiosity than necessity, sincerely, but he must do it for free, because I have no money to spend!"

However, prior to the discovery of Brugada syndrome, when he was being subjected to various medical tests, he was sent to a psychiatrist to check weather his symptoms were psychosomatic in origin, but nothing was detected and the practitioner did not prescribe any drugs to my brother. He then saw a psychologist two or three times as a routine medical practice, after implantation, Valerio was visited a second time by a psychiatrist, who investigated his experience and the presence of possible suicidal tendencies.

Fundamental for Valerio was his relationship with Dr. C., who was always able to look at the person before the disease, what negatively affected my brother the most was the lack of competence and care of the different professionals, who labeled him and attributed his illness to psychosomatic disorders or anxiety, and cost him a lot of money—"I remember a doctor, in particular" he stated "that made me talk a little bit and then attributed the first syncope to the death of my grandfather, which had taken place a month before. Come on! One hundred euros!!!".

What helped Valerio the most was the fact of having many interests and his curious nature—"I really like to read as much as I like going for a walk in the mountains, or for a drink with my friends, or staying at home", he stated. In 2004 he bought a camera and started to take pictures, developing a real interest in photography.

ICD and Relationships

Experiencing an ICD has a strong impact on personal relationships. After the first syncope, and before being diagnosed with the syndrome, Valerio's relationships were characterized by tension, worry and helplessness. He felt both physically and psychologically sick, misunderstood and in strong need of answers, but no one knew how to help him. Still, his family and friends always supported him—"During that time I was mostly sustained by my family and true friends. I am aware, it was hard for them and they were very patient. I could not even stand myself" admitted my brother "(…) and they did what my girlfriend did not do. In fact, we broke up because she was under pressure. After the operation we got back together, got married, and then decided to become parents, aware of the possible risks. Later we divorced, but the end of our marriage was definitely not caused by defibrillator issues".

Valerio always told those close to him about the ICD, not without clashing repeatedly with those who had difficulties understanding his history—"It is not possible to predict people's reactions to adverse events, in general I mean, and as far as my story is concern (…) some people seemed afraid, others were more inclusive, some treated me as a disabled (…) but, to be honest, my disease did not create any problems with my close friends, those that really matter".

Despite initially considering the defibrillator as a strong limit, the possibility of sharing the negative experiences associated with it allowed Valerio to reach complete acceptance and to be treated normally by his friends, helping him to coexist with the ICD. Social support in overcoming traumatic and adverse experiences is essential.

Progressively my brother learned to see the device as a resource. Being an ICD recipient, in fact, helps you make a selection among people, as by natural selection, you tend to surround yourself with deeper and more mature relationships.

Finally, our family had a crucial role in supporting Valerio during the entire process, particularly in making the decision to proceed with the ICD. In fact, despite his initial indecision, we did not see it as choice but as a "must", the only solution—"I never had problems, I never felt treated like a disabled (…) I never felt suffocated. I never felt tension coming from my family", he declared.

ICD and Parenthood

Another dimension strongly affected by the presence of the ICD is that of parenting. Valerio became a father nearly 5 years after the implantation, although initially the idea of having a child worried him, due to the possibility that Brugada syndrome could be transmitted genetically. Up to now, the child has never had any type of heart problems; however, the risk of occurrence of the disease is still present, and for this reason, once a year his son is subjected to diverse medical checks. In addition, the stem cells from my nephew's umbilical cord were taken at birth to preserve them. Certainly, the difficulties experienced by Valerio made him more sensitive, bringing him to do everything possible to safeguard and protect his son. Fatherhood helped my brother's acceptance of the ICD, further increasing his resilience. His son needed a father, and Valerio could no longer risk his life by choosing to remove the device.

By the time my nephew started to ask questions, my brother decided to let him everything about the defibrillator—"He explained to him that the defibrillator is there because it keeps dad well" He also tried to mentally prepare his child before the last operation—"Everyone told me to tell him that I was leaving for work for a few days, but I did not agree. He had to understand that life is not always easy". Valerio's approach had a positive outcome, my nephew appeared reassured after learning that the ICD was necessary to help Valerio's heart to function. Also, my nephew has always been careful with the defibrillator: he would play/fight with my brother without uneasiness or fear, but with great sensitivity and delicacy, being careful not to hit him on the chest.

Photography and Resilience

The way my brother reacted to the diagnosis of the disease, its consequences and then adapted to the pressures of life's events positively surprised me.

Also, none of the mental health professionals he was invited to meet, considered it necessary for Valerio to assume a pharmacotherapy or to receive a psychological support.

Engaging in compensatory activities, "trying not to be bored", in fact, helped him to accept life with a defibrillator.

Particularly, in 2004 Valerio discovered to be passionate about photography, but he seriously engaged this activity only in 2013, when he bought his first digital SLR—"I've always liked the contrast of black and white, shadows fascinate me. Photography helped me so much (…). It's my way of seeing the world, to express myself, and I am pretty sure it also helped the relationship with the woman who later become my wife, enabling me to give her my best".

Photography is now my brother's main language, a way to express feelings and emotions that are too difficult to communicate in words. It assumed a key role in his life, especially in dealing with the subsequent separation from his wife and other adverse events that characterized that period, such as inappropriate shocks, palpitations, insomnia, and impending operations—"Photography is a language, it's my language, the only one I am comfortable with. It made me laugh when I was crying (…), there are shots full of joy, others that are full of fear, others full of tension (…). Even now, people ask me where I studied photographic composition. Never! I just felt the need to shoot; and black and white pictures in particular help me tell my story".

In fact, by giving his emotions and feelings a different form, acceptable and valuable both in his eyes and in those of others, my brother transformed the ICD's presence into a strength.

"I am pretty sure something similar happened to guitarists Jimi Hendrix and Robert Johnson" said Valerio "I have no doubt that when Jimi Hendrix started playing he was profoundly disturbed, and Robert Johnson disappeared for six months when his wife and child died after childbirth. People said he went to sell his soul to the devil (…) but come on. He just took some time off and came back stronger than before which permitted him to do extraordinary things. This is compensation, isn't it?".

ICD and Birth Family

Valerio's story understandably had a major impact on the entire family, and each member reacted in a different way. Surely the first syncope was a traumatic event, and made us all feel completely powerless. I remember everything about that rainy evening: our fright due to the phone ringing, our father rushing out of the house in terror, leaving the garage and gate open, and my shocked mother in the living room. My father still recoils at the memory of seeing my brother "completely dead", pale, not breathing and with no heartbeat. That evening I was so afraid that I was going to lose my brother, I felt entirely helpless, useless and overwhelmed, I felt fear, anger and panic. Despite my mother's assurances, I was terrified, and began to tremble in my chair at the mercy of all these emotions, unable to calm down. I fell asleep at night in tears and tremors. The lack of a logical explanations for my brother's syncope and malaise from several medical tests and consultations with different professionals made us even more frustrated and desperate. We tried to be strong and to support him, but we were sick of hearing the doctors attributing all of Valerio's symptoms to anxiety. "Personally, I was in the grip of strong anger and sadness. I was sure there was a physical cause for his fainting and it was not purely psychosomatic. Soon I started suffering from anxiety, especially when the phone would ring, and auditory hallucinations that made me hear the sound of the ambulance even when there was none, even in complete silence. Also, I could not go near a hospital without feeling that I was going to faint". My family was struggling to find a new balance to this situation, but not knowing the origin of the medical problem made it harder, if not impossible. We hoped so much that the application of a coronary stent was the solution, but after a few days, my brother was diagnosed with a rare disease called Brugada syndrome, for which an ICD was considered necessary. It clearly was a shock, as we went from being told by medical professionals that there was nothing to worry about, to finding out that he suffered from a disease that affects one in a billion. Once again, we felt desperate and angry, but still solid enough to give strength to Valerio. It seemed impossible and unfair to all of us that a 25 year old boy had a syndrome that requires the implantation of an ICD in order to survive, and my brother, in fact, initially did not want to undergo the surgery. The evening before the implantation, he had a moment of crisis and phoned our mother to tell her he did not want the operation. She burst into tears and said: "But think about us? How do you think we feel? We do not want to lose you (…)". Valerio then reflected, and decided to undergo the surgery—"I agreed to the implantation only when I realized that otherwise, no one at home would have slept anymore, me neither (…) for the fear of not waking up again (…)".

The defibrillator was installed on September 21, 2004, and we like to think of it as the beginning of Valerio's second life. Those weeks were difficult and full of tension, but I am very proud of the way we have dealt with this experience, by making him feel protected and keeping his spirits up.

For the following 6 months, my brother could not exert any effort or drive. It was not easy because it seemed that everything required adaptation, but, overall, he was able to cope with the situation quite well and we tried not to overprotect him—"I did not see much difference in the relationship with my family before and after the implantation. I never had any problems, I never felt treated like a disabled or suffocated by them."

Personally, I suffered greatly from this experience, as a result of which I developed Post Traumatic Stress Disorder and started suffering from panic attacks, fortunately Valerio did not seem to perceived my discomfort at all. Furthermore, since my brother was diagnosed with Brugada syndrome I had the impression of being treated like a freak: for example, while undergoing the echocardiogram during a sport-related routine physical exam, the doctor made a phone call to another professional saying that "there was the sister of a Brugada". Shortly after the cardiologist barged into the room, and suddenly I was on the couch with the attached electrodes. I felt humiliated and even angry, because of their lack of tact. Even at the visit for the driving license, the doctor did not want to give me permission to drive in absence of further medical examinations ensuring my state of good health. I remember I cried a lot on these occasions since, in addition to the worry and pain for my brother condition, I had to emotionally cope with the incompetence and curiosity of different doctors, who often forget that in front of them there are people with their own story and emotional impairments, not only diseases.

With time, both my family and I, together with Valerio, learned to see the positive aspects of this experience, becoming even stronger and closer than before. In fact, we were lucky, because my brother survived three episodes of syncope, without any consequence.

Today, I am the same age that Valerio was at the time, and I cannot help but wonder how he could have felt in those moments and where he found the strength to fight the disease and to cope with its unavoidable consequences. He proved to be a very resilient person: he learned how to live with the ICD and to see it as a resource, turning his emotions into art.

Unfortunately, he has to face difficulties and concerns, especially when routine clinical visits or interventions occur, but what strikes me the most is the energy and determination Valerio has always shown, allowing him to find a new balance every time.

I am grateful to Valerio, because he taught me that the most powerful weapon that a person has to face adverse events and negative feeling, is the ability to laugh.

Erratum to: Neuropsychological Functioning After Implantable Cardioverter-Defibrillator Surgery

Abdullah Alabdulgader

Erratum to:
Chapter 2 in: R. Proietti et al. (eds.), *Psychological, Emotional, Social and Cognitive Aspects of Implantable Cardiac Devices*, https://doi.org/10.1007/978-3-319-55721-2_2

We received revised caption for figure 2.10 and the same has been updated in the chapter. The corrected figure caption is available below.

Fig. 2.10 (a, b) Computational tools for identifying PTSD biomarkers from "multiomic" data, illustrated biomarkers provide both a means for diagnosing new patients as well as a molecular network-level description of the PTSD phenotype. (**a**) Reproduced with permission of the Regents of The University of California (**b**) IEEE grants to Prof. Abdullah Alabdulgader, License Number 4177010395849, a non-exclusive, non-transferable worldwide license to use this image in accordance with the terms and conditions of the agreement

The updated online version of this chapter can be found at
https://doi.org/10.1007/978-3-319-55721-2_2

© Springer International Publishing AG 2017

R. Proietti et al. (eds.), *Psychological, Emotional, Social and Cognitive Aspects of Implantable Cardiac Devices*, DOI 10.1007/978-3-319-55721-2_19

Index

© Springer International Publishing AG 2017

R. Proietti et al. (eds.), *Psychological, Emotional, Social and Cognitive Aspects of Implantable Cardiac Devices*, DOI 10.1007/978-3-319-55721-2

D

E

MIX
Papier aus verantwortungsvollen Quellen
Paper from responsible sources
FSC® C105338

FSC
www.fsc.org

If you have any concerns about our products,
you can contact us on
ProductSafety@springernature.com

In case Publisher is established outside the EU,
the EU authorized representative is:
Springer Nature Customer Service Center GmbH
Europaplatz 3, 69115 Heidelberg, Germany

Printed by Libri Plureos GmbH
in Hamburg, Germany